CHILD DEVELOPMENT
AND CHILD HEALTH

CW00601236

CHILD DEVELOPMENT AND CHILD HEALTH
THE PRESCHOOL YEARS

Martin Bax DM, FRCP
Senior Research Fellow,
Charing Cross and
Westminster Medical Schools,
London

Hilary Hart MRCP, DCH
Principal in General Practice,
Hemel Hempstead,
Hertfordshire

Susan M. Jenkins MRCP, DCH
Consultant Community Paediatrician,
City and Hackney Health Authority and
Queen Elizabeth Hospital for Children,
Hackney,
London

Foreword by
Ross G. Mitchell MD, FRCP (Edin), DCH
Professor Emeritus of Child Health,
University of Dundee
and Chairman,
The Community Paediatric Group,
The British Paediatric Association

BLACKWELL SCIENTIFIC PUBLICATIONS

OXFORD LONDON

EDINBURGH BOSTON MELBOURNE

To the memory of
Ronald Mac Keith and Jack Tizard

© 1990 by
Blackwell Scientific Publications
Editorial offices:
Osney Mead, Oxford OX2 oEL
8 John Street, London WC1N 2ES
23 Ainslie Place, Edinburgh EH3 6AJ
3 Cambridge Center, Suite 208
  Cambridge, Massachusetts 02142, USA
107 Barry Street, Carlton
  Victoria 3053, Australia

First published 1990

Set by Setrite Typesetters, Hong Kong
Printed and bound in Great Britain
at The University Press, Cambridge

DISTRIBUTORS

Marston Book Services Ltd
PO Box 87
Oxford OX2 oDT
(*Orders*: Tel: 0865 791155
        Fax: 0865 791927
        Telex: 837515)

USA
Year Book Medical Publishers
200 North LaSalle Street
Chicago, Illinois 60601
(*Orders*: Tel: (312) 726 9733)

Canada
The C.V. Mosby Company
5240 Finch Avenue East
Scarborough, Ontario
(*Orders*: Tel: (416) 298 1588)

Australia
Blackwell Scientific Publications
(Australia) Pty Ltd
107 Barry Street
Carlton, Victoria 3053
(*Orders*: Tel: (03) 347 0300)

British Library
Cataloguing in Publication Data

Bax, Martin
    Child development and child health
    1. Children. Health
    I. Title   II. Hart, Hilary   III. Jenkins,
    Susan
    613'.0432

    ISBN 0-632-02048-2

Contents

Foreword

U<small>NTIL RECENT YEARS</small>, many doctors in the UK were sadly deficient in knowledge of children, their management and their disorders. The teaching of child health in medical schools was generally inadequate, with a few honourable exceptions such as the course in Child Life and Health conducted at Edinburgh University before World War II by Professor Charles McNeil. Most medical practitioners had little or no training in paediatrics and few if any opportunities for postgraduate education. Despite the work of such pioneers as Arnold Gesell, Myrtle McGraw and Ronald Illingworth, understanding of normal growth and development was very limited. Doctors entering the school health service or starting to work in child health clinics usually had no formal preparation but learned by experience: a few, such as Mary Sheridan, proved to be notable pathfinders in the practical application of theoretical knowledge.

With the establishment of the National Health Service in 1948 and the consequent rapid expansion of specialist paediatrics, there came increasing realization that a sound grasp of normal growth and development was essential to clinical practice with children. It was also recognized that the health surveillance of normal children, as well as the management of their common disorders, should largely be undertaken by family doctors and that these therefore required better undergraduate and postgraduate teaching and more paediatric experience before entering general practice. At the same time, it was appreciated that it would be a long time before all, or even most, general practitioners acquired the skills and resources to undertake this work properly and that there was a great reservoir of practical experience in the community child health services which must provide a major component of child health care for the foreseeable future. Practice involving particular interests within this field necessitates a greater degree of expertise than is required of most doctors working with children and so the concept developed of paediatric specialties such as educational medicine and the recognition and management of disability in childhood.

At present the whole field of child health and community paediatrics is in a state of ferment and change, with new ways of working being explored and new avenues of education and specialization opening up. General practitioners who wish to undertake developmental surveillance, doctors in child health clinics and schools (currently known as clinical medical officers) and specialists, including consultant general paediatricians and those with a special interest in community child health, must all acquire and maintain knowledge of child life and health at a level appropriate to their practice. There is therefore a need for an authoritative textbook on the subject, both for basic learning and for continuing reference.

This new book is written by community paediatricians of considerable experience, who are actively working in schools and clinics and have wide understanding of the problems and difficulties of child health and paediatrics in the community. They make no attempt to cover the whole of clinical paediatrics but concentrate on those aspects most relevant to child health care outside the hospital. The text deals primarily with the development of infants and young children and its variation but there is good coverage of normal health care and the childhood disorders likely to be encountered in schools and clinics. There are chapters on social and environmental factors influencing the health of children and on the use of services by children and their families. The book is written in clear and concise language, is thoroughly up-to-date and provides a useful and readable introductory text for both undergraduate and postgraduate students. It will, I believe, be accepted quickly as a standard work of reference and as a vade-mecum by all those working in community child health.

Ross G. Mitchell,
Professor Emeritus of Child Health,
University of Dundee
and Chairman,
The Community Paediatric Group,
The British Paediatric Association

Preface

Paediatrics is the medicine of childhood. Children are developing organisms. It is the aim of this book to look at children's development both in terms of physical, cognitive and social growth, and in the context of their physical health and their behaviour. The doctor who studies the young child will find that these issues are intimately connected. Thus, for example, the child whose speech and language is delayed is likely to have more common infections than other children and in addition is more likely to have behavioural problems. A child's health, development and behaviour must be assessed together if adequate plans for help are going to be developed. The primary care doctor has been aware of this intuitively for many years. Children consult her/him much more frequently than any other age group until the later decades of life. Often these consultations are for the so-called common childhood disorders — coughs and colds — but often other problems are presented at the same time.

In this book we start by reviewing the child's development in isolation and then show how this relates to his or her social and family environment. We look then at the common developmental disorders and go on to see how these relate to the physical health and behaviour problems of the young child. We end by discussing the health care of the child in the first five years of life. While discussing the management of common health problems we have stopped short of discussing the management of conditions which are well described in paediatric textbooks. We hope therefore that this book will be a useful companion to a standard textbook of paediatrics to all the doctors who see children in primary care during their first five years.

In the past, developmental paediatrics has often been taught on the basis of the doctor learning off by rote a few 'milestones'. We are uneasy about this simplistic approach to child development, but recognize that many busy clinicians need to have some outline of a routine assessment at different ages, so, while we have discussed development in general in Chapters 1, 2 and 3, we have also provided an outline of assessment at different ages. The traditional developmental examination of the child includes the assessment of functions which develop over quite a long period of time, such as the development of the upright gait, and the even more complex development of speech and language. On the other hand there are some functions such as vision and hearing where the child rapidly achieves near adult levels of function but is unable to cooperate in testing. Clearly the distinction between a problem of testing and a problem of development is an important one. Other aspects of development such as the cardiovascular system or the immune system have not traditionally been part of 'developmental paediatrics'. We believe they should be. Indeed in our view paediatrics and 'developmental medicine' are virtually synonymous.

Children are not always easy to examine, but, when the child seems seriously ill with a possibly life-threatening disease, adequate examination clearly must be achieved. When the child is not seriously ill but has a chronic problem, such as a delay in an aspect of development, assessment can often be spread over two or three consultations if this is necessary. The clinician in these circumstances will also take note of the family's report of the child's function. Again it is important for the clinician to make a distinction between what is observed and what is reported to her/him. In general mothers and fathers not surprisingly are more acute observers of their own children than even the best trained clinicians. However, there are certain instances when this may not be the case and clinicians should always try and confirm parental reports by their own observations and keep the two clearly separate in their minds.

People have queried the value of developmental checks. They have tried to apply the very quick, strict criteria of a screening test to developmental assessment and examination and this is inappropriate (Bax & Whitmore, 1988). There are three aims of surveillance of the child: to identify and deal with present problems which the child has, to identify children who are likely to have problems in the future, and to provide the occasion for health promotion and education. Surveillance should prevent or forestall health, developmental and behavioural problems. There is also an implication that if the child will 'grow out of it' it doesn't matter whether you do anything about it or not. It is true that most sleep problems which predominate around the toddler age, for example, will disappear over time and they have no long-term implications in general for behaviour problems in a child. But anyone who has had to put up with sleepless nights associated with such a problem knows that the parents are in need of present help.

That such developmental, health and behavioural problems exist in the preschool population has been abundantly demonstrated in numerous studies. In relation to the long-term outcome many studies now have looked at populations of children over a longitudinal period and show that problems recognized in the preschool period do have predictive value. The field is well reviewed in Drillien & Drummond's book (1983) (where also their own highly significant results are reported).

Our own studies (Bax, Hart & Jenkins, 1980), which we carried out at the Thomas Coram Research Unit during the seventies, allowed us to study two preschool populations in central London for a period of six years. We carried out regular health checks on the whole population and in addition other staff from the Thomas Coram Research Unit reviewed the family background of the children and particularly looked at issues such as maternal stress. Other staff again carried out a number of psychological assessments on these children. This longitudinal research study, set up by the late Professor Jack Tizard at the Thomas Coram Research Unit and in which we were privileged to participate, provided us with a rich source of data on which we have drawn heavily to write this book.

References

Bax, M., Hart, H. & Jenkins, S. (1980) *The Health Needs of the Preschool Child*. Thomas Coram Research Unit, London.

Bax, M. & Whitmore, K. (1988) Screening or examining. *Developmental Medicine and Child Neurology*, **30**, 673–6.

Acknowledgements

WE WOULD LIKE to acknowledge the help we had from many colleagues at the Thomas Coram Research Unit, but particularly Ian Plewis and Charlie Owen who helped us so much with the analysis of the data.

We would also like to express our gratitude to the health visitors who worked on the research study. Sue Rumney, June Thompson and Caroline McPherson: the staff of the Dorothy Gardiner Centre and the Thomas Coram Children's Centre always welcomed our work with the children. Both parents and children in the two research areas were amazingly cooperative and we would like to thank them for all that they taught us.

Professor Ross Mitchell gave us most valuable comments on the manuscripts and thanks are also due to various secretaries over the period the book was written; Olwen Davis, Lorraine Wilder and Joy Allsop who worked enormously hard. Thanks also to Professor Bleck for his pictures of common developmental orthopaedic problems and Mr A.J. Keniry for his table of dentition.

Finally for help, advice and support throughout the study we must acknowledge our colleague Dr Kingsley Whitmore.

1   Early Infant Development

THIS CHAPTER is concerned with the way in which the young infant grows and develops during the first six months of life. The changing features of the infant's development are reviewed in the traditional areas of gross motor and fine motor function along with early vocalization, the beginnings of understanding and social behaviour and the infant's sensory skills. Assessment of the infant abilities at six weeks is described together with history-taking from parents and physical and neurological examination. Results of our own examinations of a group of six-week-old babies are reported to illustrate the frequency of abnormal characteristics and to draw attention to important areas of concern at this age.

Development up to six months

Gross motor development

FETAL MOVEMENTS

Movement in the baby has developed well before birth. Reflex movements in response to touch have been demonstrated in prematurely born embryos as early as six weeks after conception. At this age, if the area near the mouth is touched the baby turns his head away. Later he turns his head towards the stimulus, a response which continues after birth as the rooting reflex. Using ultrasound the earliest discernible spontaneous movements can be visualized at seven weeks postmenstrual age. By eight weeks quick generalized movements, resembling the startle reflex seen in the newborn, involve the limbs, neck and trunk. The diaphragm is formed between eight weeks and 10 weeks. By nine weeks hiccups are observed which continue throughout fetal life. Episodic breathing movements begin at around 10 weeks and each episode shows a regular pattern.

Flexion and extension of the fingers occur by 10 weeks and the hand is seen to touch the face, sometimes resulting in thumb or finger sucking. The baby's spontaneous activity results in frequent changes of posture from around 10 weeks. The baby can somersault by means of alternating movements which resemble neonatal stepping. There is

1

evidence that these stepping and crawling type movements seem to maintain the fetus in the normal vertex position for birth (Prechtl, 1984).

MOVEMENT IN THE FIRST SIX MONTHS

Given this evidence of extensive activity by the baby before birth, it is not surprising to find that the newborn baby has a wide repertoire of reflex and voluntary movements. The primitive reflexes are described in detail later in this section. They diminish and eventually disappear during the early months. However, there is not always a close temporal relationship between disappearance of a reflex such as grasping and the appearance of voluntary grasping. Both patterns may exist together for a while (Touwen, 1976). For example after a baby progresses from the radial grasp to a more accurate pincer grasp both types of grasp may be used at first. The wide range of overlap in developmental sequence in infancy is striking. The motor units are the common pathway for all motor patterns but their control mechanisms undergo developmental changes. Prechtl suggests that these changes involve recruitment of new neural mechanisms rather than remodelling of existing programmes, thus allowing overlap of motor patterns.

During the first six months the infant gradually acquires control of his head and neck muscles, followed by the trunk and limb muscles. Head, neck and trunk development together with balancing and righting reactions enable him to sit upright early in the second half of the first year. Customarily early motor development is described with the infant in the prone, supine and upright positions.

Prone

The newborn infant adopts a predominantly flexed posture and older infants tend to revert to this posture when they are asleep. The arms are flexed and held close to the chest. The newborn infant lies with his head to one side, the pelvis high and the knees flexed up underneath the abdomen. When he is held in ventral suspension, that is, held horizontally with the hands under the abdomen, the head is held just below the plane of the body, the hips are semiflexed and the limbs hang downwards.

From birth he is able momentarily to lift his head off the couch and by four weeks he readily turns to face either way. The pelvis is lower and the hips and knees semi-extended. In ventral suspension (Fig. 1.1) the head is lifted momentarily with the hips and knees semi-extended.

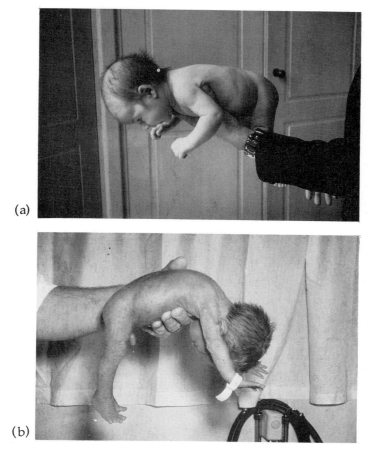

(a)

(b)

Fig. 1.1 (a) Four-week baby held in ventral suspension — note the degree of flexion in both upper and lower limbs and the way the head is held up. (b) By contrast the baby in this figure (admittedly a newborn) is totally floppy and prognosis would be worrying.

By six weeks he is able to hold his head in line with the body for a few moments. By eight weeks he can lift his head higher off the couch to an angle of about 45° and maintain it in the midline. In ventral suspension, the head is maintained for a longer period in line with the body and sometimes lifts above it.

By 12 weeks he lifts his head and upper chest off the couch, using the forearms to support himself. He lies with the pelvis flat against the couch with the legs fully extended, and in ventral suspension the head is maintained at 45–90° to the rest of the body. After 12 weeks he holds more of his chest off the couch and by 24 weeks the whole of the head and upper trunk is supported on flattened palms and outstretched arms. By 24 weeks he can roll from front to back and a month later from back to front.

Supine

The newborn infant lies on his back with the elbows semiflexed and the arms held close to the chest. The legs are semiflexed and held with slight abduction of the hips. With the head in the midline posture is symmetrical. In the first six weeks the infant sometimes adopts the posture of the asymmetrical tonic neck reflex (ATNR) (Fig. 1.2) when lying in the supine position. The ATNR is a primitive response elicited by turning the head to one side. The response consists of extension of the jaw, arm and leg and flexion of the occipital arm and leg. The response disappears by five months and persistence beyond this time indicates abnormal neurodevelopmental function.

When the infant is pulled to the sitting position (Fig. 1.3), the head lags until the body is upright when the head is lifted momentarily before falling forwards. By six weeks the infant can hold his head up for a few seconds, and by three months there is little or no head lag. By six months he is able to raise his head from the pillow to look at his feet. He will lift his head in anticipation of being picked up.

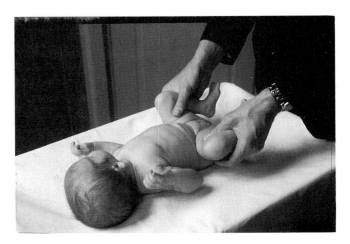

Fig. 1.2 An asymmetric tonic neck reflex seen here as the doctor is feeling the femoral pulse. Occiputal leg and arm are extended while the jaw, arm and leg are flexed. It is only partially observed in the normal neonate and a persistent response is cause for concern.

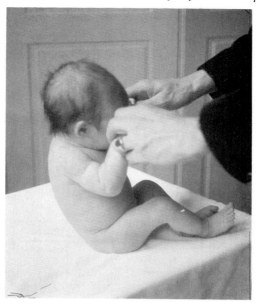

Fig. 1.3 Pull-to-sit — note the rounded back but the relative good head control in this four-week-old baby.

Sitting position

When held in the sitting position the infant's back remains rounded at four, six and eight weeks. By three months the back is straight except for a curve in the lumbar region. At 16 weeks a lumbar curve is still present and by 20 weeks the back is straight.

Held sitting at six weeks the head is held up momentarily and is maintained for a few seconds. By three months the head is mostly held steady but tends to bob forward. At four months the head still wobbles when the body is swayed but by 20 weeks there is no head wobble. By six months he can sit with support in a pram or high chair and turn his head to look around him.

Upright position

When held vertically the newborn infant demonstrates the walking and placing reflexes (Figs 1.4 and 1.5). He also extends his legs in response to pressure on the soles of the feet. At six weeks the infant still presses down with his feet, straightens the body and makes stepping movements. The primitive reflexes disappear over the first

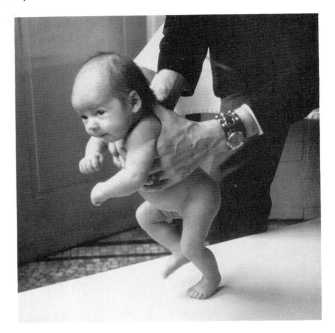

Fig. 1.4 Primary walking.

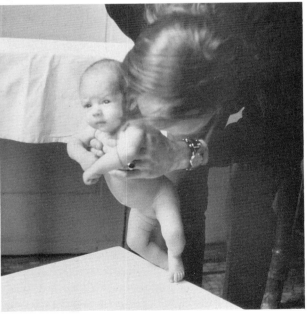

Fig. 1.5 Placing — the dorsum of the left foot has been touched on the under-surface of the table and the baby now lifts it over and places it on the surface. This response persists throughout life.

three months and the 12-week-old infant tends to sag at the knees when held standing. By 24 weeks the infant can bear almost all his weight again and bounces up and down actively.

Fine motor

The first six months of life see the transition from the strong reflex grasping and sweeping arm movements of the newborn infant to purposeful reaching and the beginning of accurate grasping. The newborn infant has a strong grasp reflex which begins to develop from the 10th week of fetal life. At birth it is actually possible to lift the infant up by the grasp. By six weeks this is no longer possible, since the grasp reflex has diminished and disappeared completely by three months. Persistence of the grasp reflex is an indication of neurological dysfunction.

By three months the infant closes and uncloses his hands and is able to hold a rattle for a few moments. Some infants can hold a bottle soon after three months if placed in the hands. At three months he begins a phase of closely watching his playful hands, known as 'hand regard'. This normally continues until 20 weeks, but it may persist longer in mentally retarded infants. Gaining visual familiarity with the hands plays an important part in the development of voluntary grasping. Blind infants, who do not know their hands visually, show marked delay in accurate prehension.

Visual and fine motor behaviours are closely related in the development of visually directed reaching. This sensorimotor skill requires focusing attention, receiving a visual signal, processing the information in the brain and selecting one of a wide variety of motor responses. This ability to reach out towards an object which attracts the infant's visual attention is a skill which is achieved fully by five months. In favourable circumstances it has been possible to demonstrate that even newborn infants attempt to reach bright objects. These early attempts at reaching are typically sweeping movements of the whole arm and cannot be adjusted during their course. However, the next attempt may be modified to try and reach the target. The three-month-old infant shows great interest in objects and takes swipes towards them. By four months the infant makes more co-ordinated attempts to obtain objects, but still tends to overshoot the mark. Between five and six months, most infants are capable of accurate reaching towards objects, and play with bricks and noise-making toys.

The five- to six-month-old gazes intently at objects and is now able to reach accurately towards them. He scoops a small object up in the palm of his hand, holding it on the ulnar side. At this age he is visually alert and well equipped to start exploring his environment with his hands.

Early vocalizations

The infant demonstrates his ability to communicate and to respond to others almost as soon as he is born. Already, the mother may have noticed the fetus's response to sound *in utero*. In the first few days of life the mother's voice is effective in soothing a crying baby and he soon learns to recognize his own mother's voice. The young infant is able to communicate his feelings to his mother with a wide variety of non-vocal actions, such as smiling, stiffening, frowning, nestling, seeking eye-contact, turning away and joyful welcoming movements. The cry is also a powerful biological means of communication and mothers soon learn to recognize the meaning of different patterns of cry, such as distress, hunger, surprise or wanting attention. Vocalizations begin at around one month, sometimes earlier than this. Initially, the infant coos and gurgles and is able to produce individual sounds, known as phonemes: these are mainly vowel sounds from the front of the mouth, such as 'oo', followed by vowels from the middle, like 'ugh' and 'agh'. After the first three months some consonantal sounds produced in the back of the mouth may be heard.

At one month the infant is able to make fine discrimination between speech sounds and this ability develops greatly during the first six months. In ingenious experiments whereby the infant learns to suck a teat in response to various voice sounds, the infant initially learns to suck in response to a syllable such as 'pa'. After a while he becomes bored and ceases sucking. Introducing a different sound 'ba' stimulates further sucking, indicating that the infant discriminates between the two sounds (de Villiers & de Villiers, 1979).

Typically, vocalization begins about two weeks after smiling, developing as a form of social interaction. The baby soon uses emotionally charged vocalizations to express his feelings and by three months the baby has pre-linguistic 'conversations' with his mother. When the mother speaks to the baby he replies with his own vocalization, which is followed by more speech by the mother. By four to six months lip and tongue consonants are developing with the production of sounds like 'ebe, pth, ele, da, ba, ka, mum'. These vowel and consonant combinations are known as 'babbling'.

Over the next few months, these sounds increase rapidly in range and complexity, and are used for social interaction and spontaneously for the baby's own amusement. The onset of babbling depends on physical maturation and the development of control over the infant's articulatory organs rather than exposure to speech sounds. Interestingly the pattern of early babble is similar across different languages so that French, Japanese and English babies all sound alike at this stage. Subsequent vocalizations, however, are moulded and reinforced by parents so that very soon distinct patterns emerge which have the characteristics of the parents' tongue. Deaf children begin to babble at about the same age as hearing children. However, continuation of babble beyond eight or nine months depends on the ability to hear oneself and others. Deaf children's babble is likely to diminish or disappear during the second six months and does not develop speech inflections later in the first year.

Retarded infants tend to have immature patterns of babble and develop speech patterns slowly. Autistic children rarely produce normal babble and produce fewer sounds with less speech intonation than normal children.

Social behaviour and understanding

The newborn infant begins to form social relationships and show an interest in his surroundings almost immediately. Already many mothers will have felt the beginnings of attachment to their infant from early pregnancy and this attachment gradually strengthens during the first nine months of life. But mothers do not always fall in love with their baby at the moment of birth. One study (Macfarlane, 1977) found that 5% of mothers did not feel love for their babies until the end of the first week of life. Sometimes it may take several months for a close loving relationship to develop.

The phenomenon of 'bonding' has been much discussed in recent years. It describes early specific behaviours which lead the baby and the mother to relate to one another socially and which were formerly believed to be innate and essential for normal attachment to develop. The evidence for these behaviours is slight and, while quite clearly very important processes go on between the mother (and father) and the young child, it is not now believed that there are specific bonding behaviours which are essential to normal social development. Rather it is seen that the process of 'attachment' is a longer phenomenon which goes on throughout early childhood and describes the intense relationship which parents have with their child. It is something which grows with the child as the child grows.

The infant has many characteristics which are attractive to mothers, such as rounded face and relatively large eyes and head. Certain features of his behaviour show variation, even in the first few days, and may influence how the mother feels and handles him. Some infants are extremely visually alert and may show keen interest in faces in the first few days and smile and vocalize early. It is likely that parents would find this sort of interaction rewarding at an early stage. Cuddliness is another behaviour which shows wide variation. The more active alert infant may be less cuddly and less readily pacified by close contact. Some infants actively dislike being held closely and may be calmed by being near to their mother, sucking, or being carried round. In contrast, the less active, placid infant is often more cuddly, likes being closely embraced and wrapped and resorts more to cuddly toys.

The infant cry is another potent biological signal which produces immediate responses in parents. The infant with a persistent, strong cry may demand and will probably receive a lot of parental attention. The weaker, less insistent cry elicits less reaction from parents and the infant may receive fewer cuddles and parental handling. What seems clear, however, is that infants vary enormously in their need for cuddling, holding and attention. The quality of attachment depends on the way a person responds to a child's individual signals for attention, rather than to the total amount of contact. Some infants may want lots of cuddling and holding and others may prefer being talked to or having a familiar face to study close by. Mothers may be surprised initially by non-cuddliness and demanding behaviour, but quickly adjust and find ways of strengthening the relationship. This demands a degree of flexibility and acceptance of unexpected behaviour in the child. A mother may need to overcome initial feelings of rejection by her infant until she finds appropriate ways of handling him. Undoubtedly, some parents find their baby's behaviour difficult to understand and accept and in extreme cases this can result in emotional deprivation or even child abuse. Hopefully, this can be minimized by a wider knowledge of the variety of behaviour, even between infants in the same family. A close relationship between parent and child develops with active interaction rather than simply caring for a child's physical needs. It is perhaps reassuring for the fathers that the time spent simply feeding an infant and changing him may be less potent in forming a deep attachment than periods when the parent plays actively with the child. Although mother–child attachment predominates in the early weeks, as she is usually the main caretaker, later in the first year the infant can become as firmly attached to father, friends or other relatives who may spend a relatively short time with the child. In one study (Schaffer & Emerson, 1964) one-fifth of the people to whom babies became attached took no part at all in their physical care.

The beginnings of understanding can be seen from the first weeks of life. The infant can imitate tongue protrusion. He watches his mother intently when feeding. Bright lights, faces and coloured objects attract his gaze. By six weeks he smiles and vocalizes in response to social overtures.

At 12 weeks he engages in playful activities like tickling and peep-boo, to which he reacts with squeals of pleasure and laughter. He recognizes familiar situations such as bathing and feeding, responding with smiles, coos and vigorous movements. He expresses dislike when parted from familiar adults.

He shows even greater interest in his surroundings by five months, reaching for objects. He begins to realize that objects are permanent and soon starts to look around for a dropped toy. He helps to hold a bottle and smiles at the image of himself in the mirror.

Development of vision

The visual system is immature at birth, yet the infant is equipped with ample visual function for his own needs. He can see objects best at nine inches away, enabling him to observe his mother's face when she is feeding him.

Eye movements have been detected *in utero* though the fetus remains in a dark environment. It is possible that when the uterine wall becomes stretched at the end of pregnancy a certain amount of light may pass through which the fetus would see as a glow. By 28 weeks' gestation the pupils react to light, though the reaction may be sluggish at first. At birth the eye is already one-third of its adult size and achieves three-quarters of its postnatal growth by the age of three. The fovea of the retina is immature at birth and develops during the first four months. The lens continues to grow throughout life, acquiring certain changes in composition as time goes on. The lacrimal gland is immature at birth. Babies rarely produce reflex tears before two months or emotional tears before four months.

VISUAL ACUITY

Visual acuity is a measure of the finest detail that can be resolved. Measurement of visual acuity in the infant is difficult and relies on obtaining certain responses to visual stimuli. However, absence of a positive response may not necessarily provide conclusive proof that the infant cannot see a given level of detail and it is not surprising that reports of visual acuity vary considerably. There are a number of techniques used to assess acuity. In 'preferential looking' the infant is confronted with a pattern and a uniform field is observed to see which one he fixates on (Fig. 1.6). Infants prefer to look at patterns rather than at uniform objects. In this way it has been found that the infant has a preference for 1/8 inch stripes over grey at birth and 1/32 inch stripes over grey at five months, equivalent to acuities of 6/120 and 6/30 respectively (Fantz, 1975). Optokinetic nystagmus, visual evoked potential and habituation/recovery are other methods used. For clinical purposes, the Catford drum is widely used in young children and indicates a higher level of acuity than preferential looking. The infant is shown a small discrete spot on a revolving drum and tracking movements of the eyes are observed. However, the infant may respond to a blur without being able to see the discrete spot and it is possible that acuity may be overestimated by this method.

Using the Catford drum visual acuity has been estimated as 6/18 at five months, 6/12 at 18 months, 6/9 at two years and 6/6 at three years (Catford & Oliver, 1973).

REFRACTION AND ACCOMMODATION

The infant is able to focus more accurately on near rather than far objects. During the first month of life the focus of the lens is fairly

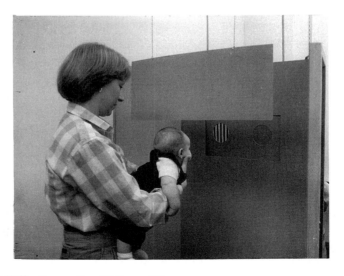

Fig. 1.6 Diffraction grating (Teller, 1986).

fixed and appropriate for objects nine inches away. Accommodation develops over the first two months, gradually increasing the infant's range of clear vision. At birth eye movements are poorly and often jerkily co-ordinated. Smooth convergence of both eyes and binocular vision develop by four to six months.

Infants are hypermetropic, using cycloplegic refraction (when active accommodation is absent). A mild degree of hypermetropia is unlikely to cause blurring of vision as this can be compensated for by accommodation. A high degree of hypermetropia may be associated with a convergent squint in older children as a result of an increased but unequal convergence in an attempt to adjust for hypermetropia.

VISUAL FIELD

The visual field of the young infant is markedly restricted. Under two months he is unable to fixate on objects introduced further away than 45° from the midline. After two months he becomes increasing able to alter his visual attention from an object he has initially fixated on to an object in his peripheral field of vision.

VISUAL PERCEPTION

A number of ingenious studies have demonstrated how the infant's perception of form and space develops. The observation that newborns prefer patterns to plain surfaces suggests that some perception of form is present at birth. Babies are attracted by complex patterns and contrasts, and will watch particularly intently the eyes of the human face. Fantz (1961) demonstrated preference for the face when he examined infants from four days to six months. He showed them three oval pictures, one of a human face, one with the same features but scrambled and one which had a solid black patch equal in area to the features of the first two. At all ages the babies looked most at the real face, somewhat less at the scrambled picture and least at the one with the black patch.

Carpenter (1974) found that two-week-old babies looked more towards their mother's face than at a stranger's face and even averted their eyes from the stranger's face.

Depth perception appears to be well developed at an early age. Fantz (1961) has shown that one-month-old infants fixate longer on a sphere than on a disc of the same diameter. The infant also reacts to an approaching object by pulling his head back at the age of one month.

Another well-known experiment employs the visual cliff to investigate depth perception. The infant is placed on a glass surface under which a step downwards is constructed. At the age of six months and later the infant refuses to crawl across the 'cliff' although it is covered by glass, an indication that he can perceive the drop in height.

The infant prefers bright colours, and is therefore more likely to follow a moving red ball than a white one during examination. Studies on colour discrimination must therefore use colours of equal brightness. There is now evidence that infants discriminate between colours. Four-month-old babies were shown one colour until they ceased to respond (habituated) to it and were then presented with a new colour, the same colour or a colour of a different wavelength which did not cross a colour boundary. The infants looked more at the new colour than at the other two colours.

The infant's ability to discriminate depth, shape and colour is important in the development of eye–hand co-ordination. Even new-born infants attempt to reach towards brightly coloured objects. By the age of six months visual acuity and fine motor co-ordination enable the baby to reach for fine objects such as threads and crumbs.

Hearing

HEARING BEFORE BIRTH

The auditory system is better developed than the visual system at birth; the newborn baby responds to sound throughout the whole range that the human ear can detect. However, *in utero* and for the first few days after birth the middle ear is filled with amniotic fluid, which dampens all sounds reaching the ear. Mothers have long been aware that towards the end of pregnancy the baby becomes more active in response to loud sounds such as music or passing traffic. Several studies have confirmed this and have demonstrated that the baby responds to sound when the mother's ears are masked, suggesting that the baby actually hears sounds and is not altering his behaviour as a result of the mother's reaction to sound.

The baby's environment in the uterus is noisy. Microphones inserted through the cervix during labour have recorded a loud rhythmical whooshing sound exactly in time with the mother's pulse. Salk played the sound of an adult heartbeat to a group of newborn babies for four days and found that they gained more weight and cried less than the babies without the heartbeat. Others have tried to use a simulated heartbeat to calm older babies with some success.

Fluid is absorbed from the middle ear during the first few days after birth. The newborn's hearing threshold is about 10 decibels higher than the older infant's or adult's. Before the age of one week the infant can recognize his mother's voice, moving his eyes more towards his mother's than a stranger's voice. Sucking is another behavioural response to sound used in a study which demonstrated that babies suck more readily to obtain a recording of the mother's than of a stranger's voice (Mills & Melhinsh, 1974).

SOUND LOCALIZATION

The young infant responds to loud sounds by blinking and sometimes with the startle or Moro response. He will quieten and listen to sound such as his mother's voice, bell or rattle and this response provides a good indication that sounds are heard. A more sensitive test of hearing involves the infant demonstrating that he can localize the origin of sound.

Testing of hearing, as of vision, presents a major problem in selecting a response. The baby is unable to give a verbal response or to press buttons in reaction to sound, and various behavioural and physiological techniques are used to indicate whether the baby can hear. Searching for sound with eyes and/or head movements is a widely used behavioural response in infants from six months onward as in the Stycar hearing test. In infants up to the age of four weeks the Linco Bennett Auditory Response Cradle measures movements and changes in respiratory rate in response to 85 dB sound and can reliably detect hearing impairment. There is plenty of evidence that infants can discriminate the source of sound at birth. However, even in controlled conditions with the infant in the ideal state, some studies have found that only 60% of infants demonstrated turning. This does not of course mean that they are unable to hear the stimulus but illustrates the difficulty of testing hearing in the infant. Turning in response to sound develops slowly in the newborn, the baby may continue turning as many as 12 times, but, by the age of five months, if turning to a sound source is not rewarded, the baby will stop responding. Another difference between hearing responses in the young baby and the baby of five months is that in the younger baby the sound stimulus may need to be presented for a longer time, say up to 20 seconds, to obtain a response. In contrast the five-month-old will react to a very short sound.

Given the right circumstances head turning to sound occurs in newborns but may occur less readily by three months, improving again by five months. By three to four months the head and eyes move together. Downward localization occurs at five to six months and is achieved by the infant turning his head to the side and then downwards. Upwards localizations happen somewhat later at about six months. At six to eight months the baby localizes upwards or downwards by turning his head in a curving arc. By eight to 10 months he turns diagonally and directly towards the sound. The older baby's head turn is based on a more sophisticated sound localization process and may represent more voluntary behaviour under intentional control. Clinically a reliable hearing test should be possible from six months onwards and there is no evidence of any advantage in leaving it until seven to eight months. (For further discussion see p. 75.)

SOUND DISCRIMINATION

The baby is born with preferences for sounds with a broad spectrum of frequencies rather than pure tones. The human voice is by far the most meaningful sound from the very beginning, preferably high pitched rather than low pitched. In a fascinating experiment, Condon (1974) filmed infants aged 12 hours to two days old and found that their movements were synchronized to human speech sounds in both English and Chinese.

Not only does the infant show a preference for the human voice but he is also able to discriminate between consonants soon after birth. One study (Eimas, 1971) used habituation techniques in which the infant, aged between one and four months, demonstrated habituation to a consonant by decline in heart rate or rate of sucking. When a new consonant was introduced the infant reacted by an increase in heart rate or by sucking more. Research into linguistic development suggests that the young child develops the ability to discriminate new speech sounds which he hears at home, indicating the importance of a wide range of early language experience.

Smell

The ability of the young infant to smell has been confirmed by a number of studies. Engen *et al.* (1963) showed differentiating responses to acetic acid, aniseed, asafoetida and phenylethylalcohol in newborns. Macfarlane (1975) showed that infants in the first week of life turned more often towards their mothers' breast pads than to those from another mother or to a clean pad. It is easy to imagine how the attraction of the smell of both breast milk and the mother helps the baby locate the nipple and begin suckling.

Taste

Two intriguing observations indicate that the baby is able to taste in the uterus. Forty years ago a doctor attempted to treat hydramnios by injection of saccharine into the amniotic fluid and found that the amount of fluid diminished as a result of the baby swallowing more of it. More recently, injection of radio-opaque substances into the amniotic fluid resulted in reduction of swallowing observed on X-ray. Taste buds begin to develop around 55 days' gestation and increase in number postnatally. The young infant does not have the adult's ability to detect subtle flavour differences. However, babies are born with preferences for certain flavours and aversion to others. In one experiment the facial expressions of neonates were photographed when they were offered their first drink after birth. A sucrose solution was followed by a slight smile, licking and sucking whereas bitter quinine sulphate solutions and sour citric acid produced expressions of dislike. Flavour preferences are modified as the child develops and experiences new tastes. Generally, familiar tastes are preferred to novel ones but repeated exposure to new foods results in increased acceptance.

The six-week developmental history and examination

The six-week examination

The assessment of the infant at six weeks not only involves detection of developmental and physical defects requiring treatment but is also an opportunity to assess how the mother—child couple are getting on together. Only 5% of babies will be found to have a developmental or physical problem at six weeks. Since early diagnosis of most of these defects, such as congenital dislocation of the hip (CDH), is vitally important, this alone would probably justify the exercise in most people's opinion. Taking a broader view of the consultation makes it even more worthwhile. It is an opportunity to begin a lasting relationship with parents. Demonstration of the baby's achievements reassures parents of the normality of their infant and may stimulate closer interaction between them.

By six weeks the health visitor will have already assessed the nursing couple and helped iron out some early difficulties with feeding and management. She will have a shrewd idea about which mothers are not coping happily with their babies and will be able to draw this to the doctor's attention.

The history

History from the mother will identify antenatal and natal factors which may predispose to difficulty in the early weeks. A stressful pregnancy, in terms of either life stress or medical complication (which may be interrelated), has been found to increase the chances of postnatal depression or a problem with the mother–child relationship. A difficult delivery provides a less than ideal beginning to motherhood and mothers may find it helpful to discuss the events at delivery with the doctor and voice their underlying fear of a further pregnancy. Mothers of preterm or sick newborns may have particular problems in adjusting to motherhood, especially if there has been a period of separation in the special-care baby unit. Several important studies have highlighted the hazards of early separation and linked it with subsequent child abuse (Lynch, 1975) and with more subtle differences in the pattern of maternal attachment and mother–child interaction (Seashore *et al.*, 1973). The mother may have left hospital without her baby, and it is not surprising that she will need additional support when the baby eventually comes home.

Most mothers will be aware if significant anoxia or delay in establishing respiration occurred after birth and this can be verified by checking on the Apgar score and discharge summary. It is important to note hyperbilirubinaemia as this could indicate the need for particular vigilance over the baby's hearing. A history of delay or difficulty in sucking in the newborn period is also relevant as it may be associated with birth trauma or neurological disorder. Developmental delay may present with disturbance of feeding, sleeping, crying or activity in the early weeks. These symptoms need careful evaluation as they are much more likely to be associated with a management problem or difficulty with the mother–child relationship than with serious brain damage. Mothers' reports of slow feeding, poor sucking or low intake of milk may reflect difficulty with feeding technique, with either bottle or breast, unrealistic ideas of normal behaviour or, less commonly, some disorder of the infant, such as immaturity, oral thrush, cleft palate, hypothyroidism or neuromuscular incoordination as in pseudobulbar cerebral palsy.

Excessive crying and difficulty in consoling is seen in babies with brain injury but is more likely to be a feature of the baby's personality or reflect underlying problems with handling. Patterns of sleeping and activity vary enormously from baby to baby as do parents' expectations of normality. At six weeks a baby may spend between eight and 18 hours asleep. Excessive sleepiness is seen in developmental delay, but it is equally worrying if a baby is just left to sleep for long hours, and is consequently likely to suffer from under-stimulation.

It is important to enquire about how the mother is feeling, if she is unduly depressed, tired or suffering from any health or emotional problems. As well as classic postnatal depression, periods of depression or mental distress occur in as many as 40% of mothers of under-fives (Brown & Harris, 1978). They may first come to light in the child health clinic or on a home visit either as feelings expressed to the doctor or health visitor or disguised as problems with the child.

Knowledge of the ages at which a child achieves certain milestones provides a valuable guide to the rate of development. The most reliable information comes from the doctor's own observation of the child, which may be supplemented and confirmed by the mother's account of what the child can do. Firstly, it is essential to make sure that both mother and doctor are talking about the same activity. Generally speaking the mother's account of the child's current abilities is fairly reliable although this is not always so. For example, sometimes a mother has not noticed that her infant can transfer objects from hand to hand, yet he demonstrates this readily in the clinic. On the other hand, parents may exaggerate their child's achievements. For example, a child may be said to be putting words together but closer examination may reveal that he is saying phrases such as 'here you are' which he has learned as one word. Ideally items on developmental examination should never be passed on mother's report alone, even if this means seeing the child for a repeat visit, e.g. if he is excessively shy. The weaknesses of some developmental screening tests such as the Denver Developmental Screening Test lie in allowing items to be passed on parental report only. A useful principle is to make it clear in the notes whether an item was observed or reported by the mother.

With regular developmental screening it is seldom that one will meet a new child for whom no previous records are available, when one has to rely entirely on the history for information about early developmental progress. However, it is important to be aware of the poor reliability of mother's recall of some developmental milestones. Although late onset of smiling is highly significant in developmental diagnosis many mothers have forgotten the event by the time the baby is six months old. In our study (Hart *et al.*, 1978), although 86% of mothers reported their babies smiling when seen at six weeks, when asked at six months only 57% remembered smiling at six weeks, 30%

said it was after six weeks and 13% couldn't remember at all. The time of walking was the most accurately remembered milestone, whereas speech milestones were poorly recalled. Interestingly, parents tended to recall the onset of single words and sentences as occurring earlier than observed at previous examinations.

Since young children are constantly learning new skills and rapidly pass from stage to stage it is perhaps not surprising that the times of past events are easily confused. Encouraging mothers to keep their own diaries to record milestones as they occur provides unique and clinically valuable data on each child.

DEVELOPMENTAL HISTORY AT SIX WEEKS

Smiling

Does he smile when you talk to him? It is important to make it clear that you refer to a smile in response to a social overture: the baby first watches the mother's face intently and then smiles in response to her talking or smiling at him. Mothers may report smiling whilst asleep or with wind, and these are not true smiles. However, genuine smiling can occur as early as three days after birth.

Soderling (1959) followed 400 normal infants closely during the first weeks of life and, using strict criteria for a true responsive smile, found that 60% of babies smiled by four weeks and 100% by six weeks. In our study (Bax *et al.*, 1980) 86% of mothers reported smiling at the six-week examination, but only 38% actually smiled during the examination although 85% were seen to regard the mother's face. Clearly, one has to rely on mother's history of smiling in many cases. Onset of smiling delayed until after the age of eight weeks in a full-term infant is significant and suggestive of developmental delay.

Vocalizations

Does he make any noises when you talk to him? Early vocalization usually begins a week or two after smiling and some mothers report it as early as two weeks. Generally speaking the infant produces phonemes at around one month which typically consist of vowel combinations such as 'ooo, aah, ooer' but some consonants may also be heard 'goo, coo'. Babies will vocalize most readily in response to parental speech and this reinforcement encourages further utterances. In contrast, the deaf baby may vocalize normally initially but as reinforcement does not occur the amount of babble diminishes over time.

Response to sounds

Does he startle or turn in response to sounds? Do you think he hears normally? By six weeks mothers will have a good idea whether their infant responds to everyday sounds. The baby may turn and jump when he hears his mother's voice. She may have noticed that he responds to a door opening or footsteps. Mothers' doubts about hearing at any age should be taken seriously and the hearing carefully tested.

Visual responses

Does he look at you? Does he follow you with his eyes? Absence of a clear history of fixating and following would be of significance at six weeks and would indicate the need for thorough visual testing.

Movements

Does he move his arms and legs equally? A mother may be the first person to notice weakness of an arm or leg in Erb's palsy or cerebral palsy.

General observations

Observation of the mother and child together can yield much information about the quality of mother—child interaction, 'mothering' and social development of the child. The baby's alertness and readiness to smile and vocalize in response to the mother are an indication of the level of social responsiveness of the infant. One may observe whether the mother cuddles her baby affectionately, whether she handles him confidently and whether she engages in eye-to-eye contact with him. Her reaction to crying or restlessness may demonstrate her concern for his welfare. A general impression of the baby's cleanliness and the appropriateness of his clothing are also valuable pointers to adequacy of mothering. Even the mother's interest in the examination may be significant in relation to the intimacy between mother and child. Kennell *et al.* (1974) in their study of early mother—infant child contact in the neonatal period noted that mothers who had experienced extended contact with their babies post-delivery were more likely to take an interest in the examination of their babies at one year, than mothers who had less contact. However, this study was carried out on a group of socially disadvantaged mothers and there is evidence to suggest that improved social circumstances can diminish the adverse effects of early separation.

Behavioural state

The state of wakefulness of the baby at the time of examination can profoundly influence the baby's response. It used to be thought that the neurological responses of young infants were so inconsistent that neurological examination was of limited value. The discovery that the intensity of the infant's responses are related to his behavioural state altered that view and enabled many valid studies of infant neuro-developmental activity to be carried out. The behavioural states have been classified by Prechtl (1977) into five main types:

1 Deep sleep, eyes closed, regular respiration, no movement.
2 Light sleep, eyes closed, irregular respiration, no gross movements.
3 Awake but drowsy, eyes open, no gross movements.
4 Alert, eyes open, gross movements, no crying.
5 Awake crying, eyes open or closed.
6 Other.

The ideal state for each examination item is one in which a response of medium intensity is consistently found. States 3 and 4 are suitable for virtually all tests. States 1, 2 and 5 are clearly impossible for vision and hearing assessment whereas some tests of motor function are possible during any state.

The behavioural state depends on the timing of the last feed and the baby is usually most amenable to testing two or three hours later. Unfortunately, it is not always possible to see a baby in an ideal state and one has to make a compromise and do the best one can. Babies may fail to show certain responses because they are in an unfavourable state for the particular test. It is worth while recording the baby's state in the notes so that a realistic interpretation of the findings can be made.

The examination can be arranged in such a way that tests which are likely to upset the baby and alter the state, such as the Moro response, and hip examination are left to the end. It is often easier to demonstrate hearing responses, visual following and smiling before the baby is disturbed by undressing.

The eyes and vision

Vision is usually tested with the baby lying supine on the couch but if his eyes remain closed he will often open them if he is held upright facing the examiner and swung gently round. On confrontation the doctor will observe whether the eyes are central or whether there is a constant or intermittent deviation or strabismus. Strabismus (squint) can be classified in several different ways. It may be *latent* or *manifest*. Latent strabismus is a tendency for the eyes to deviate under certain conditions such as tiredness, illness or stress. It may not be present on confrontation but can be demonstrated by special testing techniques. Manifest strabismus is present most of the time as the tendency to deviation is greater than the eye's ability to fixate on objects.

Strabismus may be *alternating* or *monocular*. In alternating strabismus the child uses either eye to fixate on objects. In monocular strabismus one is used for fixation and the other constantly deviates. Vision in the deviating eye may be suppressed by the brain and the child can develop amblyopia, that is, defective central vision as a result of disuse.

The direction of deviation can be described as *convergent* or *divergent* the former being most frequent.

Aetiological classification includes two major groups, *paralytic* (non-comitant) and *non-paralytic* concomitant. In paralytic strabismus the child will show deficiency of eye movement in the direction of the paralysed muscle. The external rectus muscle supplied by the sixth cranial nerve is most commonly affected.

Non-paralytic squint is more common and characteristically the angle of deviation remains relatively constant in all directions of gaze. Some children with such strabismus have an underlying ocular or visual disorder such as cataract, lesions of the macula or optic nerve or most frequently refractive errors. A high degree of myopia is often associated with strabismus. A further group of children have different degrees of refraction in each eye. Most children have a small degree of hypermetropia but if there is a marked tendency to hypermetropia an accommodative strabismus may occur. Here, in an attempt to overcome lack of accommodation, the child overconverges with resultant crossing of the eyes. This type of deviation may occur from six months to seven years, but most commonly appears at two or three years.

True strabismus must be differentiated from *pseudostrabismus*. Children with marked epicanthic folds, wide nasal bridges or facial asymmetry may give a false impression of having strabismus, particularly if the child is not facing the examiner squarely.

In the infant strabismus can be detected by shining a light directly in front of the eyes and determining whether the reflection is symmetrical in both pupils. By six weeks binocular vision predominates but monocular eye movements are occasionally seen. Thus an intermittent strabismus is fairly common but a persistent strabismus is significant and requires early referral.

In the older infant the cover test may be performed. The child is encouraged to fixate on an interesting toy. Each eye is covered in turn and the examiner looks for movement of the eye not being covered. If the eye moves to look at the toy a manifest squint is present. In a latent strabismus it is the occluded eye that tends to deviate at the moment of uncovering. If a child objects to having one eye covered more than the other it may be that that is the good eye and the other has poor vision.

Demonstration of the red reflex is carried out with an opthalmoscope. It will be absent in congenital cataract. Other gross defects such as coloboma of the iris and nystagmus can also be detected. In the 'setting sun' sign, a feature of hydrocephalus, the eyes are deviated downwards (a minor degree is seen in some normal babies).

The reaction of the pupils to light can be tested by shading the eyes with the hand and then removing it. Asymmetry in the pupil or poor response to light suggests neurological dysfunction (e.g. Horner's syndrome) or an intra-ocular lesion such as a cataract. Shining a bright light suddenly at the eyes produces the optical blink reflex, a quick closure of the eyes. This response diminishes or habituates after several trials.

Vision may be tested by first observing the baby's response to either the doctor's or the mother's face. He will first fixate and watch the face intently and will then follow the face with his eyes as it moves across his line of vision. He will also follow a moving object, preferably brightly coloured, held 9−12 inches in front of his face. The baby demonstrates 'head lag' in visual following, the movement of the head following a few moments after the tracking of the eyes. These responses can be elicited in the newborn baby, but become easier to demonstrate by six weeks. In our study 90% of babies followed visually and, in the small number of babies who did not, the usual reason for this was that they were not in the optimal state for carrying out the test. The mother will often give a clear history of visual following and one is less worried about these babies in the absence of a visual response. However, in view of the seriousness of visual handicap, vision should be rechecked at three months or immediately if the doctor is suspicious. On the other hand, it is not uncommon for the mother of a six-week-old baby to say 'he can't see yet, can he?' and the easiest way to convince her is to demonstrate his visual activity. By showing her that he can see, she may be encouraged to interact with him more.

Hearing

Hearing can be tested using the voice, rattle or bell as the stimulus. The child may quieten (still), blink, startle or cry when he hears a sound, loud or quiet. If the baby is already crying he may still in response to the sound of his mother's voice or a rattle. Movement of the eyes and the head in the direction of the sound may occur more readily if he is on his mother's lap with his head supported by her hand. It is difficult to carry out an adequate clinical assessment of hearing in the baby at six weeks and stilling to sound is the easiest response to demonstrate. This occurred in 93% of babies in our study but the noise used needs to be relatively loud at this age and the finding is of relatively low validity. Eye turning and head turning to sound are obviously much more reliable observations but these occurred in only 51% and 39% of babies respectively. Absence of any response to sound is an indication for referral of re-examination in six weeks' time particularly if there is a history of maternal rubella or hyper-bilirubinaemia or if the mother has doubts about the hearing. If the parents report their child is not responding to sound it is very worrying and must be taken seriously.

Vocalization

Vocalization heard during the consultation either spontaneously or in response to talking to the baby should be recorded. In our study over 50% vocalized during the examination and nearly all were heard to cry, usually following hip examination. The quality of the infant cry may be abnormal in certain neurological disorders, e.g. characteristically cat-like in the rare cri-du-chat syndrome, short high-pitched bursts in some infants with cerebral injury and low-pitched in the infant with Down's syndrome.

Smiling and responsiveness

The baby may be observed smiling in response to the doctor or the mother. The baby may also imitate mouth movements if the doctor is patient enough to persevere for several minutes.

Posture and gross motor performance

SUPINE POSTURE

The fetus adopts a predominantly flexed posture and after birth gradual extension occurs. By six weeks the normal full-term infant lies on his back with his limbs semiflexed. When the head is in the midline the limbs are symmetrical but when he turns his head to one side the asymmetric tonic neck reflex causes him to flex the occipital elbow and knee. If his limb posture is asymmetrical when the head is in the midline, then one should suspect hemiplegia or brachial plexus injury. The infant who lies with his legs unduly extended may have spastic tetraplegia but this posture is also seen after breech presentation with extended legs. However, the baby with spastic tetraplegia will show other signs such as increased tone and relative immobility. The child with excessive extensor tone regains a fetal position of flexion when he is asleep. The preterm infant is likely to adopt a more fully flexed posture when seen at six weeks. The hypotonic baby also tends to flex his limbs.

MOVEMENTS

The infant makes large jerky spontaneous movements of his arms and legs. The amount of symmetry of movements should be noted. One would expect the arms to be more active than the legs but a marked difference in activity might indicate spastic tetraplegia.

TREMOR

Tremor is regularly found in newborn infants and occurs in all infants who are crying vigorously. It mainly affects the arms but in some infants the legs, jaw and even the whole body may show trembling movements. It is important to differentiate a tremor which has movement of equal speed in each direction from convulsive movements which characteristically have a fast initial phase followed by a slower movement.

One occasionally sees a baby at six weeks who is still showing marked tremor and this often worries mothers. These babies are likely to have a low threshold for tendon reflexes and easily elicitable Moro responses. It is usually possible to reassure mothers that the tremor will gradually disappear and the baby is perfectly normal.

PULL-TO-SIT

The infant's hands are grasped and he is pulled slowly into a sitting position. He resists extension of the arms and keeps the elbows moderately flexed. He shows considerable head lag but is able to raise his head and maintain it in the upright position for a few seconds. The hypotonic, drowsy or developmentally delayed infant will have poor head control and weak resistance to traction.

PRONE POSITION

When the six-week-old baby is asleep he adopts the fetal position with the pelvis high and the knees drawn up under his abdomen. When he is awake he lies with his head to one side, the pelvis fairly low on the couch, and the hips semi-extended. A full-term infant whose pelvis is high or with the knees under the abdomen (the frog position) may have developmental delay, or hypotonia. However the preterm baby may still adopt this posture at six weeks.

VENTRAL SUSPENSION

The infant is held horizontally with the examiner's hands under his abdomen. The newborn baby lifts his head momentarily and holds his hips in partial extension and knees and elbows semiflexed. By six weeks the baby holds his head in line with his body for a few seconds.

The baby with hypotonia or developmental delay cannot hold his head up and the legs and arms hang down limply.

On the other hand, the infant with increased extensor tone in the spinal muscles as a result of cerebral palsy may appear advanced in the prone position and in ventral suspension. However, on 'pull-to-sit' he may show excessive head lag. Increase in extensor tone may be variable and the infant with severe cerebral palsy may be generally hypotonic at first and develop hypertonia after a few weeks.

Inherent responses

A great many 'primitive' inherent responses are described in the newborn infant; this section will concentrate on those which are most commonly observed and may have some significance in developmental diagnosis. Absence of any of these inherent responses, such as the Moro or startle response in the neonatal period, may be a sign of disordered cerebral function. Similarly, the persistence of a response after the time by which it normally disappears may be a sign of a neurodevelopmental abnormality. The method of eliciting infants' reflexes and the nature of the responses are clearly described by Prechtl in *The Neurological Examination of the Full-term Newborn Infant*.

THE MORO REFLEX

The Moro reflex was first described by Moro in 1918 and was well reviewed by Mitchell in 1960. It was originally considered to be a primitive 'embracing' or clasping movement analogous to the way in which young creatures such as the ape cling on to their mother. However, others have pointed out that the movement is essentially one of extension and is a complex response resulting from the interplay of several postural reflexes. Whatever the explanation of the Moro reflex, as Mitchell points out it must be regarded as a response of immaturity.

Moro advocated striking the table on either side of the infant so that a jolting movement is produced which acts as a stimulus for the response. However, a different method is now usually adopted involving allowing the infant's head to drop backwards. It can be elicited by holding the infant in a supine horizontal position allowing the head to drop either by releasing the head to drop a few inches or by quickly lowering the hand which is supporting the head. The head should be in the midline. A full response consists of abduction of the upper limbs at the shoulders, extension of the forearms at the elbows and extension of the fingers, followed by adduction of the arms at the shoulders and flexion of the forearms at the elbows. The baby usually cries and it is advisable to explain the procedure to the mother beforehand.

The response is easily elicited in newborn babies at six weeks and then diminishes in intensity, finally disappearing at two or three months. In our study 97% of babies had a normal Moro response at six weeks. The remaining 3% had absent responses but were thought to be normal and one child out of 350 had an asymmetrical response of possible significance.

Both complete absence of the Moro response in the infant and persistence beyond three months may be an indication of a neuro-developmental disorder. Increased intensity, usually with tremor of the hands, may be associated with a neurological disorder or with hyperexcitability. A diminished or incomplete response is seen with both increased and decreased muscle tone. An asymmetrical Moro response is also seen in Erb's palsy, fracture of the humerus or clavicle or spastic hemiplegia. The two most common reasons for an asymmetrical Moro response are the infant's head not in the midline and one thumb clenched in the baby's fist which exerts an inhibitory effect on the reflex. If both hands are in the thumb-in-fist posture there is likely to be diminished extension of the arms. A weak or absent Moro may occur if the baby is very sleepy.

STARTLE RESPONSE

This response is often confused with the Moro but, although it can be elicited by the same stimuli as the Moro, it differs in certain respects and is regarded as a separate response. Unlike the Moro response it consists of predominantly flexion movement which can involve the whole body. It is less easily elicited than the Moro in the very early weeks but, whereas the Moro reflex diminishes, the startle reflex becomes more easily elicited and eventually becomes the adult's startle or 'jump' to a surprise. Parents may be concerned that their baby jerks or startles easily in response to sounds or sudden movement or even during nappy changing or dressing. In these babies it is usually possible to demonstrate a low threshold for the Moro and startle responses. Very often the baby will also exhibit brisk tendon reflexes and such babies are often termed 'hyperexcitable'. However, parents can be reassured that this is a normal developmental pattern and that the behaviour will gradually lessen over the first six months.

PALMAR GRASP

One of the first recorded observations of the grasp reflex was made in 1891 by Robinson, who reported that newborn infants could support their own weight when suspended. The response is strongest during the first weeks of life and is easily elicited at the six-week examination. It declines to a very low level over the first six months and is gradually superseded by voluntary grasping. However, it is not until the second year that the child again achieves the capacity to support himself by grasping with his hands.

With the baby's head in the midline the response is elicited by the examiner placing his index finger in the palm of the baby's hand, taking care not to touch the dorsum of the hand as this may inhibit the grasp response. The baby should grasp the examiner's finger strongly for several seconds. If the grasp is weak it can be facilitated by the baby sucking. Differences in intensity between the two sides may signify Erb's or Klumpke's paralysis on the weaker side or spastic hemiplegia affecting the stronger side. Persistent thumb-in-fist posture of the hands may be associated with an unusually strong and prolonged grasp reflex and may indicate spastic cerebral palsy.

PLACING RESPONSE

This is carried out by holding the baby upright with both hands under the arms and around the chest. The baby is lifted so that the dorsum of the foot lightly touches the edge of a table. A cold surface such as metal is more likely to elicit a response. The infant lifts his foot by flexion of the knee and hip and places it on the table.

Placing is seen in about 90% of babies at six weeks. Most babies with an absent placing response at six weeks have a normal response when re-examined a week later. Zappella (1963) found that the placing response was absent in a group of older mentally retarded children with a mental age of less than three months and it has been suggested that a persistently absent placing response in the young baby could be significant.

PRIMARY WALKING

This response was documented by Peiper in 1929 and received extensive study. It may be difficult to elicit in the first two or three days of life but is present in most babies at six weeks. The stepping movements disappear during the fourth or fifth month, well before true walking begins. Attempts to prevent the disappearance of primary stepping by regularly exercising infants have not been successful. The infant is held in the same way as for the placing response and the soles of the feet are allowed to touch the surface of the table. The baby is moved gently forward and will usually produce two or more alternating stepping movements of the legs.

Primary walking is a variable response and cannot always be elicited, although Mac Keith's manoeuvre of elevating the chin often makes a reluctant baby walk. Primary walking was present in 84% of infants in our study. It may be absent in infants born by breech presentation who either extend or flex the legs and who may later become bottom shufflers. Rarely one may observe the asymmetry produced by a dislocated hip or the persistent extension, crossing or 'scissoring' of the legs seen in spastic diplegia.

Most of us enjoy seeing the primary walking and placing responses elicited but it is doubtful whether they are of great clinical value.

ASYMMETRICAL TONIC NECK REFLEX (ATNR)

The baby is placed in the supine position and the face is slowly turned to each side in turn. The ATNR consists of extension of the jaw, arm and leg and flexion of the occipital arm and leg. The arms adopt the fencer's position and persisting fisting of the occipital hand may suggest a hemiparesis. However, in the normal infant on restoring the baby's head to the midline a symmetrical posture is resumed. The response is variable in the newborn and is seen more consistently at six weeks. The reflex disappears by five months and persistence after this age suggests neurological abnormality.

Physical examination of the infant and young child

THE HEAD

Some degree of asymmetry of the skull is common and often gives rise to anxiety in parents. Typically, the brow is prominent on one side of the head and there is flattening of the occiput on that side. This postural asymmetry (postural plagiocephaly) is seen in the early weeks, probably because of the intra-uterine posture. Parents can be advised to alternate lying positions in the cot and can be reassured that it begins to resolve after the age of two months. It is uncommon to see marked asymmetry after the age of one year. Plagiocephaly and facial asymmetry (Fig. 1.7) may also accompany congenital torticollis (wry neck) and hence it is important to exclude this as a cause of the baby's posture. In this condition the head is tilted to one side due to shortening of the sternomastoid muscle resulting either from torsion and tearing during delivery or from persistent lateral flexion *in utero*. A sterno-mastoid 'tumour' consisting of fibrous tissue can be palpated and the

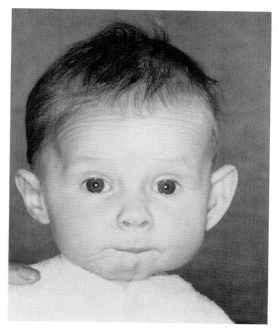

Fig. 1.7 Plagiocephaly — this actually describes the asymmetry of the skull. From the front what can be observed is bossing of the left side of the face and a flattening on the occiput can be seen from above. This finding is often associated with asymmetry of the ears. While these asymmetries are detectable in later life they are insignificant except when seen in a neurodevelopmental disorder (photo, courtesy of Dr J.K. Brown).

condition usually resolves with passive stretching of the muscle. In untreated or persistent cases the tilting may even affect the child's optic axis and occasionally surgical treatment is necessary. Other forms of head asymmetry involve premature closure of one or more sutures of the skull (craniosynostosis). When the sagittal suture closes early, the head becomes long and narrow (scaphocephaly) and a bony ridge often marks the obliterated sutures. Closure of the coronal suture results in a short head with deformity of the face and orbits (oxycephaly).

Other head shapes are characteristically, but not invariably, associated with forms of mental retardation. In microcephaly the head often slopes towards the vertex. A flat occiput may be associated with poor mental development and is also a feature of Down's syndrome.

On palpation the anterior and posterior fontanelles vary in size considerably. The posterior fontanelle usually closes by six weeks and the anterior by 18 months. If the anterior fontanelle is small at first, it generally enlarges over the first few months. Persistence of an excessively large anterior or posterior fontanelle can be associated with conditions such as hydrocephaly, preterm birth, intra-uterine growth retardation, vitamin D deficiency, rickets, rubella syndrome and a number of other rare syndromes. When measuring the head circumference, the tape-measure should be placed above the eyes and round the occiput so that it encircles the maximum head circumference. The size of the skull reflects both brain growth and the age and size of the baby. The average full-term infant has a head circumference of 35 cm at birth and the rate of increase of head circumference is 1 cm per month for the rest of the first year.

A big baby is likely to have a correspondingly large head; therefore the head circumference should be compared with the weight on a percentile chart. A baby of short gestation and one who is small for gestational age have a relatively larger head than a small full-term baby. An older malnourished infant will also have a relatively large head, as this is the measurement which is least affected by malnutrition.

A large or small head may be familial and one should look at the parents for a possible hereditary feature. A genetically small or large head by no means signifies mental deficiency. However, a clinical impression of mental retardation would be supported if the difference between the expected head circumference for the child's weight and age and the actual head circumference is more than 2 SD (2.5 cm) in either direction. Mental deficiency which is present during the first year may be associated with microcephaly with early closure of the fontanelles. An open fontanelle at nine to 12 months would suggest that the child may not have true microcephaly. Craniostenosis results in a small head with premature closure of the sutures and can lead to mental retardation if not recognized early.

Apart from extremes of normal variation of hereditary origin, hydrocephalus is the commonest cause of a large head. Megalencephaly and hydranencephaly are rarer causes. In severe cases of hydrocephalus, head enlargement occurs before birth and may prevent normal delivery. In milder cases, the head appears normal at birth and subsequently enlarges. If untreated, later clinical features include progressive head enlargement, particularly the frontal area, large bulging anterior fontanelle, palpable separation of the sutures, prominent scalp veins, and downward deviation of the eyes (setting-sun sign). Signs of increased intracranial pressure may develop, such as a high-pitched cry, vomiting and progressive spasticity of the limbs. Serial measurements of head circumference are essential for early diagnosis and assessment of rate of progression. If hydrocephalus begins later in childhood, there is no head enlargement, but instead the child has evidence of increased intracranial pressure with papilloedema, spasticity, ataxia, urinary incontinence and personality change.

EXAMINATION OF MUSCLES

Resistance to passive movements (tone) and power of active movements

Ideally, the infant should be in state 3 or 4. In state 1 and 2 he will appear hypotonic and when he is crying all movements are resisted and assessment is difficult. The arms and legs are gently moved through their full range of movements and one gets an impression of the resistance to movement and increase or decrease in the range of movements. An increase in range of movement is associated with poor muscle tone. The most common causes of hypotonia include benign congenital hypotonia, Down's syndrome, congenital muscular disease, developmental delay and early cerebral palsy. Active power can be assessed when active movements interfere with the passive movements that one is trying to demonstrate. Cerebral palsy, Erb's palsy and congenital muscle disease are amongst conditions where weakness of one or more muscle groups is found.

Muscular consistency

Palpation of the limbs and trunk muscles is useful to determine whether the muscles are unduly soft, as in congenital muscle disease or hard, as in severely hypertonic children. The infant with benign congenital hypotonia has normal muscle consistency.

TENDON REFLEXES

The tendon reflexes should be carried out in state 3 or 4, as states 1, 2 and 5 will produce misleading responses (or absence of response). The index or middle finger is the best instrument and the baby's limbs should be as relaxed as possible.

The knee jerk

The knee jerk is elicited by tapping over the patellar tendon with the hip and knee partly flexed. The examiner can also tap at intervals from the ankle to the knee. A response when tapping over the lower part of the leg indicates an unusually brisk jerk but not necessarily abnormal.

The biceps jerk

The biceps jerk is best tested by placing a finger or thumb over the biceps tendon and tapping this with the finger of the other hand. The contraction can be felt with the underlying finger or thumb and flexion of the forearm can be seen. Other commonly elicited reflexes are the triceps, supinator and ankle jerks.

Ankle clonus

Ankle clonus can be demonstrated by gentle but rapid dorsiflexion of the foot whilst the knee is partly flexed and the hip partly abducted. Ankle clonus is associated with brisk knee jerks and one often sees one or two beats of clonus. Even sustained clonus may not be of significance in the absence of other signs, such as motor delay. However, an asymmetrical response, provided the head is in the midline throughout the examination, may indicate hemiplegia.

EXAMINATION OF THE HIPS FOR DISLOCATION AND INSTABILITY

Guidelines for timing and technique of screening for congenital dislocation of the hips (CDH) are set out in a recent DHSS publication (1986).

'At risk' groups

It is estimated that in 15 to 20 per 1000 live births there is evidence of hip instability at birth. However, in a large proportion of these infants the signs resolve without treatment in the first weeks of life. About 10% of unstable hips will persist to show classic signs of dislocation during infancy while a further 10% may show evidence of dysplasia and/or subluxation. Congenital dislocation of the hip (CDH) may be familial and is also more common in babies where there has been breech delivery, caesarean section, other congenital postural deformities, oligohydramnios or fetal growth retardation. It occurs five to seven times more commonly in girls than in boys, and the left hip is more often affected than the right.

When to examine

Not all cases of CDH can be detected at birth and it is recommended that the examination should be repeated at the time of discharge from hospital or within the first 10 days, at six weeks and six to eight months and until the child is seen to be walking normally.

Examination

Inspection of the legs may show asymmetrical skin creases, notably in the groin and buttock, when the baby lies on his front. The buttock crease will be higher and less well developed on the affected side. The pelvis may appear asymmetrical and the leg may be rotated outwards and appear short. When assessing apparent shortening it is important to check that the pelvis is not tilted. In bilateral dislocation there is no asymmetry but the pelvis is abnormally wide and there is a perineal gap.

Hart's test

With the baby lying on his back, legs towards the examiner, the legs are first adducted and extended and are flexed to right angles with the trunk. With the tips of the fore- and middle finger over the greater trochanter and the leg held by the thumb around the knee, the thigh (each thigh in turn) is abducted. In the first week the thigh normally abducts to 90° from the midline and by six weeks the range of abduction is reduced to about 70°. In CDH it often stops half-way and if further pressure is applied it may then reduce with a click (Ortolani's jerk of entry) and then abduct fully (Fig. 1.8).

Barlow's test

The examiner holds the upper thigh between his middle finger on the greater trochanter and his thumb in the groin with the knees flexed. The thighs are placed in mid-abduction and then each greater trochanter is gently lifted in turn. If the hip is dislocated, the femoral head will be felt to slip into the acetabulum with a jerk. This manoeuvre also detects hip instability in the absence of dislocation. In a baby with an unstable hip and an unduly lax joint capsule, pressure with the thumb on the inner side of the thigh will cause the femoral head to slip out of the acetabulum and then slip back again as soon as pressure is released. In the early weeks decreased abduction, subluxation or instability requires immediate referral to an orthopaedic surgeon. After the early weeks of life Barlow's sign is not easily obtainable and reduced abduction is the most significant clinical sign. However, limited abduction is also seen in other conditions, such as adductor hypertonia or contracture in spastic cerebral palsy, or, if bilateral, may simply be a normal variation in muscle tone. Unilateral decreased abduction in the older

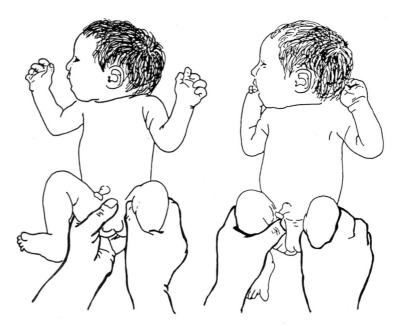

Fig. 1.8 The examiner grasps the hips in the manner indicated with the middle finger pressed on the greater trochanter. Initially the trochanter is pressed forward to relocate a possibly posterior displaced head of femur and it is felt to move forward into the acetabulum. The second part of the manoeuvre consists of pressing with the thumb on the inner side of the thigh, attempting to move the head of the femur backwards out of the acetabulum. When this happens the hip is said to be subluxible (dislocated). (Based on *Archives of Disease of Childhood*, 1986.)

infant is always suspicious and indicates referral for an orthopaedic opinion. Ligamentous clicks without instability or reduced abduction are a common finding and do not normally indicate a significant hip condition. There is no evidence that putting babies in double or triple napkins has any value. Generally, excellent results are achieved with treatment by abduction and splinting if the condition is diagnosed by six weeks. After six weeks some children may require surgery, but the final outcome is likely to be satisfactory if the condition is treated before the child walks.

EXAMINATION OF THE CARDIOVASCULAR SYSTEM

The normal cardiac rate varies with activity, crying and sleep. In the newborn the average rate of 120–140 per min can rise to 170 per min during crying and drop to 70–90 per min during sleep. The pulse rate becomes slower with age as shown in Table 1.1. Persistent tachycardia — over 150 per min in infants or 120 per min in older children — bradycardia or irregular heartbeat other than sinus arrhythmia requires further investigation.

Blood pressure should be measured with a cuff which covers approximately two-thirds of the upper arm or upper leg. In infants the flush method is the more feasible way of estimating blood pressure. The cuff is placed on the upper arm or thigh and the distal limbs squeezed whilst the cuff is quickly inflated. The cuff is then slowly deflated and the systolic pressure is the point at which the limb flushes. This gives a somewhat lower reading than auscultation methods. On older children a mercury sphygmomanometer is used in the normal way. In the legs the stethoscope is placed over the popliteal artery and readings are about 10 mmHg higher than in the arm. Blood

Table 1.1 Average pulse rates at rest.

Age	Lower limit of normal	Average	Upper limit of normal
Newborn	70 per min	125 per group	190 per min
1–11 months	80	120	160
2 years	80	110	130
4 years	80	100	120
6 years	75	100	115
8 years	70	90	110
10 years	70	90	110

pressure changes with age and varies with activity and excitement (see Table 1.2). In practice blood pressure measurement in infancy is more relevant to the work of the specialist paediatrician than the general practitioner. However, in older children the measurement is probably not carried out frequently enough and ideally all surgeries should have a selection of paediatric cuffs. For example, children with a history of renal disease or Henoch–Schoenlein purpura should have regular blood pressure checks. Palpation of the femoral pulses is an essential part of the physical examination in infancy. Coarctation of the aorta may occur as an isolated abnormality or in association with other congenital heart defects.

In the young infant femoral pulses are difficult to palpate and it may not be possible to distinguish normal from diminished pulsation. For practical purposes infants with absent pulses should be referred for investigation. In the older infant diminished or delayed pulsation may be easier to identify.

Suspicion of coarctation may be confirmed when a blood pressure difference between the arms and legs is demonstrated by the 'flush' technique. Normally systolic pressure in the legs is higher than in the arms; in coarctation it is considerably lower.

Most cardiac murmurs are not associated with cardiovascular abnormalities and are termed functional or preferably innocent. Over 30% of children may have an innocent murmur, particularly if they are examined when they are febrile, excited, active or anxious. The most frequently heard innocent murmur is a short systolic murmur at the left lower and midsternal border with no radiation to the apex or back or across the midline. Innocent pulmonic murmurs are also common in children and are heard in the second left parasternal space. The venous hum is another common innocent bruit resulting from turbulence in the jugular venous system. It may be heard in the neck and upper chest as a soft humming sound in systole and diastole and varies with

Table 1.2 Mean blood pressure (mmHg) (from Davis & Dobbing, 1981).

Age	Mean systolic	Mean diastolic
4 days	76	
6 weeks	96	
1 year	94	
2 years	100	63
6 years	97	65
9 years	106	71
12 years	115	75
15 years	119	78

the position of the head or lightly compressing the jugular vein in the neck.

Significant ejection murmurs imply increased flow or stenosis across the aortic and pulmonary valves, whereas pansystolic murmurs are heard in ventricular septal defect or mitral or triscuspid insufficiency. A continuous murmur at the upper left sternal edge is present in patent ductus arteriosus.

It is of the utmost importance to avoid alarming parents when an innocent murmur is detected, as they may become unneccessarily anxious and protective of their child. It should be explained that the murmur is simply an extra noise which does not indicate significant heart defect. Many doctors would prefer not to mention the murmur at all, but one can argue that an explanation early in the child's life may prevent anxiety should it be pointed out later on.

Physical examination should also include: examination of the mouth for cleft palate, oral thrush and tongue tie; examination of the chest; examination of the abdomen (the liver extends to 2 cm below the costal margin); examination of the genitalia to detect undescended testes, ectopic testes, hypospadias, inguinal or femoral hernia or labial fusion; examination of the back for spinal bifida occulta and scoliosis.

Summary of findings at six weeks (Table 1.3)

In our study, out of 355 babies at six weeks, the number reported as possibly abnormal on developmental examination was very small and there were no babies with a definite abnormality of development. These findings correspond to the level of developmental delay to be expected in a population sample. Severe disability occurs in one in 400 children and was not present in our sample.

Physical conditions were noted in 18% of infants. Some, such as heart murmurs and abnormal hips, needed further investigation, whereas others merely required observation to determine whether they resolved naturally. For example, four babies were thought to have increased muscle tone at six weeks but were normal at six months. Other conditions, such as plagiocephaly and umbilical hernia caused considerable parental concern and reassurance was possible at an early stage.

Nine out of 10 parents reported observing their babies smile.

Wind, colic and crying were common complaints at six weeks and are examples of a wide spectrum of behaviour and management problems which came to light whilst talking to mothers and observing the

Table 1.3 Results of examination at six weeks (355 babies).

	Normal		Possibly abnormal		Definitely abnormal
	n	%	*n*	%	
Developmental item					
Posture/gross motor	346	97	9	3	0
Primitive responses	352	99	3	1	0
Vision	346	97	9	3	0
Hearing	342	96	13	4	0
Crying	352	99	3	1	0

Physical
One or more physical conditions $n = 64$, % $= 18$
Conditions identified — plagiocephaly, eczema, heart murmur, umbilical hernia, undescended testes, hypospadias, abnormal hips, metatarsus varus, syndactyly, increased muscle tone, sternomastoid tumour

	n	%
Behaviour problems		
Wind or colic most days	61	17
Wind or colic most feeds	43	12
Cries most days	22	6
Problem to mother	22	6

mother–infant couple. Many mothers, especially those of first babies, experience a high level of anxiety in the early weeks and welcome the opportunity to discuss these informally with a doctor in a relaxed setting. Despite the low yield of developmental abnormalities a broad approach to the consultation covers a wide field of parental concerns and potential problems. The six-week assessment enhances the relationship between parents, infant and doctor, forming a valuable base-line to the further consultations, both routine and non-routine, which will doubtless follow during the next few years.

Summary of development

Gross motor

NEWBORN

Prone: arms and legs flexed, pelvis high, knees under abdomen
Ventral suspension: head held just below body
Supine: arms and legs semiflexed, head to one side

Pull-to-sit: complete head lag
Held upright: legs extended, stepping and placing reflex

4 WEEKS

Prone: pelvis lower, lifts head off couch
Ventral suspension: lifts head momentarily
Supine: arms and legs semiflexed
Pull-to-sit: lifts head momentarily
Held sitting: rounded back, lifts head momentarily
Held upright: stepping and placing reflex, legs extended

6 WEEKS

Prone and ventral suspension: holds head in line with body for a few
seconds
Supine and pull-to-sit: holds head up for a few seconds, intermittent
ATNR posture

12 WEEKS

Prone: lifts head and upper chest off couch, pelvis flat, legs extended
Ventral suspension: maintains head 45–90° to body
Pull-to-sit: little or no head lag
Held sitting: lumbar curve still present, some head wobble
Held upright: sags at knees, stepping and placing reflex disappeared

Fine motor

4 WEEKS

Grasp reflex
Drops object immediately
Hands mainly fisted
Sweeping movements towards objects

12 WEEKS

Little or no grasp reflex
Opens and closes hands
Watches objects for few seconds

Holds bottle for a few moments, but seldom capable of regarding it at same time

Hand regard begins — watches movement of own hands

20 WEEKS

Accurate reaching

Palmar grasp on ulnar side of hand

Hand regard ceases

Language

4–6 WEEKS

Coos, gurgles

Phonemes — oo, ugh

12 WEEKS

Long streams of babble

Conversations with mother

16–24 WEEKS

Babbling — ebe, ele, da, ba, ka, mum

Social behaviour and understanding

4 WEEKS

Can imitate tongue protrusion

Gazes at bright lights, faces, coloured objects

Recognizes mother

12 WEEKS

Laughs at playful activities

Recognizes familiar situation — bathing, feeding

Dislikes being left

20 WEEKS

Looks for dropped toy

Holds bottle
Smiles at mirror image

Vision

4 WEEKS

Pupils react to light
Focuses at 9 inches away
Looks at faces, bright light, coloured objects
Prefers mother's face to stranger's
Appreciates depth
Follows moving objects and faces up to 45° from midline

12 WEEKS

Visually very alert
Looks at small objects
Smooth convergence and binocular vision developed
Discriminates between colours
Follows moving objects through 180° vertically and horizontally

Hearing

4 WEEKS

Turns eyes and head to sound
Prefers voice sounds to pure tones
Startles, blinks, cries to loud sounds
Quietens to mother's voice or rattle
Recognizes mother's voice

12 WEEKS

Eyes and head move together to sound

5−6 MONTHS

Downward localization of sound

References

Bax, M., Hart, H. & Jenkins, S. (1980) *The Health Needs of Pre-school Children*. Thomas Coram Research Unit, London.
Brown, G. & Harris, T. (1978) *Social Origins of Depression*. Tavistock Press, London.

Carpenter, G. (1974) Mother's face and the newborn. *New Scientist*, 21 March, 742–4.

Catford, G.V. & Oliver, A. (1973) Development of visual acuity, *Archives of Disease in Childhood*, **48**, 47–50.

Condon, W. (1974) Speech makes babies move. *New Scientist*, 6 June, 624–7.

Connolly, K.J. & Prechtl, H.F.R. (1981) Maturation and Development. *Clinics in Developmental Medicine* **77/78**, MacKeith Press: Blackwell Scientific Publications, Oxford.

Davis, B.B. & Dobbing, J. (1981) *Scientific Foundations of Paediatrics*. William Heinemann, London.

de Villiers, P.A. & de Villiers, J.G. (1979) *Early Language*. Fontana/Open Books.

DHSS (1986) *Screening for Detection of Congenital Dislocation of the Hip*.

Eimas, P.E. (1971) Speech perception in infants. *Science*, **171**, 303–6.

Engen, T., Lipsitt, L.P. & Kay, H. (1963) Olfactory response and adaption in the human neonate. *Journal of Comparative Physiology and Psychology*, **56**, 3–5.

Fantz, R.L. (1961) The origins of form perception. *Scientific American*, **204**, 66–72.

Fantz, R.L. (1975) Early visual selectivity. In: Cohen, L.B. & Salapatek, P. (eds) *Infant Perception — from Sensation to Cognition*. Vol 1. Academic Press, New York.

Hart, H., Bax, M. & Jenkins, S. (1978) The value of a developmental history. *Developmental Medicine and Child Neurology*, **20**, 442–52.

Kennell, J.H. *et al.* (1974) Maternal behaviour one year after early and extended postpartum contact. *Developmental Medicine and Child Neurology*, **16**, 172–9.

Lynch, A.M. (1975) Ill health and child abuse. *Lancet*, **ii**, 317–9.

Macfarlane, J.A. (1975) *Olfaction in the Development of Social Preferences in the Human Neonate in Parent–Infant Interaction*. CIBA Foundation Symposium 33 (new series), Applied Science Publishers, Amsterdam.

Macfarlane, A. (1977) *The Psychology of Childbirth*. Fontana/Open Books, London.

Mills, M. & Melhinsh, E. (1974) Recognition of mother's voice in early infancy. *Nature*, **252**, 123.

Mitchell, R. (1960) The Moro reflex. *Cerebral Palsy Bulletin*, **2** (3), 135–41.

Moro, E. (1918) Das erste Tremonon. *München Medischer Wochenschrift*, **65**, 1147.

Peiper, A. (1963) *Cerebral Function in Infancy and Childhood*. Consultants Bureau Enterprises Inc., New York.

Prechtl, H. (1977) *The Neurological Examination of the Full-term Newborn Infant*. Blackwell Scientific Publications, Oxford.

Prechtl, H. (1984) Continuity and Change in Neural Development. *Clinics in Developmental Medicine*, **94**, SIMP, London.

Robinson, L. (1891) Infantile atavision: being some further notes on Darwinism in the nursery. *British Medical Journal*, **5**, 1226–7.

Schaffer, H.R. & Emerson, P.R. (1964) The development of social attachments in infancy. *Monographs of Social Research in Child Development*, **29** (94), and in *Mothering* (ed. R. Schaffer). Fontana/Open Books,

Seashore, M.J. *et al.* (1973) The effects of denial of early mother–infant interaction on maternal self-confidence. *Journal of Personality and Social Psychology*, **26** (3), 369–78.

Soderling, B. (1959) The first smile: a developmental study. *Acta Paediatrica*, **48** (suppl. 117), 78–82.

Teller, D.V., McDonald, M., Preston, K., Sebris, S.L. & Dobson, V. (1986) Assessment of visual acuity in infants and children: the acuity card procedure. *Developmental Medicine and Child Neurology*, **28**, 779–89.

Touwen, B.C.I. (1976) Neurological development in infancy. *Clinics in Developmental Medicine* 58, Blackwell Scientific Publications, Oxford.

Zappella, M. (1963) The placing reaction in the newborn. *Developmental Medicine and Child Neurology*, **5**, 497–503.

2 Physical Growth and Systems Development

IN THIS CHAPTER physical growth is considered both in normal infants and in those displaying differing growth patterns such as the light-for-dates or preterm infant. A brief summary of the development of the body systems in the first five years is included to provide some physiological and anatomical background to the more detailed accounts of development, health and behaviour throughout the book.

Physical growth

Measurement

In clinical practice growth of the infant and child is generally measured by estimating the weight, length, head circumference and in certain circumstances skinfold thickness.

WEIGHT

Weight changes are a non-specific measurement of growth as they reflect the composition of all body components including fat, water, muscle, bone and viscera. However, in young children weight is the most widely used measurement and is a more sensitive index of acute episodes of ill health and nutritional status than length or head circumference. For maximum accuracy babies should be weighed on regularly checked scales without a nappy and at the same time in relation to a feed. In some clinics babies are weighed with their clothes on, to save time or because it is feared that the baby will get cold. Whilst heating in some clinics is undoubtedly inadequate, as far as possible weighing undressed is to be recommended. Weighing with clothes should be recorded as such in the notes. Weighing unclothed also offers the opportunity for the health visitor to observe the amount of subcutaneous fat and look out for any other abnormalities.

Although growth charts have great value, paediatricians recognize that simply looking at an infant can be equally informative; it is not uncommon to see a baby whose weight gain is at the lower limit of normal but a glance at chubby arms and legs reassures both doctor and mother that the infant is thriving.

LENGTH

Measurement of the crown−heel length provides the best measure of skeletal growth since, unlike weight gain, it is not influenced by the accumulation of fat and water. A baby's length can be measured accurately in a special length measurer such as the Pedobaby[1] or the Starter baby mat. This is an inexpensive device suitable for use in the general practitioner's surgery or a child health clinic. Admittedly we do not routinely measure infant's length at each visit but would recommend measurement at three months, six months and 12 months and more often if there is any question of failure to thrive or growth disorder.

Routine height measurement is practicable from the age of two and a stadiometer such as the Harpenden Stadiometer gives the most accurate measurement. Wall charts such as the Oxford Growth Charts[2] are valuable for use in the surgery to give a rapid indication of whether the child's height is within the normal range for his age or whether there is cause for concern.

HEAD CIRCUMFERENCE

The measurement of the head circumference provides a clinical indication of head growth. However, there is no simple relationship between head growth and brain growth. Nevertheless deviations in head circumference are of clinical importance in assessment of growth disorders and intracerebral pathology. Head circumference can be measured by a steel or paper tape placed over the maximum circumference around the supra-orbital ridges and the occipital protuberance.

SKINFOLD THICKNESS

The thickness of a skinfold in the mid-triceps or subscapular region can be measured with skinfold callipers and gives an estimate of the amount of subcutaneous fat. Its clinical importance lies in assessing nutritional status. It has been used widely in assessing nutrition of

[1] Pedobaby is available from Infant Growth Foundation, 2 Mayfield Avenue, Chiswick, London W4 1PW. Tel. 01-994 9625.
[2] Available from Castlemead Publications, Swains Mill, 4A Crane Mead, Ware, Herts SG12 9PY.

preterm and full-term infants. However, this is not normally a routine measurement in the general practitioner's surgery or child health clinic and is used more for research.

The pattern of growth

Generally speaking growth proceeds in a continuous fashion rather than in stops and starts. However, acceleration and deceleration occur in response to events such as illness or changes in nutrition or environment. Changes in activity such as when the infant starts to crawl can affect weight gain. Interpretation of growth problems involves looking at the infant together with the growth chart.

The growth of an individual child can be plotted as various kinds of growth curves. The curves most commonly used represent the height or weight attained at successive ages (Appendix 1). This does not necessarily show how growth is proceeding at any one time but reflects growth in all the previous years. Increments in height or weight from one age to the next are expressed as growth rate or velocity and represent the child's recent growth activity. After birth the rate of weight gain and growth in length accelerates to reach maximum velocity between four and six weeks (Fujimura & Seryu, 1977). The velocity of growth then declines rapidly until the age of four or five years and then more slowly until there is a marked acceleration of growth — the adolescent growth spurt. Typically this reaches its peak at age 12 years in girls and 14 years in boys although the range of normal is wide.

Weight has a similar growth curve to height, as do most structures of the body such as bone, muscle, liver, spleen and kidneys. However, certain organs, notably brain, skull, the reproductive organs, the lymphoid tissues of the tonsils, adenoids and intestines, and subcutaneous fat, show variations in growth curve (Fig. 2.1). The reproductive organs show slow prepubescent growth followed by a large adolescent spurt. The brain and skull grow most rapidly in the early postnatal years and do not show an appreciable adolescent growth spurt.

Lymphoid tissue on the other hand reaches its maximum amount before adolescence and then declines, probably under direct influence of sex hormones.

Individual variation in growth

There is a wide variation amongst children in actual heights and weights and in velocity of height and weight increase. Percentile

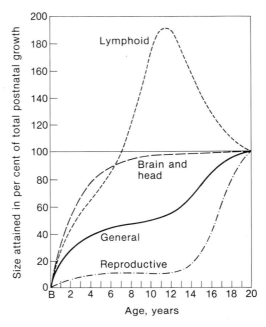

Fig. 2.1 The growth curves of different parts and tissues of the body, showing the four chief types. All the curves are of size attained, and plotted as percentage of total gain from birth to 20 years, so that size at age 20 is 100 on the vertical scale (Tanner, 1978).

charts make possible comparisons of a given child with the rest of the population. A typical growth chart shows the heights of boys at successive ages. Each line represents a centile. In a normal population the heights of 97% of children lie below the 97th centile and only 3% of children are taller than this. Correspondingly, looking at the smaller children, 97% of children will have heights above the 3rd centile, and 3% will be shorter than this. Children's heights at any age follow a normal distribution and the 50th centile corresponds to the mean height. The outside centiles are taken as 3rd and 97th, which are rounded forms of the 2.5th and 97.5th corresponding to minus and plus two standard deviations from the mean.

Conventionally children whose heights and weights fall outside the 3rd and 97th centiles are considered possibly to have some physical abnormality. However, many children in the bottom and top three percentiles will be perfectly normal and represent extreme variations of normality. Furthermore, because of ethnic differences in size, the growth charts used should ideally be standardized on children of similar backgrounds.

Relationship between height and weight

Comparing a child's centile positions in height and weight gives a good idea of his relative weight for height. Since weight reflects the level of nutrition and the sum of so many different tissues it is not surprising that there is quite a large variation in weight and height percentiles in normal children. Generally if a child's height is on the 50th centile his weight should be between the 10th and 90th centile. Weight is a good and easily measured indication of physical health and nutrition but not a reliable indication of linear growth. For example, in growth hormone deficiency a child's weight may be within normal limits but his height may be well below the 3rd centile.

Parental height

One additional useful piece of information to help decide whether a child's growth variation is significant is the height of the parents. In the absence of illness or adverse environmental factors height is genetically endowed.

Parental height can be used provided there have been no environmental or health reasons why the parents have not fulfilled their growth potential. As both mother and father exert an equal effect on the child's stature the average of the parents' heights is used (mid-parent height). Using a parent-allowed-for chart the child's height centile allowing for mid-parent height centile can be plotted. For example, if a child's height is on the 3rd centile and he has parents who are also small with mid-parent height also on the 3rd centile, when plotted on such a graph the boy's height will be on the 15th centile, well within normal limits for his family.

Prediction of adult height

From the age of two years, when the child has reached nearly half his adult height, until the beginning of puberty, the correlation between the child's present height and his adult height is between 0.8 and 0.85, which means that in 95% of cases height can be predicted within about 7 cm either side of the predicted height, not a very high degree of accuracy in the individual case. One reason why prediction is relatively inaccurate is that children vary in the rate they progress through various phases of growth and the time when they begin the adolescent growth spurt. A method has been devised for prediction of adult height which incorporates skeletal maturity scores, occurrence of the menarche in older girls and allowance for mid-parent height. This increases the level of prediction to within 6 cm for premenarcheal girls aged four to 11 and within 3 cm for postmenarcheal 13-year-old girls (Tanner *et al.*, 1975).

Crossing percentile channels

As well as looking at the weight and height which a child has attained and their position on the percentile charts, the trajectory of growth along percentile channels provides further information about the individual child's progress. Commonly, in normal infants, growth pathways deviate from the percentile channels in which they were born. This reflects the maternal influences which regulate intra-uterine growth and affect the size of the infant at birth. After birth these influences are removed and the infant can grow in its own genetically determined direction. During infancy this shifting growth pattern results in infants crossing the percentile channels on the growth chart. Generally, the infant will reach his genetically determined growth channel by 12–14 months (range four to 19 months). The smaller infants who are destined to 'catch up' do so earlier in infancy than the larger babies who 'lag down' later in infancy (Smith *et al.*, 1976).

Whilst it is generally accepted that young children's growth curves may cross percentiles before getting on to a genetically determined path, if a channel is crossed too rapidly, particularly in a downward direction, it may indicate cause for concern for a variety of reasons. These changes are seen in weight measurements. Changes in length velocity are less acute and are not generally monitored in young children. The commonest cause of deceleration of weight velocity is an episode of illness and if weekly weight measurements are made a change in rate of weight gain may be observed before the child has overt symptoms of illness. If the illness is acute, such as gastroenteritis, there follows a period of 'catch-up growth' in which the child rapidly regains his former percentile channel. In chronic illness, such as renal disease or malabsorption, velocity may continue to decline; this decline may be seen on the growth chart before it is clinically obvious that the child is ill. Some recent studies have identified a decline in weight gain as an antecedent factor in the sudden infant death syndrome (SIDS). This may occur in cases where there is an identifiable physical illness culminating in SIDS but also where no definite pathology is found. It also may be associated with changes in feeding pattern and with emotional deprivation.

The Sheffield weight chart (Emery *et al.*, 1985) has been constructed so that a healthy child's weight is not expected to move up or down more than one channel width over a period of two weeks, or two channel widths in eight weeks. Significant fall in weight gain as judged by these charts was accompanied by illness in over 99% of cases. The illnesses ranged from relatively minor conditions such as colds to more serious illness such as pyelonephritis.

In practice these charts require careful plotting and interpretation and can be used in conjunction with symptom charts to alert health visitors and doctors to the possibility of illness or marked change in feeding patterns so that treatment can be initiated at an early stage. The evidence suggests that regular weighing in the early months is going to be a useful aid in monitoring babies with an increased risk of SIDS, particularly when parents are anxious for some kind of intervention. Weekly visits by the health visitor also play a vital part in intervention and support, probably exceeding that of weighing alone (Emery *et al.*, 1985).

Prenatal growth

Intra-uterine and postnatal growth is a continuous process. At the time of birth it has been said that the baby is 'unfinished'. The event occurs midway in the process of myelinization of the nervous system. Not surprisingly, the pattern of fetal growth in the latter part of pregnancy influences the pattern of postnatal growth and affects the well-being of the preterm infant. The rate of intra-uterine growth depends on the genetic potential of the fetus and on the immediate uterine environment. This is in turn dependent on the mother's ability to supply nutrients and oxygen via her circulation and on placental function. The fetus will grow abnormally if his growth potential is affected by chromosomal abnormalities or congenital infections or malformations, or if his growth support is compromised as in the placental insufficiency syndrome. Maternal and environmental factors which reduce fetal growth rate include maternal malnutrition, high altitude, maternal ill health (cyanotic heart disease, thyrotoxicosis), hypertension, pre-eclampsia, toxaemia, small stature, smoking, alcohol consumption, rubella and drugs. Tallness, maternal diabetes and high parity enhance fetal growth.

There is wide variation in birthweights of different ethnic groups which seems unrelated to prosperity. In one study of different ethnic groups living in the same area, the order of sizes of the neonates from largest to smallest was Irish, British, Jamaican, Barbadian and Cypriot.

GENETIC INFLUENCES

Monozygotic twins are actually less alike in size at birth than dizygotic same-sex twins. This is probably partly because there is unequal splitting of the ovum and one twin receives slightly more cytoplasm than the other and partly due to varying positions in the uterus. However, the situation rapidly changes and by three months monozygotic are more alike in size than dizygotic, same-sex twins (provided they are brought up in the same environment).

By the age of four years the correlation in height of monozygotic twins is 0.95 compared with 0.6 in dizygotic twins. The correlation in height between non-twin sisters is about 0.57, between brothers 0.54.

HEAD CIRCUMFERENCE AND BRAIN GROWTH

The brain consists of neurons (nerve cells) and neuroglia (support cells). Neurons are formed during the period from 10 to 18 post-menstrual weeks. Axons and dendrites, consisting of drawn-out cytoplasm of the nerve cell, develop in size and complexity during the latter half of pregnancy along with the neuroglia. This accounts for the rapid increase in brain weight during the second half of pregnancy, which continues well into the second postnatal year (the brain growth spurt).

Head circumference growth velocity reaches a peak at 30–32 weeks of gestation and then decreases until 40 weeks. After birth the velocity increases to a peak just below the peak intra-uterine velocity and then decelerates quite swiftly. However, although the external linear dimension of the head follows a similar growth pattern to length and weight, Dobbing & Sands (1978) have shown that brain weight does not necessarily follow the same path and shows little sign of slowing in growth at the end of pregnancy.

The brain growth spurt precedes the period of maximum growth of other organs; in other words there is a 'cerebro-somatic' sequence of growth. At birth the brain is already 25% of its adult weight and by four years 50% of adult weight.

There is now convincing evidence of the vulnerability of the developing brain during its phase of rapid growth. Intra-uterine growth restriction and under-nutrition in infancy have been found to be associated with physical brain deficits such as reduction of brain size, loss of cerebral cortical neurons, deficit in brain lipids and reduction in the numbers of synapses per cortical neuron. A study of Jamaican children demonstrated a reduced level of intellectual performance in children malnourished during the first two years of life. These findings are clearly relevant to antenatal care and to maternal and infant nutrition. But other studies suggest that the child's home environment can add to or compensate for physical consequences of brain growth restriction. Studies in Third World countries have found no detectable behavioural consequences of severe infant malnutrition in a minority of children who had good home care and emotional relationships. Similarly children who suffered severe starvation due to childhood disease but whose home environments are advantaged show no behavioural effects of malnutrition. Nevertheless there is no doubt that good early nutrition promotes optimal brain growth. The relatively recent findings that the human brain growth spurt is more postnatal than was formerly thought are a stimulus for providing an ideal nutritional environment for every infant, in both the developed and the developing world.

Preterm infants

The average duration of gestation measured from the first day of the last menstrual period is 280 days or 40 weeks. There is considerable variation in the normal duration and, conventionally, babies born before 37 weeks (259 days) are considered to be preterm. About a third of preterm babies are light for dates (LFD) and may have a reduced growth potential. However, about two-thirds of preterm babies have not experienced intra-uterine growth deprivation and eventually attain a similar size to full-term babies.

In the first week or so the preterm infant grows very little as he adjusts to extra-uterine nutrition. When feeding is established there is a marked increase in head growth velocity so that by the expected date of delivery (EDD) the head circumference is either on, or higher than, the centile at birth. Weight and length show less of a spurt and at EDD the preterm infant is likely to be lighter and shorter than the full-term infant.

The preterm infant's weight curve crosses the centiles during the first few months and by the end of the first year the length of the average preterm infant is around the 50th centile. The smallest infants may not reach normal centiles until after the second year.

Light-for-dates (LFD) infants

Various criteria are adopted for defining light-for-dates (LFD) infants. The term small for dates (SFD) is also used synonymously. Most LFD infants are born at term but by definition their weight must take into account gestational age. Generally a baby is considered to be LFD if his birthweight is below the 5th or 10th centile or less than 2.0 kg at 38 weeks' or later gestation.

Congenital malformation or infection and chromosomal abnormalities are often associated with poor fetal growth and subsequent reduction in postnatal growth. Most LFD infants show some degree of intra-uterine malnutrition with signs of wasting with loss of subcutaneous fat and muscle bulk. Some LFD infants are so-called 'perfect miniatures'. They have no obvious clinical signs of under-nutrition. These infants may be genetically small. However, studies using skinfold thickness measurements found that the majority of LFD babies show some evidence of reduced deposits of subcutaneous fat. LFD infants are similar in appearance to preterm babies of similar weights and are generally smaller in all dimensions than babies whose weight are appropriate for gestational age.

LFD infants show varying degrees of 'catch-up' growth after birth, which is most marked during the first six months of life, resulting in attainment of percentile channels approximately between the 10th and 25th for weight and length by the age of two years. However, in one study 35% were under the 3rd percentile at six years with only 8% over the 50th centile (Fitzhardinge & Stevens, 1972). In other words, the vast majority of light-for-dates infants will attain heights within the normal range, of whom a few will be in the taller half of the population but most will be below the 50th centile. Their average height will be around the 25th centile.

This phase of 'catch-up' growth is accompanied by an increase in the infant's appetite for milk in the early months. Infants who experienced slow fetal growth rate before 34 weeks are likely to remain smaller than those in whom growth retardation was confined to the last six weeks of pregnancy. Head circumference also shows a period of 'catch-up' growth after birth which suggests that some degree of restriction of overall brain growth occurs in these infants. Dobbing's hypothesis (Dobbing & Sands, 1978) is that the brain may be irreversibly harmed if its growth is impaired during the latter part of pregnancy. This is a period of growth by hyperplasia of glial cells, which may be irreparably harmed by under-nutrition. Studies which have shown an increased incidence of minor neurological and behavioural disturbances in LFD infants support this view. On the other hand, fulfilment of physical growth potential might be possible in these infants. Davis suggests (Davis & Dobbing, 1981) that, as growth of the main viscera occurs by cell hypertrophy rather than hyperplasia in the latter half of pregnancy, catch-up growth is more likely to restore the infant close to his genetically determined growth channel.

Development of the body systems

Cardiovascular system

FETAL CIRCULATION

The embryonic circulation is established at around the fourth gestational week and by the eighth week it has evolved into the form which prevails during the remaining fetal life. The fetal circulation is organized so that the blood with the highest oxygen content is delivered to the myocardium and the brain, and the lungs are, to a large extent, bypassed. This is achieved by arteriovenous shunting and by a high pulmonary vascular resistance.

Oxygenated blood from the mother returns to the fetus via the umbilical vein. About 60% of blood enters the inferior vena cava via the liver and ductus venosus whilst the remainder travels directly to the heart. Blood enters the left heart through the foramen ovale and leaves in the ascending aorta. After giving off branches to supply the head and upper limbs the aorta is joined by the ductus arteriosus carrying blood from the right ventricle and lungs. Circulation continues along the descending aorta to supply the viscera and lower trunk and returns in the umbilical arteries to the placenta (Fig. 2.2).

EVENTS AT BIRTH

At birth the umbilical circulation ceases and the pulmonary vascular resistance falls on expansion of the lungs, resulting in changes in the fetal pattern of circulation. Pressure in the right atrium falls as a result of loss of umbilical input and pressure in the left atrium rises with increased flow from the pulmonary veins. The ductus arteriosus contracts in the first 24 hours after birth in response to rise in oxygen tension and then obliterates permanently. Failure of duct closure at birth may lead to cardiac failure in early infancy. However, in infants with certain types of congenital heart disease patency of the ductus may be life-saving by maintaining pulmonary blood flow or by bypassing an aortic obstruction. There is continuing debate on the timing of umbilical cord ligation since about 30 ml of blood per kg is available for neonatal transfer. Maximum transfer is not necessarily advantageous and it has been suggested that 30−45 seconds is an appropriate interval when half the transfer is completed. The ductus venosus closes

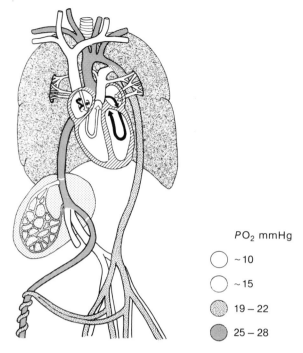

PO₂ mmHg

○ ~10

○ ~15

◍ 19 – 22

● 25 – 28

Fig. 2.2 Fetal circulation (adapted from Davis & Dobbing, with permission).

during the first few days of life as a result of drop in pressure following cessation of umbilical flow.

RESPONSE TO HYPOXIA

Towards the end of gestation the fetus responds to hypoxaemia by vasoconstriction of peripheral vascular beds in order to maintain placental blood flow and oxygenation. Tachycardia occurs to maintain perfusion and is usually the first indication of fetal distress. If hypoxia affects the myocardium in the fetus or newborn the tachycardia is followed by bradycardia, heart block and eventually cardiac arrest. Bradycardia during late labour in response to a uterine contraction (type 2 dips) has been shown to be associated with hypoxaemia and to correlate with poor fetal outcome and acid—base disturbance.

HEART RATE DURING CHILDHOOD

The normal heart rate averages 120 per min at birth and increases after birth, reaching a maximum at one month after which there is gradual slowing, reaching adult levels at between 12 and 16 years. It may increase by as much as 50 per min in the crying infant (see Table 1.1, p. 37) and decrease by as much during sleep.

CARDIAC OUTPUT

Cardiac output is greater per kg body-weight in the fetus and newborn than in the adult. Output rises during the first 10 days of life and then gradually falls. The infant cardiac output is three times adult level and is related to a higher oxygen consumption than in the adult. The infant requires a larger oxygen consumption to maintain temperature control as he has a larger surface area in relation to body mass than the adult. However, cardiac size follows a similar growth curve to other organs. Boys have larger hearts than girls though girls temporarily overtake boys in heart size at the time of the adolescent growth spurt.

BLOOD PRESSURE

Fetal blood pressure is low as a result of the low vascular resistance in the placental circuit. Systolic blood pressures of around 76 mmHg are found at birth and levels rise to 96 mmHg by six weeks. There is hardly any change between the ages of six weeks and six years and after this the blood pressure rises until adult levels of 120 mmHg are reached at adolescence. Exercise, excitement, coughing, crying and straining can increase the child's systolic blood pressure by as much as 40−50 mmHg above his usual levels. An infant would be considered hypertensive if his systolic blood pressure, awake but not crying, is above 95 mmHg at four days of age or greater than 115 mmHg between six weeks and six years (see Table 1.2, p. 38).

Development of the respiratory system

PRENATAL DEVELOPMENT

The primitive lung bud develops during the first five weeks after conception and begins to branch at five weeks. The bronchial tree acquires the number of branches found in the adult by the 16th week of gestation. As the fetus grows the diameter and length of the bronchi increase and bronchioles and primitive alveoli develop. The alveolar phase begins at 24−26 weeks' gestation and at this time the alveolar region becomes adequate for gas transfer, making the fetus viable. At birth around 70 million primitive alveolar sacs are present, though true alveoli do not develop until after birth.

During fetal life the lungs are fluid-filled and there is no gas interface. Pulmonary vascular resistance is high and pulmonary blood flow is low. Respiratory movements occur from an early stage of gestation without much movement of fluid in and out. Before 24–26 weeks the lungs are unable to retain gas as they collapse because of high surface tension in the primitive alveoli. After about 26–28 weeks inflation is possible due to presence of surfactant, a phospholipid which is present in the alveolar lining and lowers surface tension. Although surfactant can be detected in lung extracts from the 23rd week, its quantity increases greatly towards term. Deficiency of surfactant gives rise to respiratory distress syndrome, in which there is widespread collapse of air spaces, leading to hypoxaemia and respiratory failure in severe cases.

POSTNATAL DEVELOPMENT

During establishment of respiration after birth, fluid is removed from the lungs and is replaced by air. Some fluid is expelled through the mouth, assisted by pressure on the thorax during vaginal delivery. The rest is absorbed via the pulmonary lymphatics during the first 24 hours of life. The first breath requires a large pressure to open the terminal airways and overcome the initial stiffness of the lungs. Over the first few hours of life lung compliance increases and the effort of breathing is considerably reduced. Overall lung growth has been measured in children using annual radiographs. Lung width and length follows a similar growth curve to overall height with an adolescent growth spurt. Boys are on average larger than girls in all lung dimensions but the pattern differs from other organs in that girls do not temporarily exceed the boys in lung size due to the earlier timing of their growth spurt. At age six the lung length and width are 66% and 62% respectively of their adult values.

The number of alveoli increases after birth, reaching 90% of its adult number at age four years and virtually all its adult complement of 200–600 million at age eight years. The amount of air–tissue interface more than doubles between then and adulthood but remains roughly the same in relation to body surface area. The conducting airways compared with the respiratory part of the lungs are proportionately larger in the infant than the adult but the small absolute size of the infant's air passages renders them more susceptible to obstruction and collapse of the supporting walls. Since smooth muscle is present throughout the lungs at birth bronchospasm can occur even in the very young infant.

The mechanics of respiration change during childhood. The infant's breathing is mainly abdominal, in which the abdomen distends, the diaphragm contracts and the thorax expands. After the age of five costal breathing plays a larger part. In this type of breathing the ribs move first, followed by bulging of the abdomen. The maximum inspiratory pressures generated by the infant and child are similar to those in the adult. However, since the chest wall is softer in the infant retraction during respiratory distress is greater in infants than in older children.

RESPIRATORY RATE

The normal resting infant's respiratory rate is about 30 per min. By the age of five it decreases to a level of about 25 per min as tidal volume and body size increase. Adult rates of around 20 per min are reached at adolescence.

PEAK EXPIRATORY FLOW RATE (PEFR) (Table 2.1)

This simple clinical test measures the maximum flow achieved in expiration after a maximum inspiration. The flow achieved reflects not only the size of the airways but also the effort which the child exerts. It is an excellent practical method of monitoring asthmatic children but the level of co-operation required means that it is mainly of value over the age of five. PEFR is size-and age-dependent, an average five-year-old achieving 150 per min, a 10-year-old 240 per min and a 15-year-old 400 per min.

Immunological and lymphatic development

The newborn baby is well equipped with an immunological defence system which protects it against invasion by infectious agents. Although levels of circulating immunoglobulins are low during the first three

Table 2.1 Peak expiratory flow rates at different ages.

Age (years)	Average height (cm)	PEFR (per min)
3	95	110
4	100	120
5	110	150
10	130	400

months of life compared with later on in childhood, the young infant is capable of producing antibodies in response to antigenic stimuli. The major components of the immunological defences are the cellular and humoral systems, along with other blood components such as the complement system, lysozyme and interferon.

BIOLOGICAL PROPERTIES OF THE IMMUNOLOGICAL SYSTEM

The cellular system comprises lymphocytes that are known as T cells because of their association with the thymus gland. Certain T cells, the T helper and T suppressor cells, are involved in the synthesis of immunoglobulin by the B cells. Others function as 'killer' cells when they combine with antigens to destroy invading organisms. T cells are primarily active against viruses such as measles, varicella, herpes, cytomegalovirus, EB viruses and slow viruses, fungal infections, live *Candida*, protozoa, and acid-fast bacilli. They are also involved in contact dermatitis, the delayed hypersensitivity reaction and graft rejection.

Humoral or circulating antibodies are immunoglobulins produced by plasma cells derived from B lymphocytes. Immunoglobulins protect against bacterial infections such as *Staphylococcus*, *Streptococcus*, *Haemophilus* and *Pneumococcus*. They are important in neutralizing viruses to prevent initial infection but can do little to control a virus disease once established. There are five classes of immunoglobulins, each of which is produced by a different cell line (Table 2.2).

IgG forms the largest part of circulating antibodies. It has a long half-life and is the only class to cross the placenta. IgG antibodies are involved in passive immunization, as occurs in the fetus and newborn baby, and in recall immunity.

Table 2.2 Characteristics of immunoglobulins.

Type	Placental passage	Function
IgG	Yes	Circulating antibodies (from mother to infant)
IgM	No	First line of defence, enhances agglutination, complements fixation, opsonization
IgA	No	Protects secretory surfaces, e.g. gastrointestinal tract and eyes
IgD	No	Lymphocyte receptor, binds antigen in initial immunization
IgE	No	Involved in allergic reactions, eliminates parasites

IgA comprises 20% of total serum immunoglobulins. It is known as secretory IgA as it is present in body secretions such as colostrum, milk, saliva and intestinal and bronchial fluids. It protects mucosal surfaces against undesirable micro-organisms by combining with mucus and antigen to release mucus which sweeps away unwanted molecules. Recent studies have suggested that a transient low level of IgA in infancy may be implicated in the aetiology of food allergy and eczema. Lack of protective secretory IgA is thought to increase the permeability of the gastrointestinal tract to food molecules which may act as antigens, resulting in the production of antibodies to foodstuffs, particularly milk and egg protein.

IgM constitutes 8% of total immunoglobulins and can be considered the first line of defence. It forms first in reaction to antigen and is mostly distributed in the vascular space. Certain specific antibodies are associated with IgM, such as cold agglutinins and rheumatoid factors. IgM assists in the function of the complement system, in agglutination and in opsonization. Neonates with congenital rubella may have elevated IgM levels at birth, derived not from the mother but as a result of the fetus's own immune response to intra-uterine infection.

IgD occurs in small amounts and its function is to bind antigens to B-cell surfaces to accomplish initial immunization.

IgE antibodies, normally present in concentrations of between 66 and 1830 ng/ml, cause the release of pharmacologically active agents from mast cells and are active in asthma, anaphylaxis, hay fever and immediate-type hypersensitivity reactions. Levels are increased in about 50% of people with allergic disease.

THE DEVELOPMENT OF LYMPHOID TISSUES

Stem cells from the embryonic yolk sac are the primary source of the B and T cell system. Cells destined to be T cells migrate to the thymus, which begins to develop as an active lymphoid organ after seven weeks' gestation. By 14 weeks mature T cells are present in the thymus gland and function immunologically in the fetus. Lymphopoiesis also begins in the spleen at about 12 weeks' gestation and early lymph nodes begin to develop at around six weeks. After leaving the thymus gland, where primary differentiation occurs, T cells circulate freely through the major lymphatic channels, lymph nodes, thoracic duct, spleen and vascular tree but do not re-enter the thymus. Final differentiation into the various kinds of T cells occurs in the spleen (Fig. 2.3).

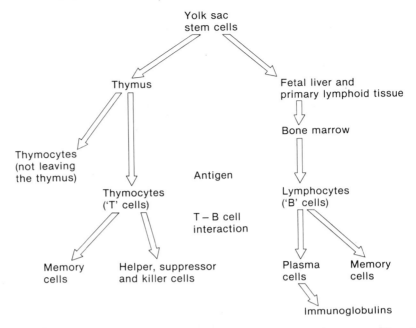

Fig. 2.3 Migration of yolk sac cells and their differentiation into thymocytes (T) and bone-marrow-derived cells (B) (Davis & Dobbing, 1981).

The total amount of lymphoid tissue in the body, including the thymus, lymph nodes and lymphoid tissue of the gut, increases throughout childhood, reaching its maximum at adolescence, after which it declines to adult levels.

B-cell precursors initially enter the fetal liver at about six weeks of gestation. They pass into the bone marrow before developing into B lymphocytes which eventually differentiate into plasma cells and memory cells. Circulating B cells have been detected as early as 13 weeks' gestation. Secretory capability is present for all classes of immunoglobulins by 20 weeks. Extensive synthesis of immunoglobulins does not occur *in utero* due to the relatively sheltered antigenic environment of the fetus. However, following intra-uterine infections increased levels of IgM may be found in cord blood.

The normal newborn infant's blood contains mainly IgG with small amounts of IgM, IgA, IgD and IgE. Most of the IgG is derived from maternal circulation by placental transfer and confers a degree of immediate passive immunity. The other four types of immunoglobulins do not cross the placenta. The level of IgG falls rapidly during the early postnatal weeks as maternal IgG is expended, reaching a trough as physiological hypoglobulinaemia at three months. Subsequently levels of IgG rise and reach adult levels by about four years of age. There is a striking difference in the pattern of maturation of IgM globulin as compared with other classes of immunoglobulin. The levels of IgM increase sharply during the first months of life, in contrast to the slow rise of IgA and IgE. IgM reaches the adult level by one year, in contrast to IgA, which attains this at adolescence.

Complement is synthesized from around the 15th week of fetal life; newborn levels are about half maternal levels and not augmented by placental transfer. Lysozyme is also synthesized from early fetal life. This enzyme is released by macrophages in plasma, saliva, tears, colostrum and milk and acts on infectious agents.

Interferon, an anti-viral factor, is produced by lymphocytes from 18 weeks of fetal life.

ANTIBODY PRODUCTION IN YOUNG INFANTS

The very young infant has been shown to produce antibodies in response to various agents including adenoviruses, enteroviruses, typhoid vaccine, polio vaccine and pertussis, diphtheria and tetanus antigens. The newborn baby is capable of responding to antigens such as polio vaccine but the synthesis of specific antibodies may be suppressed by the presence of specific maternal antibodies in the newborn circulation. If the level of these antibodies is low immunization at a young age can produce satisfactory antibody levels.

Development of the digestive system

The digestive tract develops early in fetal life and is relatively mature in even the smallest preterm baby. The primitive fore- and hind-gut are recognizable in the four-week embryo and form a complete tube by 10 weeks. Development involves a complex series of steps including elongation, rotation and joining of the caudal end with the cloaca. Most of the congenital structural abnormalities result from delay or aberration in this process.

Peristalsis begins at eight weeks of fetal life but is not fully co-ordinated until term. By 20 weeks intestinal villae and deep crypts are well formed and around this time the fetus begins to swallow liquor amnii along with lanugo hair and desquamated epithelium. Liquor is absorbed from the fetal intestine and oesophageal or intestinal obstruction may lead to hydramnios.

The secretory function of the digestive tract begins during fetal life and continues to develop during infancy. Initially the infant's digestive

Table 2.3 Approximate average age for eruption of primary dentition.

Incisors	6−9 months
Canines	16−19 months
1st molars	10−15 months
2nd molars	16−27 months

system is designed for milk feeding alone and adaptation to cope with a wider variety of foodstuffs occurs at various stages during the first year.

THE TEETH

The range and ages at which the teeth erupt in young babies is enormously variable (Table 2.3) and as a marker of other aspects of development it is not very helpful. Occasionally a baby is born with an incisor which may interfere with breast-feeding. In general, however, the first deciduous teeth do usually appear at about five or six months. It is, however, normal for them to appear at any time between four and 36 months. The incisors tend to erupt roughly between four and 14 months with the generally accepted average of six to nine months being the norm. The canines tend to appear some 10 months after the incisors while the first deciduous molars appear some four to six months after the incisors and the second molars some six to 12 months later. It is interesting that early or late development tends to occur within families.

Hypoplastic enamel may occur in small babies and is sometimes associated with the use of tetracycline in either the mother or the young infant. It is also seen in certain congenital syndromes but may occur as an isolated phenomenon. It is not usually significant in relation to the development of the second dentition but a paediatric dental opinion may be advisable if the mother is very anxious.

The issue of teething is discussed in Chapter 7.

THE STOMACH

At birth the stomach contents are alkaline and acid secretion increases rapidly initially but falls again by 10 days. Gastric acid production reaches appreciable levels from three months onwards. Pepsin secretion follows a similar pattern to that of acid. Intrinsic factor rises slowly after birth whereas gastrin levels are extremely high in the neonate.

The stomach largely acts as a reservoir for food in the infant. Acid and pepsin coagulate the casein in milk, thus slowing its passage into the small intestine.

THE INTESTINE

Most breakdown of food occurs in the small intestine. In the young infant food reaches the caecum in about four hours.

DIGESTION OF PROTEIN

The breakdown of protein into large polypeptides is brought about by pepsin and hydrochloric acid. Subsequent breakdown into amino acids occurs by the action of the pancreatic enzymes, trypsin, chymotrypsin and polypeptidases, and by enzymes derived from the small intestinal mucosa, such as enterokinase.

There is evidence that the newborn infant can absorb some whole protein molecules, such as lactalbumin and antibodies. The antibodies in colostrum and milk, however, act mainly in the lumen of the bowel against viruses and bacteria.

DIGESTION OF STARCH AND SUGARS

The young infant is poorly equipped to digest starch since pancreatic amylase production is minimal until one year. Small amounts of amylase appear in the saliva from three months and some amylase is also derived from the small intestinal mucosa. Young infants can only tolerate small amounts of starch; therefore it seems logical to delay introducing starchy foods until three or four months. Disaccharidases, responsible for the breakdown of sugars, are produced by the brush border of the villi of the small intestine. They are detectable in the 12-week fetus but the lactase system becomes maximal only at the end of normal gestation. Thus some preterm infants may not be able to digest lactose in milk.

Usually, after breakdown into monosaccharides (Table 2.4), sugars are absorbed in the small intestine. In disaccharidase deficiency, either occurring as an inborn error of metabolism or more commonly due to preterm birth or damage to the intestinal mucosa following gastro-enteritis, some disaccharides are absorbed whole. Some are then excreted in the urine and some will pass into the colon. Water retention and fatty acid formation occurs, distending and irritating the bowel, resulting in the frequent passage of watery acid stools.

Table 2.4 Disaccharide metabolism.

Source	Disaccharide	Enzyme	Monosaccharide
Milk	Lactose	Lactase	Glucose and galactose
Weaning foods	Sucrose	Sucrase	Glucose and fructose
Starch	Maltose	Maltase	Glucose and glucose
Glycogen	Isomaltose	Isomaltase	Glucose and glucose

DIGESTION OF FATS

Young infants have poor tolerance of fats, principally because bile salts and pancreatic lipase are at low levels during the first three months of life. Bile salts help emulsify fats, which are then split into monoglycerides, glycerol and fatty acids by the enzyme lipase. Absorption takes place into epithelial cells or lacteals (as globules of fat).

ABSORPTION OF MINERALS AND VITAMINS

In the proximal small intestine iron, calcium, magnesium, sodium, potassium, ascorbic acid, folic acid and water-soluble vitamins are absorbed. Vitamin B is absorbed from the terminal ileum.

References

Davis, B.B. & Dobbing, J. (1981) In: *Scientific Foundations of Paediatrics*, 2nd edn, Heinemann, London.

Dobbing, J. & Sands, J. (1978) Head circumference, biparietal diameter and brain growth in foetal and postnatal life. *Early Human Development*, **2**, 81.

Emery, J.J. et al. (1985) Apnoea monitors compared with weighing scales for siblings after cot death. *Archives of Disease in Childhood*, **60**, 1055–60.

Fitzhardinge, P.M. & Stevens, E.M. (1972) The small for dates infant: later growth patterns. *Pediatrics*, **49**, 671

Fujimura, M. & Seryu, (1977) Velocity of head growth during the perinatal period. *Archives of Disease in Childhood*, **52**, 105.

Smith, D.W., Truog, W., Rogers J.E., Greitzer, L.G., Skiner, A.L., McCann, J.J. & Harvey, M.A.S. (1976) Shifting linear growth in infancy. *Journal of Paediatrics*, **89**, 225.

Tanner, J.M., Whitehouse, R.H., Marshall, W.A. & Carter, B.S. (1975) Prediction of adult height from height, bone age and occurrence of menarche at ages 4 to 16 with allowance for mid-parent height. *Archives of Child Disease*, **50**, 14.

Tanner, J.M. (1978) *Foetus into Man*. Open Books, London.

3 Development from Six to 18 Months

IN THIS CHAPTER we discuss the development of the baby from six months to 18 months. Certain aspects of development which have been discussed in Chapters 1 and 2 are not reviewed here again. Thus it is important to monitor the child's height and weight throughout the first five years of life and any significant variation in a smooth increment of either height or weight needs consideration. The use of the percentile chart was explained in earlier chapters. Equally we do not review the main systems of the body such as the cardiovascular–respiratory system, but it is important to reflect that development is going on within these systems during the early years of life. The child is acquiring his own specific antigens to various diseases following naturally occurring infections, and the artificial introduction of antigens during the process of immunization takes place at specified times.

We are mostly concerned, however, with the maturation of the central nervous system as displayed in the development of function. It is important to remember that these functional changes reflect in part morphological changes in the central nervous system. There is a relationship between these changes and the stimuli the child has from his social and physical environment. Thus it is not clear to what extent exercise can affect the age at which the child achieves independent walking. The programme is probably largely genetically determined. On the other hand without input of human speech the child will not develop speech and language, but the way he does it is influenced by the changes within the central nervous system.

Motor development

By six months of age a baby has good head control; if you pull him into the sitting position from supine, he will make an anticipatory lift of the head off the surface, the head remaining in line with the body as it is pulled up. Placed prone, he will lift his head up to look round with the head in the vertical position. It seems as if he is aware of the importance of the stable position of the head in order to use his visual and auditory senses efficiently. He can sit at six months easily with

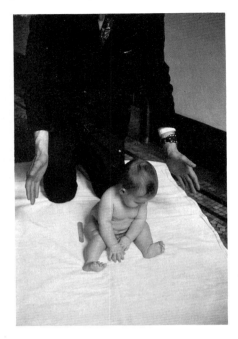

Fig. 3.1 Sitting at six months using forward propping reaction to maintain stability.

minimal support such as a high chair or simply with a cushion behind him and this means he can use his hands to manipulate objects freely. At six months we found that 70% of the babies we examined ($n = 329$) were sitting freely (for 30 seconds) on a flat floored surface although we allowed them to use their hands for support if necessary (Fig. 3.1). This may account for the fact that this rate is rather higher than others have reported. Thus Bryant *et al.* (1979) found 50% of babies sitting without support by 6.8 months, and 75% by 7.5 months, but did not specify whether the child was allowed to use his hands to support himself during the 30 seconds free sitting required by their study. These propping actions by the hands are important in maintaining balance. They are sometimes referred to as 'parachute reaction' or 'protective reaction' and they simply consist of putting out an arm and a hand to stop oneself falling over. They develop forward first and very quickly to the side (Fig. 3.2). Backwards propping, that is, reaching a hand behind oneself, does not develop until a month or six weeks later. A seven- or eight-month baby apparently sitting very stably may suddenly fall over backwards if he is distracted by a noise or something behind him because he has not yet developed this response.

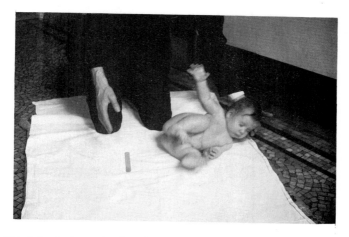

Fig. 3.2 This baby had not developed lateral propping (or parachute reactions) and consequently his sit was unstable. The lateral parachute reactions will develop shortly.

Having achieved free sitting, the next step in gross motor development which one sees in many babies is the development of crawling (by this we mean movement on hands and knees, described as creeping in some of the American literature). Very soon after six months many babies will be seen on hands and knees rocking to and fro, but not quite moving. Most babies start crawling around seven or eight months. Capute *et al.* (1985) found crawling present by a mean age of 7.8 months. There are a number of babies who will never crawl and who move about in another way. A very small proportion start walking very early and are not seen to have a crawling stage at all. There are a small group of children who do not crawl but actually quite like rolling around, a skill which the baby usually acquires at about four months. Other babies drag themselves along on their bellies for some time, but most children who have these habits find by seven or eight months that crawling is a faster way of getting around. Another group who don't crawl learn to shuffle along on their bottoms. This bottom shuffling, in which the baby puts his hands down and then punts himself forward with one leg, is a dominantly inherited mode of movement (Robson, 1970, 1984) and occurs in about 10–12% of children. In our study we found, however, that half the bottom shufflers also crawled and only 6% of babies at one year were not crawling at all. Children who are bottom shufflers walk late and may still not be walking at around two and a half years but be quite normal. Robson (1970) records 82% of children as crawlers, 9% bottom shufflers, 1% creepers, 1% rollers and 7% who just stand up and walk.

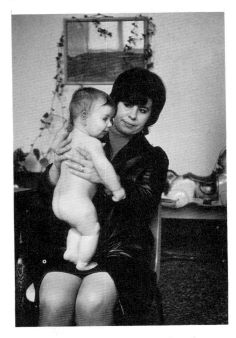

Fig. 3.3 Baby standing on mother's knee at six months of age.

This intermediate method of movement, crawling or bottom shuffling, precedes the normal adult method of locomotion, walking. In
order to walk the child obviously has to stand first. Around about
three months the baby will often not support his weight very willingly,
bending at the knees and hips. By six months he will stand happily on
his mother's knee (Fig. 3.3), although it is noticeable that hip and knee
are still slightly flexed. The child prefers slightly flexed postures although
he can stand perfectly straight. Certain babies may have some resistance
to standing on their feet. Babies born by breech delivery often keep
their hips flexed almost at a right angle and their acquisition of standing
may be delayed. It is our impression that babies who bottom shuffle
stand less readily too. The sitting-on-air posture of the breech-born
baby is seen around seven or eight months but we would anticipate
that it would have disappeared at 10 to 12 months and the baby would
be making standing movements, if not standing independently quite
well, at this stage.

A most important development for the child is the ability to stand
by himself and this requires him to pull himself up into the standing
position from sitting. This the child will do in his cot or using a low
table or chair, and round about eight months we see the child standing

holding on. Very soon after this he can cruise, which means he moves round holding on to the furniture, using his hands to support himself. About this time too, one will see him standing at a low table, leaning against it and using elbows to support himself while playing freely with his hands on the table. The child may now walk, initially reaching from one support to another, which requires him to take a step. He may walk pushing an object and he may also walk in a baby walker. He will be encouraged by his parents to walk first with both hands held and then with only one hand held and then finally he walks independently.

In our study seven steps scored as independent walking. There is some evidence that children are perhaps walking a little earlier than they used to. In our study 46% of the children were walking alone by one year (total $n = 275$) while the mean for the population studies by Capute *et al.* (1985) for walking was 11.7 months. Earlier studies, such as that by Hindley *et al.* (1966) (a multi-centred European study), showed that 50% of the babies were not walking until the age of 13 months. There is a considerable spread in the age at which independent walking is achieved and it is quite normal for a child not to be walking at 18 months. Two per cent of the children in our study were not walking by this age, while others have reported 3% of children. Many of the children who are not walking at age 18 months are late normal groups or babies who bottom shuffle. It is important to know why a baby is not walking by 18 months. There is something to be said for Gardner Medwin's recent suggestion (1979) that any baby not walking at this age should be screened for muscular dystrophy; a small minority may also be found to have cerebral palsy (Hardie & MacFarlane, 1980). Of the normal babies the bottom shufflers are often the late walkers — some as late as two years. Robson (1984) has provided some predictive tables which allow one to estimate when the baby will based on the age he started shuffling. At whatever age the child first walks, he tends to have bursts of steps and then a pause. The gait is uneven, which means to say that one pace may be longer than the other, and the legs tend to be held rather more widely apart initially, although in part this is often an artefact because of the nappies the child is wearing. When the child first walks the hands are held high about shoulder level (high guard) and they are thus ready to push the child up again should he topple forward on to his hands. Within a month, they will be held about waist-high and reach the side in about two to three months.

It is hard to make a distinction between walking and running at these early ages. The child seems almost to run as soon as he walks.

Running involves both feet being off the ground at once. Capute (1989) in his parental reporting series describes how about 15% of children are active climbers, and, as soon as they can crawl, they will work their way up stairs and clamber from chairs on to tables. Some developmental tests make great play of the age at which the child climbs up steps one step at a time, and brings both feet on to one step before proceeding to the next, as opposed to the so-called adult modes of alternately placing one foot on one step and one foot on the next. This, however, is an artefact relating to the child's height and the height of the tread of each stair. Peiper (1963) demonstrated that the primary walking baby will walk alternately stepping up a flight of stairs providing the steps are small enough.

Fine motor development

The six-month baby is using both hands freely, reaching out and picking up objects and subsequently transferring them from hand to hand and exploring them with the mouth (Fig. 3.4). Objects, however, are grasped with the whole hand and if he is given a small sweet (e.g. a Smartie) he will scoop it up with the fingers against the palm, and eventually eat it by licking if off the bottom of his hand. By 10 months, however, he will have developed the pincer grasp, in which small objects are picked up between the opposed thumb and forefinger. He can pick up a piece of food therefore and put it quite neatly into his mouth. This progression from the whole-hand grasping of the six-

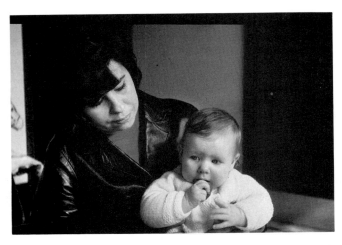

Fig. 3.4 This six-month old baby 'chews' one of the examiner's bricks which he has successfully picked up.

month-old to the pincer movement of the 10-month-old is a gradual one involving the child using fingers at first against the base of the thumb before full opposition develops. Also at the six-month stage, one can see that the grasping of objects involves movement of the whole forearm and arm and swiping movements at objects may be misdirected. Movements become more discrete once the upper arm is more stable and objects close to can be manipulated with movements of the forearm and hand, or hand and wrist only. This stability of the upper arm is seen at about eight months.

Initially the child when he first holds on to things around five months can only hold in one hand at a time, but soon he learns to pass an object from one hand to the other (a process known as transferring). Around six or seven months he spends a lot of time handling, sucking and manipulating objects. This period is when he is probably developing a sense of texture and the 'taste' of objects. At about 10 months he enjoys throwing or dropping objects, a behaviour called 'casting'. At home one will see the baby in his high chair with objects on the table which he throws with pleasure to the floor, waiting for someone else to pick them up. Again this is a behaviour which should diminish by round about one year of age. It is at this age that the use of his index finger allows him to poke into objects and explore them in rather more detail than he did earlier on (Fig. 3.5). He will now look at a toy car with great interest, though it won't be until around 15 months that he will treat it as anything but an object. But at 13 months he'll push his finger through the windows, open the doors (if this is possible) and play with the wheels.

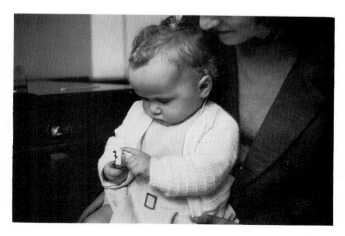

Fig. 3.5 Exploration of a toy car with a prehensile forefinger (one-year old baby).

Once the pincer grip is achieved, the child is capable of making fine discrete movements of the hand and when he moves an object from one place to another the movement is delicate and controlled. However, when he is involved in approximating one object to another the movement becomes clumsy again and can even be described as ataxic. At about 15 months he can be persuaded to put one brick upon another. This operation requires the co-ordination of vision, and the hand movement to make the necessary approximation of the bricks. Initially this is difficult for him and there is some uncontrolled wobbling as the building hand approaches the first brick; tidy placement of the second brick on the first is not achieved until 18 months or older. Initially one may observe the child having difficulty 'letting go'. He places the brick correctly but then takes hand and brick away again.

Vision

By six months the child's visual acuity is about 6/12, but it is difficult to test and examine its discriminatory function. The child's visual world still tends to be fairly close to and he will pay more attention to objects within about 10 feet in an ordinary environment than he will to more distant objects. However, given a suitably neutral room and the ability to attract the child's attention it is easy to see that he will follow a small object, and focus on it at 20 feet. Sheridan (1979) developed a range of tests of vision for the young child which are clinically useful in picking up severe problems of visual acuity in a child and allow one to observe the child's visual function. The test involves moving small white balls, either by rolling them or by mounting them on black sticks across a dark surface, and watching the child follow them. The smallest ball in the set is a 16th of an inch in diameter and a child will readily follow this at 10 feet. This function can be watched from behind a black screen with an eye slit in it. In the visually handicapped child another observation which can be useful is to see if he can locate a small sweet (Smarties or hundreds-and-thousands). Be careful to drop the sweet with a sweep of the hand and not so that the alert child can locate the object by watching the arm movement.

As ever, the child is perhaps more concerned with interesting objects and the face remains the most potent object. The child will follow movement of the adult face close to and at a distance. Recently tests have been developed in which the child is shown a card with a graded grating. He looks at the patterned card rather than a plain card and by reducing the size of the grating an equivalence to visual acuity can be made in infants (Teller *et al.*, 1986).

The child should have achieved binocular vision by this age and one should see both eyes moving together as they study objects of interest to the child. One can also observe convergence as an object is brought closer to the child.

Hearing

It has recently been shown that there are two levels at which auditory functions develop. First, the most primitive level allows the organism to track a sound through changes in intensity, and head and body movements are made in the process of locating the sound. This process requires a fairly long signal duration and is probably present at birth. Secondly, a more sophisticated response allows the organism to identify brief sounds at durations of 25 microseconds or less: this allows for more accurate localization. This is a later evolutionary development and dependent on an expanded auditory neocortex, so that the older baby's more sophisticated loud sound localization process was seen fully developed at six months. The baby at six months will localize sounds left and right although a sound made at 45° above the horizontal line between the ears is localized first by turning laterally and then looking upwards towards the sound's source. Localization of noises made immediately above the head continues to be quite difficult for the child even up to the age of five. The hearing response at five to six months is not so rapid as that seen at seven to eight months. The child may first pause, apparently alert to the sound and then turn towards it (Fig. 3.6). At eight months, he will turn more rapidly around and turn away again after the briefest glance. At five or six

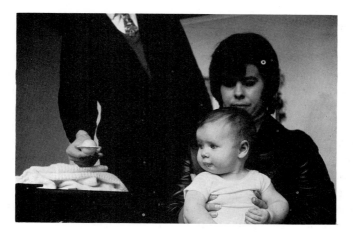

Fig. 3.6 Sound location at six months. A good persistent turn to a sound-making object.

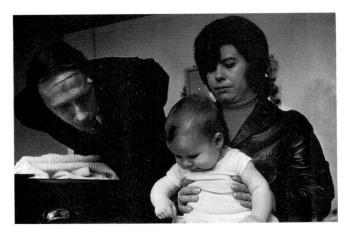

Fig. 3.7 The baby has caught sight of his toes and is visually 'involved' with them, so ignoring the sound that the examiner is making.

months a child will sometimes not attend to sound when he is engaged in other activities, particularly visual activities (Fig. 3.7). Therefore the child playing and examining an object in his hands may ignore the sound. Again, although he can certainly localize sound well at a distance, the baby's auditory world is close to him; he attends to people speaking to him who are within four or five feet, but seems to ignore sounds made far away from him.

The way the child ignores sound may seem puzzling to the inexperienced examiner, but while the baby is *in utero* (see Chapter 1) he is exposed to a very noisy environment and he has to learn to ignore sounds before beginning to pay selective attention to them. All these factors mean that at any age the child may not apparently respond to sound even when he has perfectly normal hearing, and therefore clinical testing is bound to produce some non-responders.

In our own study we tested hearing in babies at six months and had 10% non-responders at this age. These non-responders included (a) some children with conductive hearing loss associated with upper respiratory tract and ear infections, (b) children who are slow to develop localization, and (c) children who were irritable for some other reason and from whom we were unable to get a response at the time we tested. All the non-responding babies were retested and had normal responses at some time within the next two months. Thus all our conductive 'losses' under one year showed spontaneous recovery though they may have had further episodes of hearing loss associated with glue ear in the second year of life.

Our non-responders rate is similar to those reported at around eight months. We favour the earlier testing at six months, which we think is just as easy as testing at eight months, and it does mean that the child with a potential hearing loss is identified earlier and should reach specialist attention earlier. Early detection of hearing loss and fitting of appropriate aids has been shown to result in improved language acquisition. The characteristic response of stilling before turning at six months is helpful when one is assessing a child on one's own without an observer. The child's lack of knowledge of object permanence (see p. 82) also makes him easier to test at this age, as, when the examiner 'hides' behind the baby, the child does not look for him. (For a review of the development of auditory localization see Muir & Clifton, 1985.)

Vocalizations

Around about five or six months the sounds which the child makes, which have been largely vowel sounds up to that time, are varied with the introduction of the first consonantal sounds. These are usually gutturals made at the back of the throat, the 'g' and 'k' in the 'gars', or 'kars', but soon other sounds appear, 'd' being an important one in most English-speaking societies because it is quickly encouraged by the parents, who see it as the start of 'dad' or 'da'. The type of consonantal sounds that the baby develops varies very much from child to child, and shows no particularly consistent pattern. By one year the child is making a wide range of noises. By 15 to 18 months he has expressive speech so that he can make many words. It is perhaps easiest to remember those sounds which are quite often acquired late, although individual children will have some of them earlier; these include 's', 'l', 'r', 'th', 'sh' and sometimes the hard 'k' as in 'cup' (usually substituted by children with a 't'). Two or three consonantal sounds may not be required until the child is around five and indeed the voiced 'th', as in thumb, not until after that (in Cockney children never!).

First words acquisition

Towards the end of the first year, a child produces the first words. There is considerable debate as to whether this should be distinguished from the larger flow of words which begins somewhere around 15 months or so. Usually these first words are naming words, that is 'mum', 'dad', 'gran' and so on, and sometimes later on a word which has been used apparently consistently to say 'daddy' will be extended in the second year of life to a very much broader use, i.e. the word 'dad' being used to refer to all men. These first words are rather different from later words. They are used more inflexibly for specific people and they don't have the flexibility that words used later have (see Yule & Rutter, 1987 for a recent reference).

Semantics, transmission and syntax

In order to understand the development of speech and language in the young child, it is necessary to understand some of the elements of language development. There are three elements in our communication system. These are semantics, the transmission system and syntax.

SEMANTICS

Semantics describes the use of a word meaningfully in the acquisition of a labelling or classifying process, and it is unique to the human species. What is fascinating about this is the speed with which the child seems to grasp very complicated symbolic notions. Thus the child around 15 months will begin to use a sound or word to represent 'car'. It might actually be 'car' or it might be 'brm brm'. He will not only use it for the real object, which he sees parked outside his parents' house, but also of one- or two-inch models of a toy car or, again, luridly drawn pictures of it in modern children's books. This emphasizes that the actual expression of the word in spoken language conceals the ability to think in symbols and to classify objects in a distinctly human way. Another good example of this ability is the use of the word 'dog' by a child, particularly one brought up in a rural district. He or she will apply the word correctly to a vast range of four-legged animals, from a Pekinese to a wolfhound, and discriminate all dogs from sheep. This again emphasizes that somehow he has got hold of the notion of 'dogginess' as opposed to the characteristics of a sheep. Later on, if he proceeds to study biology in school, he will write essays describing how this complicated classification is made, forgetting that subconsciously he made it himself when he was two. (Many children will go through a period of calling all four-legged animals dogs at an earlier stage.)

There is evidence that the child acquires the inner language or symbols which he thinks in, which we have just discussed, before he produces them in spoken language. Thus it is easy to demonstrate that a child will often point at objects correctly when he has not yet been heard to say the word. He can demonstrate the existence of an inner

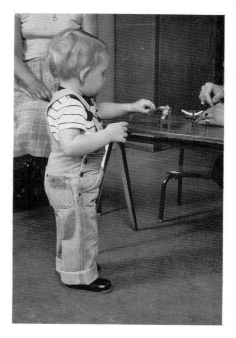

Fig. 3.8 An 18-month-old child has been asked without any demonstration to offer the doll some food in his own language (e.g. 'give dolly din-dins').

language by using models appropriately. For example, if shown a picture of a brush and comb, he may pretend to pick the comb off the page, and make combing movements in his hair. This clearly indicates that he recognizes the illustration for what it is and has a knowledge in his head which distinguishes comb from another shape, such as a knife. Symbolic play, therefore, which one can often observe in children under two, demonstrates the existence of this inner language. Play with dolls or teddy bears for example, where 'blankets' are pulled over them or toy cups are offered and dolls are fed from spoons and so on (Fig. 3.8), implies that all the objects which are models of the real things are recognized and classified correctly within the child's brain. The development of this ability occurs very rapidly, during the second year of life, and can easily be demonstrated with a simple toy like the toy car. A one-year-old will usually take a toy car and explore it with his forefinger, rolling the rear wheels round and poking into the doors and so on. The 18-month-old, will take the object at once, put it down and proceed to 'drive it around'. A useful but somewhat simplistic notion is to talk of his receptive language (semantically) and his expressive language. The one he demonstrates by vocalizing, the other by pointing at named objects. While this distinction is sometimes helpful it may also be confusing. What is the child doing when he *plays* with a toy silently?

TRANSMISSION SYSTEMS

The inner language described above is transmitted to the outside world through a medium of expression. In the young child, this medium is usually the spoken voice, but there are other mediums, such as the written word, Morse code and many sign languages, which are potentially available to the child. There is even some evidence that children can acquire a signing language rather earlier than they would a spoken language. Children will parrot words or imitate them, before they know what they mean. Very occasionally one sees a child who has considerable speech but no inner language. For example a blind child said 'ba ba black sheep' when he was two, but had no concept of black or sheep.

Although the transmission system is therefore distinguishable from inner language, it usually plays an important part in its development and indeed plays a part in getting over meaning. There are two elements to it, the first being the phonetic element — which describes the actual sounds made. Quite clearly to signal 'cat' as opposed to 'cap' we must make different consonantal sounds. The phonological system means using the phonetic system appropriately in relation to the spoken language being used. A native English speaker will rarely if ever achieve full phonological competence in Chinese. Different languages have different phonological systems, and as the child grows he acquires one or more. In later life he may have difficulty learning accurately another phonological system; thus most of us who learn foreign languages in adult life find that we are unable to acquire certain phonological elements of these languages, so we always speak with a 'foreign' accent.

Another element in the system is the use of inflection or prosody to imply meaning. Thus the young children can say 'dad' expressing affection or fear, and a considerable amount of meaning is implied in the tone in which we say things. One can say 'yes' quickly and delightedly or one could say 'ye-es' when one actually means 'no'.

SYNTAX

The third element in the development of human language is syntax. Clearly the extension of human communication involves the combination of symbols together, which allows more complex messages to be composed. Very simply, the sentence 'dog chase cat' means exactly the opposite to 'cat chase dog'. The arrangements of words into sentence structures allows us to develop our highly sophisticated communication system. It has been possible to train some other primates to produce single words, but not produce sentences. The child begins to use sentences towards the end of the second year and this development will be discussed further in Chapter 4.

PRAGMATICS

Sometimes a child will say a sentence which seems to be semantically and syntactically correct, but is inappropriate in relation to the situation the child is in at the time. An autistic child said 'he cleans his teeth' but only when in a particularly therapeutic situation when shown one picture. He said no other sentences at all.

Social and emotional development

The child of six months has very relaxed social responses to other human beings. He or she is friendly and if a stranger makes an approach to him he will usually respond in a friendly fashion. He is certainly developing close attachments to his immediate family and, from the age of five or six months onwards, separation experiences, such as admission to hospital or a procedure without his parents, are disturbing to him and may have short- or even long-term consequences. Although the very much younger child (as described in Chapter 1) will certainly recognize aspects of his mother, for example turning preferentially to her voice from a very early age, it is only around about five or six months that he probably begins to identify her as a person and others as distinct people, and can 'think of them' as individuals whom he needs. During the next two or three months he will develop some fear of strangers. Different children have very different temperaments, but nevertheless the 10-month child may cry, if a stranger approaches him rapidly. Indeed, as the second year proceeds, he may show a tendency to cling tightly to his parents. This does not mean that he necessarily has to spend all his time with his parents, and he will relate well to other caretakers, such as grannies or daily minders, although probably the number of individuals he can happily associate with on an emotional level are small.

The development of the concept of the individual as a unique and separate person is probably associated with the cognitive development in the child of the sense of object permanency, first described by Piaget. The six-month-old child will not search for a person or an object which is concealed and leaves his direct line of sight. If, for example, you walk round behind a six-month child, seated on his mother's lap, he will follow you with his eyes until you disappear from view; he will not then crane round to see whether you are coming back the other side, which a one-year-old child will do, an ability acquired around eight months. A ball hidden under a cup has gone for the six-month child, but the nine- or 10-month-old child will search for it under its concealing cup.

Many of the ways we signal our social responses are acquired during these second six months of life. For example, a six-month child will stare at a face for quite long periods of time, and his social responses are still quite slow (Fig. 3.9). He will look at a stranger for a moment and then smile. By one year, the child glances (as do adults) at strangers and does not maintain direct gaze fixation with them for long periods. These may be superficial indicators of the developments of feelings and affections, but they are useful to the clinician because they are observable and, in the retarded or disturbed child, they can be abnormal. The autistic child avoids gaze fixation, and the mentally handicapped child is often, although not invariably, slow to respond to social advances. Some mentally handicapped children never develop the fear of strangers. The Down's syndrome child is classic in this respect and, at very much later ages, will (like a six-month-old child) smile willingly at complete stranger, a promiscuity which can be both embarrassing and sometimes of more serious consequence.

After the age of six months or so, the child begins to develop his own personality, although all parents will recognize this from earlier on. However, for the observer more distinct characteristics begin to appear at this time. How long does it take a stranger to relate to the child? Some one-year-olds can be in the clinic for 10 minutes or more before they will allow anyone to approach them without crying; others will settle down much more quickly. Parents will tell you that some children seem very happy and chuckle and laugh a lot, whereas others seem more serious and more difficult to stimulate. Rapid mood swings are, of course, a feature of young children. The child will cry when something is taken away from him but, distracted by noise such as a bell ringing, will stop at once and seconds later be happily chuckling. A child whose moods are difficult to interrupt in this way can be difficult for the parents to manage, and again should be a cause of some concern to the clinician. With the infant under the age of five or six months, the clinician can pick up the baby and soothe him himself. With older children one watches how rapidly the mother is able to

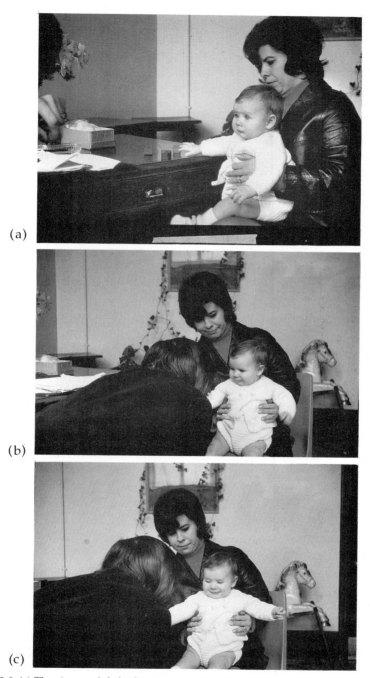

(a)

(b)

(c)

Fig. 3.9 (a) The six-month baby has just come into the room and his mother has just sat down with him. (b) He stares fixedly at the examiner's face, ignoring other interesting objects such as the daffodils. (c) When the examiner bends down he looks at him with interest and then breaks into a friendly smile.

soothe the child, say following an injection, and with what skills she distracts him from the pain on to some other activity.

Another important feature of early social response which is useful clinically is the child's facial expression. The six-month baby, once settled opposite the examiner on his mother's lap, will often stare quite fixedly at the examiner; if the latter now smiles at him quite slowly, the baby will usually respond with a similar response. This type of interpersonal reaction contrasts with the quick visual contacts which are exchanged between adults and indeed, if one stared at an adult as long as a baby does, one would be making very intimate contact. Equally it takes the baby some time to work out how to respond to things. For example if you place a stethoscope on the six-month-old baby's chest (which most young children dislike) it will be 10 seconds or so before he starts wriggling to free his arms. By one year of age, however, he will be responding much more quickly to adverse stimuli and examination is consequently more difficult (Fig. 3.10).

The one- to two-year-old child will still stare at a stranger's face for much longer than an adult will. He will also, through the three and four years, wish to watch the face of somebody who is talking to him, because he uses visual cues to help him understand their speech. The use of gesture can also be important in social relationships and the child points at his father delightedly, saying 'da' perhaps. All these indicators of social response are available to the clinician as he tries to decide whether the child is developing socially as he should.

Gesture develops significantly once the child has acquired pincer grip and is using the forefinger prehensively. He now begins to point at objects he wants or to emphasize the vocalization he is making by using the forefinger as a 'debating instrument'. Characteristically, we are looking at an item of behaviour which is involved in social development, language development and, of course, fine motor development, thus emphasizing how all parts of development go along together.

Mouthing

Around five or six months the baby indulges in a lot of mouthing activities, that is, putting everything he gets hold of in his mouth. Some babies suck their fingers from very early on and this may develop into thumb sucking. At about three months when the baby is lying on his back and watching his fingers as he moves them, he will

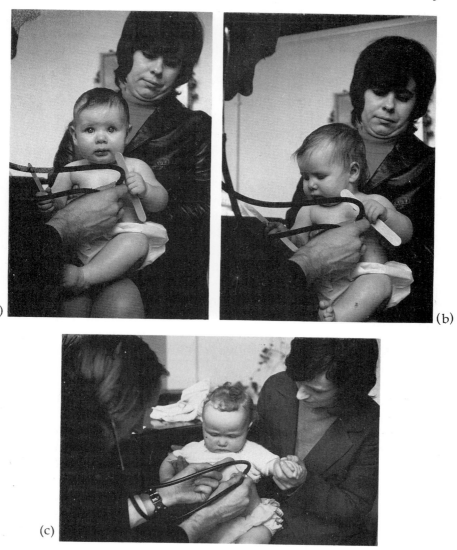

Fig. 3.10 (a) The examiner places his stethoscope on the child's chest, to which he objects as his slightly alarmed stare indicates, but he is unable to use his hands to remove it because they are occupied. (b) He looks at them and then discards the stick from the right and then the left hand; then he reaches for the stethoscope which is just being withdrawn. (c) By one year this trick will no longer work and the child's hands must be gently restrained.

also tend to put them in his mouth, but once objects are being picked up competently he begins to mouth them and this behaviour reaches its maximum at this time. It used to be interpreted by psychoanalytical writers as oralism and related to the child's emotional development. It seems rather to be more of an exploratory behaviour. The child uses his fingers and his tongue to explore shape and texture and most importantly taste. As adults we know what a lump of coal, earth or fluff would taste like although we have not stuffed such objects in our mouths for many years. Equally the intimate knowledge of texture, the feel of velvet as opposed to canvas, is probably partly acquired during this period. Whether this is the correct explanation or not, the behaviour begins to decrease around seven or eight months and is much less common at one year. Under stress the child may put something in his mouth again, but he does not do it very readily. At this time too the child's dribbling is at its maximum. He doesn't keep his mouth shut or swallow his saliva. Control is activated over the next two or three months.

The relationship of this mouthing behaviour to finger or thumb sucking is problematic. Undoubtedly babies like to suck and get some comfort from this. They certainly get pleasure from sucking the breast, and they will suck a teat which is not delivering milk — a dummy or pacifier — which they obviously find comforting. This behaviour can go on for many years, even into adult life.

Parents tend to worry about these sucking behaviours and there is no very firm basis for advice on what to do about them. In general, however, sucking behaviours are so common during the first year that they are best accepted, but as the child gets older it seems reasonable to try and reduce them, particularly as the child of 18 months to two years who has a pacifier attached around his neck on a piece of string is not likely to be an early talker. One hopes to get rid of the dummy by around this age, or at least restrict its use to when the child goes to sleep. Thumb sucking continuing when the secondary dentition is appearing can cause some mild deformity of the mouth, protrusion of the upper incisors with the reverse effect on the lower ones.

Cognitive development

As indicated under fine motor development, by 10 months the child has developed the pincer grip of an adult, and he can now use his fine motor skills to explore objects. There is plenty of evidence of developing cognitive skills between six and 18 months. Early on objects are picked up and their texture examined in great detail.

This early interest in shape and textures is followed by an exploration of the properties of objects, such as whether they float or not. A 10-month-old infant will sit in his bath endlessly bobbing an object up and down. Objects which make a noise are interesting, and the way things relate to one another. He will pick up a toy car at this age, look at it as described in the language section, and explore its properties. This exploration of shape will allow him during the second year of life to carry out simple matching tasks. For example, sometime after age one he will begin to pick up an object with a hole in it and put it over a rod. At this age, also, with considerable difficulty initially, he will push shapes through a letterbox. Often, early on, he will persist endlessly trying to get something too large through a hole. The properties of materials will be explored. He will bang and rattle objects. Endless repetition is a feature of this stage of development and is important to the child.

He will also use objects in developing his relationships with other children. For the 10-month child, a favourite game is to throw objects away from him, encouraging an adult to give them back. Sitting at a chair with a table, he will throw all the objects on the table off it. This activity is known as 'casting'. Again, this is behaviour which is seen very commonly around the five-month to one-year period, but should recede in the 13- to 15-month period as he becomes more sophisticated and wants to use objects given to him.

At about 15 months he may actually place one brick upon another, and by 18 months, in our sample, we managed to persuade 40% of children to build us a tower of four or more bricks. By two years old 70% were building six-brick towers. At 15 months or so the child's play, as discussed under the language section, begins to indicate that he knows what the objects are, and complicated play structures can develop: driving cars round to get them fuel, setting out a dolls' tea-party. Initially, the sequences of play will be quite short, but they rapidly build up.

The young child's attention span is noticeably short compared with an adult's, and the parent will get to know how long a child will explore one thing before he must be moved on to another. Again, a 10-month baby will stand happily exploring knobs, say on a radio set, for 10 to 20 minutes or more, but then he will move off around the room. A lot of his time can be spent, as he begins to crawl and walk, in exploring the environment, crawling around the room behind chairs, up on to sofas, and so on. The energy within these explorations seems almost limitless, although the child can move very rapidly from rushing around the room to exhaustion and be found quietly curled up in a corner asleep.

Imitation and learning

Although all learning is not imitation or copying, copying quite clearly does play a major part in the child's development of all sorts of skills. It is important therefore to observe the child developing this ability to copy. A very young child will in fact copy those around him. It has to be remembered that the baby has some difficulty making precise movements and it would be impossible for a three-month-old baby to copy the examiner picking up a brick and placing it on top of another one. At this age he lacks the fine motor skills. At this early age baby's most skilled 'tool' is his tongue and a six-week-old baby will protrude his tongue imitating his mother or other adult if he sees this done to him. Equally he will imitate the babble of those around him, so that he can transfer from an 'ah' sound to an 'oo' sound quite early on, and, by five or six months, similar imitation will be taking place with 'd's and 'g's. He will suddenly say 'da, da, da' for you and it may be possible to get him to transfer to the 'g' sound — 'ga, ga, ga'. At seven or eight months, now that he has a stable sit and good control of his hands, he is able to carry out imitative games much more easily and this is the age at which one sees the child enjoying repetitive, imitatory games. He waves 'bye-bye' when instructed to; he claps his hands copying other people; if the doctor picks up a pair of one-inch bricks the baby will bang the bricks together in imitation. Often when a child is in front of you, and you try and get him to bang the bricks he will not do it, but will sit looking at you holding his two bricks but not moving them (Fig. 3.11). When you stop doing it yourself and take your attention away from him, he may suddenly carry out the manoeuvre himself, and it seems therefore that he is thinking about what has gone on and then tries out to see whether he can do what you can do — he has learned something.

Examination of the child

When the child reaches the age of six months one begins to need some equipment in order to examine him and it seems useful at this point to review some of the material which developmental paediatricians (from the time of Gesell onwards) have developed for use in examining a child.

The problem facing the clinician is that the easiest way to assess a child's function is to watch him over a period of time and the assessment that the clinician is trying to make is an unusual, if not an abnormal, social event for the child. The clinician wishes, as rapidly as possible,

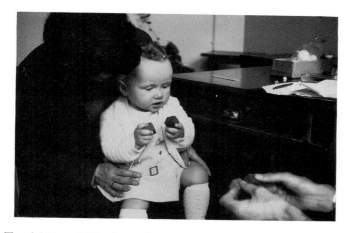

Fig. 3.11 The child is watching intensely as the examiner bangs his bricks together and will imitate him (one-year-old child).

to assess all aspects of the child's function and in order to do this he tries to get the child to carry out a series of tasks for him. It is worth emphasizing that this is not the natural way that a child plays. The clinician's aim is to try and persuade the child that this is just a normal social event while at the same time rapidly taking him through a series of fairly standardized tests. Clearly the approach must be flexible so that advantage can be taken of the child's spontaneous activity.

The very way the room is organized may be important in this connection. A confrontation across a desk means that at a certain point the clinician must get up and stand over the young child and may consequently appear to threaten him. The arrangement of the room is discussed in Chapter 4 but we always like to have a low table at the side of the mother and baby, on which as he reaches the toddler age the child can manipulate objects. It is not sensible to have too large a number of toys displayed, because the child flits from one to another. We tend to put out one rather interesting toy to start with, offering new toys as appropriate, but simultaneously removing others.

For testing fine motor function one-inch bricks have been tradition-ally used. Around six months common objects such as wooden spoons, small saucepan and unbreakable plastic cups are objects with which a six-month-old child may play. Sticks and bits of grass are examined by a six-month child who plays outside. For older children symbolic objects, that is, toys which represent something in the adult world, are obviously useful and toy cars, toy cups, dolls, and dolls'-house furniture have particular appeal. With children from different cultures it is necessary to find out what are familiar household objects. We prefer to avoid rather confusing objects which to adults and older children may represent something but which may be difficult for the young child to understand. We have in mind things like plastic monsters which an older child may recognize from television, but may simply be seen as objects by the young child.

For testing hearing there are two rattles available, one made by the Manchester audiology unit and one by the Nuffield,[1] which deliver a high-pitched sound when shaken gently. Recently a warbler[2] has been developed which should prove useful clinically. Bells are often used, but produce rather loud sounds even when gently shaken. Increasingly with the toddler age group, we believe that most examiners wish to carry out their own impedance audiometry. We have also found it useful to have a free-field audiometer and a sound-level meter. Hearing is such an important element in the child's development that it seems unfortunate that some people are not, for financial reasons, adequately equipped. Ordinary audiometers, which one begins to use with children of four or five years, where the child has the sound delivered through earphones, are not recommended for use with children under the age of three or four, who actually find the removal of all ambient noise and the application of the earphone quite alarming.

Vision testing

Equipment to test the vision of young children does present particular problems between the ages of six months and about two and a half years. The Catford Drum, to elicit optokinetic nystagmus, has been described in Chapter 1. The late Dr Mary Sheridan developed a series of balls with which to test the vision of normal and young children and older handicapped children. Unfortunately (Hall *et al.*, 1985) it seems unlikely that the test is sufficiently accurate to allow one to identify the problems of visual acuity at this age. We in fact use a modification of this test (Bax *et al.*, 1981) in which we watch children of six months, one year and 18 months follow a small ball mounted on a stick as it is moved through an arc. Although we found the test quite practical to carry out, the results were negative in so far as no problems of

[1] These rattles are obtainable from The Department of Audiology, Manchester University; The Nuffield Hearing and Speech Centre, Gray's Inn Road, London.
[2] Obtainable from Meg Instrumentation Ltd, PO Box 32, Sharrow Mills, Ecclesall Road, Sheffield, S11 8PL (cost £64 plus £12.00 for battery charges — 30, 50, 70 dB, 500–2000 Hz frequency — price accurate at September 1989).

visual acuity were identified by this method. We nevertheless find the balls are useful objects to have if a parent is concerned about a young child's vision and the equipment again can be extremely helpful with the handicapped older child and to demonstrate severe visual defects.

A new development has been the use of acuity gratings (Teller *et al.*, 1986). In this situation the baby is sat facing two screens on which a striped pattern can be displayed. As the stripes get smaller and smaller they can no longer be distinguished and the child feels that he is looking at a homogeneous grey background. The child will look preferentially therefore at a striped pattern as opposed to a grey pattern and by observing his eye movements through a peep-hole it is possible to decide whether he is detecting the stripes or not. While this technique is rather time-consuming and not in wide use clinically, it is helpful to be aware that it is now possible to make a good assessment of the child's visual acuity at early ages.

A still more recent development which is not in regular use yet is photorefraction, which involves the six-month-old child having a flash photo taken of his eyes. This allows one to identify the child who has an abnormal lens, which may subsequently cause him to develop a squint and allows treatment to begin at a really early age.

As the child begins to be able to name objects, it is possible to get him to look at and name small toys at a distance (a test developed by the late Dr Mary Sheridan): small toys such as a car, brick, chair, doll, knife, spoon and fork are customarily used for this examination. The spoon, fork and knife are very small and have been related to the Snellen letters. A problem often arises that the child, at least at early ages, refers to all cutlery as spoon ('poon') and particularly the knife and fork are not discriminated very readily at ages under two, although sometimes the child can be trained to match them.

Equipment for testing vision and hearing of older children is described at the beginning of Chapter 4.

The early examination of speech and language uses real objects such as chairs and tables, toys and picture books with common objects in them from the house and from the garden. We prefer to use fairly orthodox drawings and avoid books which have fantastic objects or cartoons in them because this makes the child's performance difficult to understand.

If possible we do like to have bigger toys such as a dolls' house in the examining-room. It is quite useful to have it hidden away, so that it is something which can be brought forward to interest and stimulate a child.

Examination at six to eight months

HISTORY

Ask the mother if the baby is sitting; whether he can pick things up and transfer objects; whether he sees well; whether he hears well; what noises he is making. McCormick (1986) has a simple question sheet for parents (Table 3.1) which has proved valuable in helping identify babies with hearing problems.

It may be necessary to prompt in order to get a history of a consonantal sound ('g' and 'd') but one should try to obtain the information without suggesting it. Ask how he is feeding; solids will usually have been introduced by this age and the mother will tell how easy this has been. Ask if he is chewing small lumps. One can review his weight with the parents. Ask about what illnesses the child has had since the six-week examination. It is more than likely he has had colds by this age and it is useful to discuss how ill he was and if the mother feels at ease handling these mild infections or whether she worries that the cough with the cold represents more serious illness (of course he may have had a significant illness).

In terms of behaviour we talk about how the child is eating and how he is sleeping. We also ask how he is socially relating to his family and others around him. One would anticipate hearing at this age that, if he had been a colicky baby, this symptom of early evening restlessness had disappeared. We ask if he is generally happy or whether he cries a lot.

As we have indicated under hearing, we prefer to examine children as near six months as possible, but at the moment there is a vogue (based we believe on an inadequate understanding of hearing responses) for recommending eight months as the age at which children should be examined. We indicate here some of the tests which would be used during the six-, seven- and eight-month period.

GROSS MOTOR FUNCTION

Sit the child on a flat surface and observe him. Many children will sit at this age; some may need some minimum support. Sitting on the mother's lap will provide this minimum support and the child ought to be able to hold the head up well and use his hands freely.

Observe the baby standing with support on the mother's lap. The baby can fully extend both hip and knee but will often prefer to

Table 3.1 McCormick's parental questionnaire (with permission from Dr Barry McCormick).

Here is a checklist of some of the general signs you can look for in your baby's first year:

Yes/No

Shortly after birth
Your baby should be startled by a sudden loud noise such as a hand clap or a door slamming and should blink or open his eyes widely to such sounds

By 1 month
Your baby should be beginning to notice sudden prolonged sounds like the noise of a vacuum cleaner and he should pause and listen to them when they begin

By 4 months
He should quieten or smile to the sound of your voice even when he cannot see you. He may also turn his head or eyes toward you if you come up from behind and speak to him from the side

By 6 months
He should turn immediately to your voice across the room or to very quiet noises made on each side if he is not too occupied with other things

By 9 months
He should listen attentively to familiar everyday sounds and search for very quiet sounds made out of sight. He should also show pleasure in babbling loudly and tunefully

By 12 months
He should show some response to his own name and to other familiar words. He may also respond when you say 'no' and 'bye-bye' even when he cannot see any accompanying gesture

maintain some flexion at hip and knee. He will take his weight on his legs but cannot balance yet.

FINE MOTOR FUNCTION

Observe the child reach out and pick up an object. A one-inch cube is fine for the purpose — he should be able to transfer the object to the other hand, often via the mouth. At six months the baby may well fail his first attempt to reach a brick on a flat surface, knocking it off, but he should succeed in getting hold of something eventually. Quite often he drops things. Towards eight months he will be able to scoop up a pellet in his palm.

VISION

Visual acuity cannot very easily be tested at this age (see p. 74). However, one can usefully watch the child look at objects both near and far. The eye movements should be followed in all directions, particularly upward gaze, to see that eyes move well together and there is no suggestion of a squint. Reaching for a pellet demonstrates useful visual functioning. Shine a light at the eyes and check the light reflex, which should be central in both pupils and also observe pupillary contraction and some convergence of the eyes as an object is moved towards them.

HEARING

Hearing should be most carefully tested at six months. It is best to have an observer present who can watch the infant's head turning and visual attention towards sound. It is also helpful to work in a sound-damped room. If one is not in such ideal circumstances, watch how the child does respond to interrupting noises but don't assume because he turns to a noisy vehicle outside that his hearing is normal. Babies will quite quickly ignore ambient noises such as noisy central heating but will attend to novel sounds. One has to adjust oneself to ambient noise level and be careful not to increase the stimulus level because of the ambient noise. A sound-level meter is useful to check ambient noise levels and stimulus levels. The chief danger in testing at any age is that a movement the examiner makes attracts the child's attention visually and is misinterpreted as a hearing response. The examiner must therefore be behind the child, and ensure that his sound-making objects are 18 to 24 inches from the ear and that he doesn't move them in front of the line 90° to the ear, which effectively makes it certain that he is behind the line of the child's vision. Beware of mirrors and shadows. Ask the mother to gently occlude the ear that is not being tested by placing a finger over the ear lobe and external orifice. (Some babies may not tolerate this very well; one often has to proceed to testing without occlusion.) Observe the baby turn to the human voice and specifically make a pure 's', a high-pitched sound and a low-pitched 'oo'. We like to see a good response to at least four other sounds. Quietly shake bells and lightly scrape a spoon around the inside of a cup. A high-pitched rattle (either the Nuffield or the Manchester) and a rattle or other sound-making objects in a more general frequency can be shaken more accurately some 10 inches from the ear to deliver a really quiet sound around 10–20 decibels. 'Stir' rather than shake the rattle. It might be desirable to use a low-pitched sound-making object but in practice, as high-pitch hearing loss is far commoner than a loss in the low pitches only, one tends to concentrate on the high-pitched sounds with pure tone sounds. We use the spoken-voice tests to quantify the very rare hearing loss in the low frequencies.

At six months the baby will usually still pause (that is stop making any movements he is making) and then turn towards the side that the sound is coming from. In our view this rather measured response makes the baby easier to test at this age than at seven or eight months when he will turn more rapidly without stilling, and if one is alone it is sometimes more difficult to be certain, when observing from behind, that the head turn is in response to sound and not random activity. This is where a second adult is extremely helpful.

SPEECH AND LANGUAGE

At this age one can try to stimulate a child to make noises by smiling and babbling at him oneself, but vocalizations may not be heard when the baby is in the clinic room, so one may be very dependent on the history. Hopefully one will hear (a) vocalizations and (b) the use of one or two consonantal sounds like a 'g' or a 'd'.

EMOTIONAL AND SOCIAL ASPECTS

Observe the baby's friendly response to the examiner. Observe the way the mother comforts the child if he becomes distressed (e.g. following an injection).

PHYSICAL EXAMINATION

The child should be physically examined including auscultation of the heart, palpation of the abdomen and examination of the testes. Height and weight are reviewed. Until he is standing and walking the hips should be examined. Look in the mouth and review the child's dentition. The age at which teeth erupt is very variable but many children have acquired their first tooth round about this age (p. 64).

Examination at one year

Many people do not carry out a developmental examination at this age, but wait until 18 months or two years to do a second one following the six- to eight-month examination. However, a clinician must be able to carry out a developmental examination of a child at any age.

HISTORY

Ask the mother if the child can sit freely, crawl or move about in some other way, stand and cruise or walk. Ask again about vision and hearing.

Ask whether he is picking up objects, such as small sweets or raisins; whether she thinks he sees and hears; how he responds to close relations and to strangers; if he is happy or if he cries a lot; how he sleeps and how he is fed. Make specific enquiries about the vocalization he is producing now, whether he has the naming words and whether he is producing long streams of sentence-like structures with many different consonantal sounds coming into play. Usually he should be imitating sounds at this age. Ask if he plays imitative games such as waving bye-bye or pat-a-cake.

As before, make enquiries about any illnesses the child has had, particularly checking on whether he has had ear infections, and also question now at this and subsequent ages whether he has had any significant accident.

EXAMINATION

Gross motor function

Usually the child will walk (cruise) round a small table if he is not walking alone. One may observe him crawling or bottom shuffling.

Fine motor function

Observe him pick up a small pellet of paper with both right and left hand. He should have a pincer grip. Watch him manipulating bricks and try and get him to carry out some imitative tasks like banging them together.

Hearing

This is more difficult at this age than it is at six months, but one can only test by distraction again. Use a similar technique to the six-month examination. The child will watch to see what the examiner is doing, so great care must be taken that he is not looking when the examiner shakes or uses a sound-making toy. Secondly he will quickly become uninterested in the noise and his non-response may simply represent a lack of interest (Fig. 3.12).

Vision

Look at the eyes moving in all directions. Check for squint by observing the light reflex.

Speech and language

This is entirely dependent on the child making some noises and some one-year-olds will be inhibited and not say anything during their clinic visit. Note if you hear sounds or not. If sounds, noises or words are heard, these can be recorded.

Social and emotional responses

Observe the way the child behaves when he comes into the room with his parents. Very often there may be some mild distress at first and he will insist on sitting on his mother's knee. Hopefully he will be quite quickly interested in a toy placed on the low table beside him and reach out and point to it. As soon as possible move him on to the floor from his mother and observe how easy or difficult it is for the examiner to come into contact with the child and play with him. Watch the way he responds to his siblings if they are in the room.

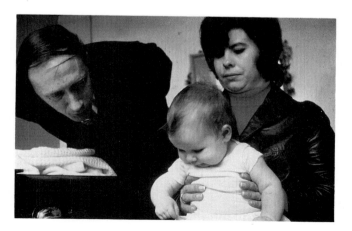

Fig. 3.12 The child is looking at his toes so takes no notice of the sound the examiner is making.

Examination at 18 months

In many health districts an assessment of the child is not carried out at 18 months. It is an important age in terms of gross motor function and any child who is not walking by this age needs a fuller examination. Also there should now be good evidence of speech and language having begun to develop and it is important to obtain evidence of this. There is often a problem that at 18 months one may not oneself hear a great deal of language from the child but depend upon history.

Ask similar questions to those asked at one year. For a child who is not walking explore the early forms of motor development in more detail and ask if there is a family history of bottom shuffling. Enquire about fine motor skills — one should hear that the child not only explores objects with his fingers but is now using them meaningfully, driving cars around and picking up small toys and playing with them. This leads into a discussion on speech and language development. Ask how many words the child is saying with meaning and then explore what words he understands. Will he point, for example, at his shoes, will he go and get his nappy? Some children will have been taught to point at their hair, nose and mouth already by this age. However, one is exploring what the child's own language understanding and output are, not trying to check that he uses a particular word because children and their parents will use different words.

EXAMINATION

Gross and fine motor examination

As at one year, the examiner watches the child walk and would expect him now to be able to run. For the late walkers a fuller examination and a neurological examination will be necessary and a decision will be taken as to whether the child should be referred; this should be done unless there is a strong family history of late walking associated with bottom shuffling. The 18-month-old will build a tower if one demonstrates it with three or four bricks. Again watch particularly the quality of the movement. He will be using his forefinger to gesture and point at things.

Vision and hearing

These are tested as described under the one-year-old examination.

Speech and language

Ask the mother which words the child does say, and if for example he is reported to say 'car-car', show him a car. If he says 'shoes' does he point to or look at his shoes. Does the examiner actually hear him say words? He may look at pictures at this age and some children will say words when they see pictures in books, but he may be inhibited in the presence of the examiner and it is often a good idea to get the mother to show him things. Conversing with her, the child may produce the appropriate words. Provide him with some toys and see what he does with them. Does he drive the car, pick up the doll and look at it the right way up? Then begin to make suggestions such as 'would he like to feed the teddy bear?' A hairbrush is a useful object. Ask him if he will brush the dolly's hair. Quite often a child will make a slightly inappropriate response such as brushing his own hair rather than teddy's but he displays that he has some understanding of what you are saying to him.

Summarized research data from the Coram study

Six months

MOTOR DEVELOPMENT

Sitting on a flat surface for 30 seconds — 70% achieved this.
97% of children were observed reaching for objects.

HEARING RESPONSES OBSERVED

	Yes		No	
Hearing	*n*	%	*n*	%
HP* rattle L	295	89	35	11
HP rattle R	299	91	31	9
LP rattle L	303	91	30	9
LP rattle R	306	92	27	8
Voice 'ss' L	302	92	29	8
Voice 'ss' R	303	92	28	8
Voice 'oo' L	300	92	28	8
Voice 'oo' R	297	91	31	9
Bell/cup L	300	92	26	8
Bell/cup R	303	94	21	6

* High pitched 'Nuttfield' rattle.

The table indicates that a positive response was obtained from 90% of the sample and it was felt that these were normal. Responses to different sounds are shown in the table. Most of the hearing loss was conductive. There was one child in the study who had a sensory neural loss but the loss was not identified at six months.

BEHAVIOUR PROBLEMS

Just 1% of children were reported as crying or miserable most days but a further 7% were reported as being sometimes miserable and crying two or three days a week.

SUMMARY OF DEVELOPMENTAL FINDINGS

	Normal		Possibly abnormal		Definitely abnormal		
	n	%	n	%	n	%	n
Gross motor	328	98.5	5	1.5	—	—	333
Fine motor	323	97	11	3	—	—	334
Vision	323	96	13.4	4	—	—	336
Hearing	295	87.5	40	12.5	—	—	335
Vocalization	322	96	13	4	—	—	335

One year

Some of the motor responses at one year are given above right. The categories are not necessarily mutually exclusive. A child can bottom shuffle and crawl.

MOTOR RESPONSES (total $n = 267$)

	Yes		No	
	n	%	*n*	%
Gross motor				
Sits alone	275	99.5	1	0.5
Crawls	254	94	16	6
Bottom shuffles	30	12	221	88
Stands holding on	259	98	9	2
Cruises	244	91	23	9
Walks alone	126	46	149	54
Fine motor				
Finger-tip approach	268	98	6	2
Picks up fine objects	269	99	2	1
Matches cubes	250	94	17	6
Imitates	242	93	19	7

OVERALL DEVELOPMENT

	Normal		Possibly abnormal		Definitely abnormal		
	n	%	*n*	%	*n*	%	*n*
Gross motor	266	97	9	3	—	—	275
Fine motor	265	98	6	2	—	—	270
Vision	266	97.5	6	2.5	—	—	272
Hearing	269	97.5	7	2.5	—	—	276
Vocalization	265	98	6	2	—	—	271

BEHAVIOUR

Only three children were reported as being miserable at one year most days, that is, 1% of the sample. More than 20%, however, were waking most nights.

	Camden ($n = 188$)		Westminster ($n = 89$)	
	n	%	*n*	%
Crying				
Usually happy	180	96	83	93
Sometimes miserable or cries				
two or three days	5	3	6	7
Settle to sleep				
Easy	153	82	75	84
Sometimes difficult	10	5	5	6
Difficult most nights	25	13	9	10
Night waking				
Hardly ever	130	69	71	80
2 to 3 nights a week	13	7	4	4
Most nights	44	24	14	16
Appetite				
Good	175	93	76	85
Sometimes poor	11	6	6	7
Always poor	3	2	7	8
Food fads				
Not faddy	168	89	74	85
Few fads	15	8	9	10
Very faddy	5	2	6	7
Not on solids	1	0.5	0	0
Problem to parents				
No problem	172	91	83	93
Problem	17	9	6	7
Doctor's assessment				
Mild problem	8	4	3	3
Moderate	3	2	2	2
Severe	0	—	0	—

Eighteen months

MOTOR DEVELOPMENT

98% of children were walking by this age.
40% could build a tower of four bricks or more.
96% had *meaningful* manipulation.
92% had stopped casting.

SPEECH AND LANGUAGE

89% carried out a simple command.
72% pointed at objects or pictures such as a doll or a cup.
37% said no words at all.
31% said 1–5 words.
20% said 6–10 words.
12% said more than 10 words.

OVERALL DEVELOPMENT

	Normal		Possibly abnormal		Definitely abnormal		
	%	*n*	%	*n*	%	*n*	*n*
Gross motor	245	98	2	1	—	—	249
Fine motor	239	95	9	4	3	1	251
Vision	243	97	4	2	3	1	250
Hearing	244	97	7	3	—	—	251
Speech — prelanguage skills	218	87	27	11	4	2	249
Vocalization	203	82	39	16	5	2	247

BEHAVIOUR

	Camden (*n* = 170)		Westminster (*n* = 81)	
	n	%	*n*	%
Crying				
Usually happy	162	95	75	94
Sometimes miserable or cries				
two or three days	7	4	3	4
Settle to sleep				
Easy	138	81	73	91
Sometimes difficult	11	7	2	3
Difficult most nights	21	12	5	6
Night waking				
Hardly ever	113	67	70	86
2 to 3 nights a week	20	12	3	4
Most nights	35	21	8	10
Appetite				
Good	140	82	64	79
Sometimes poor	22	13	10	12
Always poor	8	5	7	9
Food fads				
Not faddy	147	87	65	80
Few fads	21	12	9	11
Very faddy	2	1	7	9
Not on solids	—	—	—	—
Problem to parents				
No problem	160	94	76	94
Problem	10	6	5	6
Doctor's assessment				
Mild problem	4	2	6	8
Moderate	4	2	1	1
Severe	0	—	0	—

References

Bax, M., Hart, H. & Jenkins, S. (1981) Clinical testing of visual function of the young child. *Developmental Medicine and Child Neurology*, **23**, 92−5.

Bryant, M.B., Davies, J.D. & Newcombe, R.G. (1979) Standardisation of the Denver Developmental Screening Test for Cardiff Children. *Developmental Medicine and Child Neurology*, **21**, 353−64.

Capute, A.J., Shapiro, B.K., Palmer, F.B. & Ross Wachtell, R.C. (1989) *Normal Gross Motor Development, Growth, Sex and Socio-economic Status. Developmental Medicine and Child Neurology*, **27**, 636−44.

Gardner Medwin, D. (1979) Controversies about Duchenne Muscular Dystrophy. (1) Neonatal screening. *Developmental Medicine and Child Neurology*, **21**, 390−2.

Hall, S.M., Pugh, A.G. & Hall, B.M.B. (1982) Vision screening in the under fives. *British Medical Journal*, **285**, 1096−8.

Hardie, J. de Z. & MacFarlane, A. (1980) *Health Visitor*, **53**, 466.

Hindley, C., Filliozata Clackenberg, G., Nicolet-Meister, D. & Sand, E. (1966) Differences in age of walking in 5 European longitudinal samples, *Human Biology*, **38**, 364−79.

McCormick, B. (1986) Screening for hearing impairment in first year of life. *Health Visitor and Community Nurse*, **22**, 199−203.

Muir, D. & Clifton, K.C. (1985) Infants orientation to the location of sound sources. In: *Measurement of Audition and Vision in the First Year of Life* (ed. Gottlieb, G. & Krusnegar, N.A.). Ablex Publishing Company, New Jersey.

Peiper, A. (1963) *Cerebral Function in Infancy and Childhood*. Consultants Bureau Enterprises Inc., New York.

Teller, D.Y., McDonald, M.A., Preston, K., Sebris, S. & Dobson, Y. (1986) Assessment of visual acuity in infants and children − the acuity card procedure. *Developmental Medicine and Child Neurology*, **28**, 779−89.

Robson, P. (1970) Shuffling, hitching, scooting or sliding − some observations in 30 otherwise normal children. *Developmental Medicine and Child Neurology*, **12**, 608−17.

Robson, P. (1984) Prewalking locomotor movements and their use in predicting standing and walking. *Child Care, Health and Development*, **10**, 317−30.

Sheridan, M.D. (1979) The clinical assessment of visual competence in infants and young children. In *Visual Handicap in Children* (ed. Smith, V. & Kean, P.). SIMP, London.

Yule, W. & Rutter, M. (1987) *Language Development and Disorders*. Blackwell Scientific Publications, Oxford.

4   From 18 Months Onwards

I N THIS CHAPTER we review the child's development from the age of 18 months to five years — from the so-called toddler age to the preschool period. All but a small percentage of children are walking and running by the age of 18 months. They have also just begun to speak, but over the next two years these communication skills are going to develop extensively. It is also the period during which the child, from having social relationships largely restricted within the family, develops relationships outside the family and particularly with his own peer group. Other developmental milestones are the achievement of continence, the ability to feed himself and the ability to dress himself (providing he is not asked to tie shoe-laces and do up cuff buttons). His ability to solve problems and learn increases tremendously so that by the age of five or six he is able to cope with formal instruction and is thus ready to go to school. This involves not only the ability to learn, but the ability to concentrate and to sustain himself socially for periods of the day without the support of his parents. Development throughout these periods will be discussed and suggested examination schedules at various ages given at the end of the chapter.

Gross motor development

Gross motor development is easy to observe but by no means the most important of the developmental functions. As mentioned in Chapter 2, only 2 or 3% of children are not walking by the age of 18 months. For this small minority the reason for their failure to walk at this age has to be sought and diagnostic possibilities are discussed further in Chapter 7. However, it is worth noting here that most non-walkers of this age are normal.

Sutherland *et al.* (1988) has recently provided us with detailed studies from his gait laboratory of the development of walking in the young child from the early stages onwards. What is remarkable about these studies is how rapidly most children walk in an adult way, that is, rhythmical movements of the leg accompanied by alternating swinging arm movements. Paces should be even within two or three months of starting to walk and there should be good heel strike after the swing through from stance phase (Figs 4.1 and 4.2). Note that the arch of the forefoot does not develop until four or five years and the foot is relatively flat at earlier ages (see the orthopaedic section, Chapter 7).

The child at two, therefore, who can walk and run has better motor abilities than most older physically handicapped children and these abilities alone are all that are needed for adult motor activity. However, improvement in gross motor skills can be observed throughout early childhood. It has already been mentioned that climbing stairs is not a good developmental test since it is dependent on the height of the child and the height of the stairs. Children walk upstairs alternate foot at a time before they walk down with alternate feet. This pattern of one step at a time walking downstairs will persist in older children who are ataxic. The next milestone is the ability of the child to stand on one foot. Three-year-olds can stand on one foot momentarily but

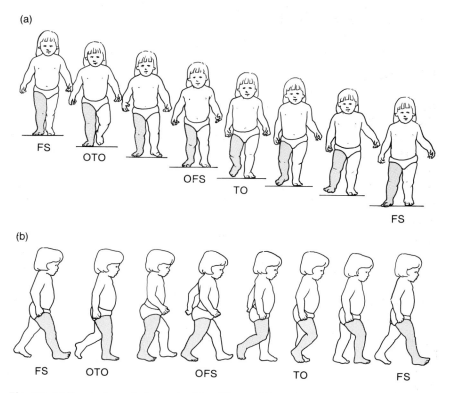

Fig. 4.1 (a) Front view of 18-month-old toddler walking. (b) Lateral view. While there are differences from the mature adult gait — notice for example that the foot strikes the ground rather flatly — nevertheless these gait cycles indicate how good the child's walking pattern is at this age.

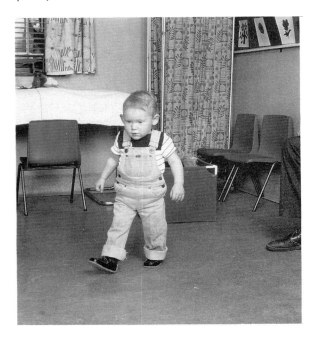

Fig. 4.2 Normal walking at 18 months.

cannot sustain this for more than four or five seconds. Until they can hold this posture, kicking is difficult and fathers who are anxious to get their children started off on football find it a frustrating task with a two-year-old. On the other hand circular movements of the legs on a small tricycle, often with pedals driving a front wheel, can be managed readily by a two-and-a-half-year-old, although the bigger-geared tricycle is not easily ridden until four or five. Hopping is something which is not usually achieved until four and a half or five. Girls in general hop a little earlier than boys, and our data on this at four and a half are given. At four and a half most children can begin to carry out heel−toe walk along a line on the floor but quite a number still can't do this (backwards heel−toe walk is not achieved until seven). Touwen (1979) lists a number of other tasks, such as toe-and-heel walking (achieved from three onwards), which one can use at appropriate ages.

Catching and throwing a ball is an achievement which develops around three. Throwing is obviously easier than catching. The three-year-old will stand with hands held out and only hold on to the ball if it drops into them. He is unable to watch the ball and move his hands. He either looks at his hands or at the ball. Over the next couple of years he begins to be able to move his hands to the appropriate position without visual control. Another motor development at this age is the disappearances of associated movements (sometimes called mirror-movements). These are movements in another part of the body unrelated to parts involved in the specific task being undertaken. An easy way to demonstrate their presence is to ask the child to alternately supinate and pronate the wrist (diadochokinesia). Children under three will find this task very difficult; over that age they may be able to carry it out, but there will be both homolateral and contralateral associated movements. The importance of this development is that stability of other parts of the body allows better control over fine movements.

Fine motor movements

Pincer grasp as previously described develops from 9 to 10 months onwards and the child can make discrete hand movements from this age, but his ability to carry out intricate tasks is limited because he lacks experience. Round about 18 months most children will make their first attempts with a crayon, a pencil or a piece of chalk; the writing implement is first picked up and held in the fist with the point protruding beyond the little finger and stabbing or circular movements are made at the blackboard or on to paper. Very quickly, however, the child realizes that this is not a good way to control the tip and he begins to develop 'tripod' grip. First the pencil is held protruding beyond the fingers with the whole hand clasping it, and the pencil running up inside the palm. Later it is realized that it is more effective to have the pencil protruding between the forefinger and thumb, although initially it is held high up, until he finally modifies his grip to hold the pencil between the thumb and the second and third fingers. This is known as the tripod grip (Figs 4.3, 4.4 and 4.5).

A small number of normal adults hold a pencil a different way (from casual counts in classrooms, we estimate about one in twenty). A common variant is to allow the pencil to protrude between the index and middle finger; it has been said that this is a position favoured by artists as it allows one to draw a steadier line (but we have no idea whether this is true!). There is considerable variation in the age at which the tripod grasp is developed and there is no question that practice with pens and pencils and indeed paint-brushes plays a part in the age at which this is achieved. In studies comparing children from a deprived part of inner London and from the Isle of Wight, we found striking differences in the number of children who had a clumsy grip at the age of five. In the deprived area nearly 10% of children's

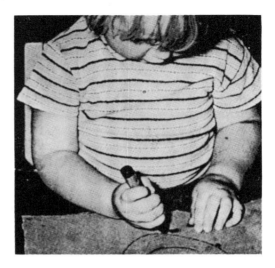

Fig. 4.3 This is the earliest grasp of young children when the crayon is held supinate (Rosenbloom & Morton, 1971).

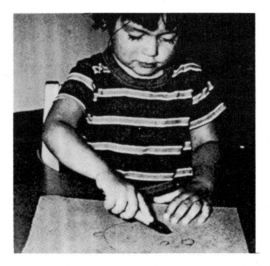

Fig. 4.4 An immature grip often seen around the age of two-and-a-half years (Rosenbloom & Morton, 1971).

grip was rated as clumsy. In general we would regard a fisted or high clumsy grip at this age as abnormal, but with three-year-olds we would accept any grip except a fisted grip as normal.

Banging clumsily with a hammer can start from 14 or 15 months onwards but twisting movements, such as undoing jars or using even

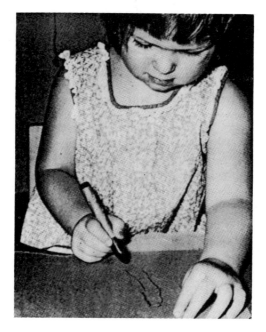

Fig. 4.5 The mature tripod grip (Rosenbloom & Morton, 1971).

a large screwdriver, are much later and we don't expect the child to be able to demonstrate these skills until after the age of three.

The smaller bricks (standard Lego) are too difficult for most two-year-olds to manipulate effectively and they should be reserved until the child is over the age of three. The standard wooden one-inch bricks are manipulated effectively at two when most children will build a six-brick tower. However, in observing the activity a smooth, non-jerky performance and effective eye–hand co-ordination are more important than the number of bricks in the tower. In all fine motor tasks practice certainly makes a difference for the age at which the skills develop, as we have indicated with the development of pencil grip. In trying to decide whether a child is clumsy or not it is important to check with the parents what sort of experience of play and drawing materials the child has had. In studying movements we found just over 1% of children at two, three and four and a half years who we felt had abnormal fine motor control. Our assessments correlated well with the Griffiths developmental tests carried out by a psychologist who was blind to our assessment. Most children who are simply clumsy and have no other developmental problem do well, but when clumsiness is associated with other abnormal findings the child may well have learning difficulties. Clumsy children should therefore be followed up, carefully reassessed and given appropriate early help.

Vision

As mentioned in Chapter 3 the child's visual acuity is near adult levels at 18 months but testing is difficult until about the age of two and a half. At this age the child acquires the ability to match shapes, this preceding his ability to recognize letters. It is easier for him to have a single shape held up and to match it than to match a letter within a row of letters, as in the traditional Snellen chart. Nevertheless, if you show him a single letter and he matches it this may give a rather optimistic view of the child's visual acuity and as soon as possible he should be asked to identify a letter pointed out to him in a row of five to seven letters. With younger or handicapped children naming small objects (toy, spoon, fork, chair) held up at a distance eliminates serious visual problems.

Hearing

Hearing by this age is at adult levels, but there will still be some further development in the ability to locate sound (Fig. 4.6). This is done well from side to side by six months and by nine months sounds made at 45° to the horizontal are promptly identified. It is not until five years that the child can immediately locate a sound made directly over

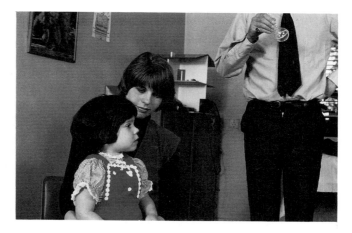

Fig. 4.6 Distraction test in two-year-old child showing instant localization at an angle of 45° from the horizontal.

his head, so clearly some fine tuning of the system is still going on. In the second year of life the child is very prone to upper respiratory tract infections, leading to ear infection or obstruction of the middle ear and some hearing loss. As children lip-read very readily the parents may not be aware of the hearing loss even when it is quite substantial. Equally, the child may not be very attentive and the parents may complain that he doesn't seem to hear; when this happens one needs to make a distinction between the child who *listens* and the child who *hears*. Hearing, of course, simply implies the conversion of sound signals to nervous impulses and their receipt at the auditory cortex, whereas listening implies attending to and understanding it, and this attention to sound is something which continues to develop during this period. A child of three who is by this time well able to talk will, when faced with a telephone, find that he cannot interpret the sounds he hears. He holds the receiver out to an adult and says it is 'talking', but fails to recognize the short remarks his father is making down the phone. The child continues to use vision to help his interpretation of spoken language and in a crowded room a three-year-old will have difficulty attending to what is said to him, until you bend down and look at him. Consequently, unless children are seated quite close to the adult, story time can be difficult; nursery teachers understand this and arrange their group very close to them.

Speech and language

From 18 months onwards the great development which is most apparent to the child's family is the ability to talk. The three elements of language have been described: semantics, the transmission system and the syntactical system or grammar. It is usual also to draw a distinction between receptive and expressive language, the receptive describing the child's ability to understand what is said to him while the expressive side involves being able to produce words with meaning. Generally the two develop alongside each other, but it is common to find children whose expressive language is somewhat behind receptive language. They will point at different objects named by the examiner but will not say the words themselves. It is hard to tell sometimes if they cannot or will not. Equally one sometimes sees children with speech they do not understand. They use abstract words like 'apparently', and one wonders if they comprehend the meaning. All children may learn rhymes whose meaning they are not certain about; for example a blind child of two who knew 'baa baa black sheep' by heart had no conception of what black or what a sheep was.

In terms of semantics, the problem of deciding how many words a child knows is extremely difficult because it is very time-consuming to obtain an adequate spontaneous output. The receptive side can be tested by asking the child to point out named objects in pictures but this again is time-consuming. However, it is usually stated that children know 50 words by 18 months, 200 by two years and 500 by five. In terms of syntax the use of two-word sentences begins sometime around two with most children, although at two only 40% of utterances are classified as sentences. The sentence must not be two words automatically joined to mean one thing, such as pick up, but a new combination of two words to give a unique meaning, e.g. daddy's car, daddy's brush, daddy's hat, etc. As time goes on the child begins to make more complex sentences. The number of words per sentence can be counted (mean length of utterance) and this simple assessment remains one of the best measures of development. There are not many words in a sentence at these early ages and three-year-olds are usually using only about five words in a sentence. Five-year-olds are beginning to manage sentences of seven words or more. Note the period between two and a half and three when 'and' is used continually to link up sentences e.g. 'daddy outside *and* daddy got a spade *and* daddy digs holes, *and* daddy got potatoes', describing the sequence observed by a child of his father planting potatoes.

In terms of syntax and construction, a child's speech is often described at this age as telegrammatic, a curious idiosyncratic structure which cannot be copied from adult speech. The existence of this 'child' language was one of the reasons which led Chomsky to suggest there must be some innate language structures within the brain which enable humans to develop language. The child between two and three years is handling all sorts of complex language tasks. A common problem which observers note is the difficulty of the personal pronoun. A child may be confused because she is both 'I' when she is talking about herself and 'you' when you are talking about her. Sometimes the child will use her proper name to avoid the ambiguity, so when she talks about herself she will say 'Sarah go upstairs' meaning 'I go upstairs'. 'I' and 'you' are usually sorted out around the age of two and a half or three. The child may use language to help organize her world. So Sarah might be overheard whispering 'You go upstairs now'. Past and present tense are a further complication which the child struggles with initially and gets right after the age of three, but misconstructions like 'I goed' are again normal.

The understanding of children's speech and language development is an enormously complex subject and the clinician may feel a bit overwhelmed as he tries to assess it. It is worth remembering that, although psycholinguists don't fully understand how we develop language, we as adults do know how to use it and we can use that subconscious knowledge to help us assess children's language. Also the clinician is looking for the grosser degrees of abnormality rather than the great range of normal development. We found in our studies that we correctly identified children clinically as slow developers when compared with a study of the same population by two psychologists who used a standardized development language test (the Reynell, see p. 125).

Around 18 months to two years, most children are beginning to speak but some will not be comprehensible to people outside the family. If the family understand him that's usually a good indication that in time the child will become comprehensible to others. There are children who have *phonological* problems; phonology describes the use of a sound in relation to a particular context, that is to say, the ability to make the appropriate sounds within a particular language. Our inability as adults to grasp the niceties of phonology of a foreign language means we speak with an accent. Sometimes a child miscodes sounds, so that he consistently gives the wrong sound for another one; he might consistently say a 't' instead of saying 'c', so he talks about a 'tup' instead of a 'cup'. Most of these simple phonological errors correct themselves with time and are normal, being called substitutions. Reversals are also common, e.g. 'goddie' for 'doggie'. Again these errors in the preschool child are common and unless the problem is severe no interference is necessary. Even over the age of four, three or four reversals or substitutions are quite common and should be accepted as normal. Table 4.1 from Ingram (1969) gives ages of consonantal acquisition and also the most commonly substituted consonants. Children who are still totally incomprehensible beyond the age of three need a fuller assessment by a speech and language therapist.

Another 'error' in the transmission system which is common around three or four is a mild degree of stuttering (or stammering — the words are synonymous). The child may get stuck on a particular letter — classically 's' — and sound it repetitively, or he may have 'blocks', i.e. he may be unable to initiate the sound at all for some seconds. Persistent stammerers often have a family history of the problem.

Social and emotional development

By 18 months the child has formed strong affectional bonds to his immediate family including his siblings. Depending how much contact

Table 4.1 Most frequently mispronounced, substituted or omitted sounds in 80 children with specific developmental speech disorders (Group 1) and 112 unselected children aged 3½ years (Group 2). (From Ingram, 1969.)

Sounds	% With defective sounds	
	Group 1	Group 2
r	78	37
sh	74	15
th (thing)	66	31
s	63	5
l	62	1
k	36	12
t (church)	34	13
d (hedge)	34	13
g	26	9
f	20	6
v	17	—
p	17	1
b	17	—

he has had with his extended family (grandparents, uncles and aunts) he will have similar attachments to these people. Usually, however, in nuclear families in the developed world attachment to the parents now has a major priority for the child. In the eighteen-month to two-and-a-half-year age-group the child may have great anxieties about separating from his parents, particularly when he is away from home. The attachment can be so strong that the toddler will barely leave his mother alone, standing outside the door of the toilet, for example, and banging until she comes out. However, providing the mother settles the child in, which under the age of three may take some time, he will go to a well-known neighbour or child-minder although quite often he will show distress when his mother leaves and also when he is picked up. Longer detachments from the parents are often the cause of disturbance and it is difficult to explain to children of this age anything about the departure of their parents. Children over three or four can tolerate and understand the necessity for parents to leave them for short periods of time. Children who are brought up in nuclear families often get a strong feeling of home and become very attached to the environment they live in. Changes of environment for some children can seem almost as disturbing as changes in the adults who are around them.

These behaviours which we see in many developed countries may differ in other societies. For example, children brought up in the

Israeli kibbutzim have quite limited contact with their parents and share a range of caretakers and there is no real indication that this different pattern of child-rearing affects the child adversely. Similarly the travelling people, although they may have the same van or caravan, move their children frequently from one geographic site to another. It is very difficult to talk about immutable patterns of behaviour because there is so much variation. One can recognize, however, that at these early ages separation from parents, such as hospitalization or putting into care, does have disturbing effects on the child's behaviour. These effects can last for six months and longer-term effects have been identified. Again, the way a child reacts will reflect his previous experience.

Single children have very different behaviour patterns from children with siblings and the older child is inevitably a single child to start with. While siblings make similar demands on parents, they are also likely to spend large amounts of time in each other's company and the three-year-old will often have good relations with a younger sibling and play with him quite happily.

Very detailed studies have now been made of the effect of the arrival of a second sibling on the previous one. The incursion of a new baby may give rise to jealousy and other difficulties. Despite the parents' efforts, the amount of time that the older child has with them is dramatically reduced by the new arrival and inevitably the older child is going to feel somewhat neglected and deserted. It is not a time therefore to introduce other changes, such as putting into day care because the new baby has arrived. Nevertheless, it is reassuring to know that the major study that has been done on this topic (Dunn & Kenrick, 1982) showed that two-thirds of children accepted the arrival of a new sibling without major disturbance.

Numerous other aspects of the child's emotional and social development can be observed during these ages. The child's temperament becomes firmly established. Is he a light-hearted, extrovert person joining in easily with new people, not shy of new situations or faces, or is he rather the opposite? The latter child is sometimes described as sensitive by parents, referring to the difficulties they have taking him out socially, but it's worth pointing out to parents that sensitivity and awareness are characteristics which many of us admire in older people. They should therefore try to recognize the strength of the child's personality and behaviour rather than compare him adversely with another. Some children are very equable, others cry but become excited and 'uproarious' just as easily, so that one can identify underlying characteristics in the child.

Activity level is another feature of the child's social and emotional responsiveness at these ages which it is important to observe. Activity may be linked very closely with attention span and distractibility. The over-active preschool child may spend much of his time running round the house. He climbs and explores and loves going outside, finding the constraints of a small flat almost unbearable. He (and it often *is* a he) may not find it easy to settle to a game of bricks or such-like for any period of time and any interruption such as somebody coming into the room will cause him to break off the game. Other children are the reverse. They are very happy to stay indoors playing with cars or dolls for seemingly hours on end, providing they know their attendant adult is near at hand. They don't seem to need all the gross activity that other children need. These different children clearly warrant different patterns of management and a flexible approach by their parents to these issues. It is important to try to see each child's behaviour not as a problem but as a spur to the adaptation that adults have to make to their children in the normal process of child-rearing.

Play

One of the activities which all children engage in is play and by watching children play insight can be gained into the development of the child. The word 'play' is used to define an enormous range of activity from board games like 'Monopoly' to blowing bubbles in a bath, and it is difficult to identify exactly what characterizes an activity as play, a problem which has concerned writers for many centuries. Play as classically defined lacks any apparent functional purpose (see, for example, Huizinga, 1974, and Tizard & Harvey, 1977). That is to say, playing with toy cars achieves apparently nothing for the child except pleasure and any purposeful nature of the activity is internal to the play itself. However, paradoxically the child clearly can acquire all sorts of skills while playing, from the ability to use a screwdriver to the ability to mix socially with other people from widely differing social and ethnic backgrounds. Play, Aristotle believed, is one of the highest of human activities and it is often highly structured. Rule systems develop which are essential to the game: 'you've ruined the game' a seven- or eight-year-old complains when an adult intervenes and 'breaks' a rule.

Play around the age of one

The word 'play' is used to describe lots of early childhood activities such as the baby lying on his back playing with his toes, which will occur at around three months, finger play with the hands at about the same age and later play with objects, which begins at about four to five months, when he begins to hit out at mobiles and slowly grasp on to things. At this age the child explores toys with both hands and mouth, and when he is a little bit older at nine or 10 months he begins to poke his fingers into things in a more purposeful way and explore them. He may do all sorts of things with objects such as repeatedly throwing them on to the floor for an adult to pick up for him and this is described as a 'game'. Other types of play in the first year of life are 'peek-aboo' and 'pat-a-cake' games.

It can be argued that none of the above activities should be described as play. They don't involve imagination, fantasy or rule systems but they link up as we have indicated with the developmental functions of the child. Some people would prefer therefore to describe play as beginning in the second year of life. Early on the child likes posting games of putting objects into letter boxes, and banging with bricks on to pegs. Then some time around 15 months symbolic play begins, using models of real objects — driving little motor cars about, feeding dolls with doll's 'food', putting dollies to bed, changing their nappies, pretending to cook. This type of play obviously involves motor skills initially but language skills are also involved. Play sequences become more and more elaborate as the child gets older. Ways of recording play have been developed; for example, Kalverboer (1977) has systematically analysed the levels of complexity of play with a car and toy garage over the age of two.

These types of play with toys go alongside other types of play, some involving equipment and some not. Playgrounds with climbing-frames and swings (not easy for young children to use) and slides can form part of the child's play. Of course, he may be happy playing by simply running round and round the dining-room table to the growing irritation of the family, explaining that 'it's only a game'. As indicated under motor development, the equipment that the child can use for this gross motor play begins, after the age of two, to involve tricycles or pedal cars, rocking-horses and other contrivances which adults provide.

Another set of materials which begins to be used with much pleasure even from under the age of one, but more positively from over that age, is sand and water, and children will spend hours happily in a sand-pit. Some of their play with this can appear to be abstract but involves the child beginning to make shapes and investing the objects he makes with some relationship to the real world.

Play over the age of two

While the types of play we have been discussing obviously continue over the age of two, a most significant change which begins soon after this age is the involvement of other people in play. Many two-year-old children will not play together, although they will play side by side, one perhaps picking up words from the monologue that the other child is chanting as he drives his car around or whatever. There are exceptions to this of course. The two-year-old will often play with siblings or indeed with a child who may have been brought up with him, but if he is introduced to a day nursery or play group at this age he may be seen watching other children rather than joining in.

At two and a half to three years, however, play begins to be enjoyed in the company of others, although the problems of sharing toys with others involve squabbles at first. However, games mimicking the adult world are very common at this age, e.g. playing 'schools' which older siblings are involved in and 'mummies and daddies'. The 'Wendy' corner and paddling pool are very popular in the nursery. The more complicated childhood games like hopscotch or skipping are not enjoyed very much by preschool children although balls begin to be used from over the age of three in a more effective way and games that involve chasing also start (Fig. 4.7).

Over the age of two 'paper and pencil' play develops. The child initially will just scribble, first a linear scribble and then often in a circular fashion, but by three he will begin to copy. At three he should copy a circle and a cross, at four he will copy a square and at five a triangle. Drawing a person is something most children will try. Paints

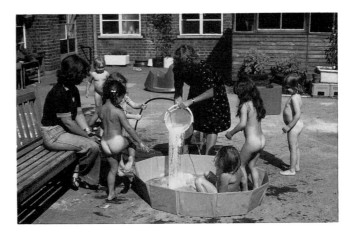

Fig. 4.7 Preschool children at play in the paddling pool.

and colours will also be used once he can handle a pencil and brush. At first the child tends to mix all the colours up by painting over those he has already applied. With judicious advice he learns to use the colours separately.

In watching play one often sees the child use many of the developmental skills one wants to assess — gross motor and fine motor function can easily be assessed in this way. Spontaneous language too can be assessed and this may often give one a better view of what the child is doing than the more formal tests we rely on in assessment situations, which are described towards the end of this chapter. Time is never wasted, therefore, when one is in a nursery because one can simply go and watch the children. It is useful to try to be somewhat methodical in making observations, in order to increase understanding of what children do at different ages when they play.

Intelligence

With children over two we can begin to ask how intelligent they are going to be and doubts as to whether a child is mentally normal may arise. Intelligence is very hard to define, but what we generally mean by intelligence is the individual's ability to solve problems and deal with the world around him in a competent manner. The intelligent person is able to handle new situations and solve 'novel' problems. Some psychologists think that insight is an essential element in intelligence and that it implies that the person is aware of the relevance of his behaviour in terms of achieving goals and its effect on other people.

There is as yet no physiological or anatomical understanding of the nature of human intelligence beyond some awareness that certain parts of the brain are concerned with different activities. Thus in most people the left side of the brain is involved in language function while the right side is involved in pattern recognition and other visual perceptual activities. Psychological theories of intelligence mostly involve recognition of the general intellectual ability (sometimes referred to as 'g') and then specific intellectual ability, although how easy it is to distinguish one from the other is a matter of debate. Specific ability is sometimes related to numerical ability, spatial ability, memory, musical ability and so on. Intelligence is shown by the child learning things in general and not just doing a test. A good example would be counting. A child may be taught to count by rote at around the age of two-and-a-half, but he does not actually count bricks very accurately until over this age. In testing intelligence and the ability to perform particular tasks, a whole range of tests is used, some of which are bound to be novel to the child.

Intelligence is obviously a developmental function and its assessment must be age-related. It is often difficult to decide if the child is simply developing slowly or whether his poor performance indicates he is always going to be slow. In general, the older the child the more accurate the prediction (not surprisingly). One tends to assess aspects of the child's functioning independently and, for example, talk about his language as being delayed but the rest of his function as being normal. However, all aspects combine to make up 'intelligence'. Thus language is an important element in the child's ability to handle a new situation, describe home life and give an account of his nursery school. These descriptions will all display elements of the child's intellectual development, as well as the language used itself.

Visual perceptual function develops early in children and relates to their later intelligence. Shape perception can be demonstrated by asking the child to do puzzles; one of the earlier ones is the letter box with different shaped holes for the shapes to be matched up with and posted. The child achieves this type of skill around the age of 13 or 14 months, often getting the objects in by trial and error. From 18 months the child will attempt to do a simple formboard, that is, a frame into which shapes have to be fitted. One of the simplest consists of a circle, a square and a triangle and this should be achieved by two. Notice that, if the child has not seen the puzzle before, he may achieve a result at first attempt by fitting the objects one by one into each of the spaces, but after two or three trials he identifies each object and puts it straight into the appropriate space in the frame. At two and a half and

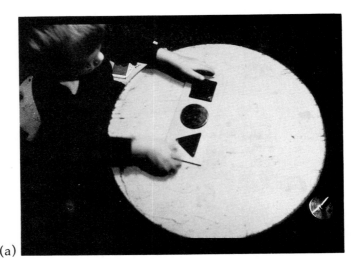

(a)

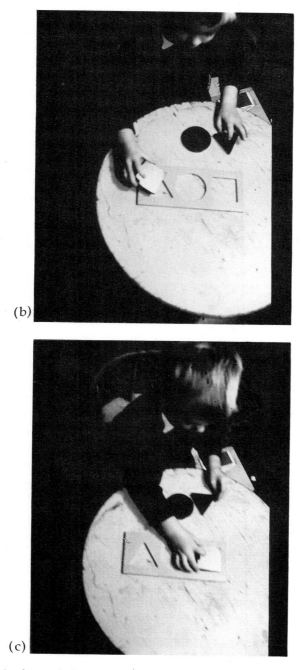

(b)

(c)

Fig. 4.8 A simple puzzle for a two-year-old. (a) When the pieces are opposite the right holes it can be done easily. (b, c) If the pieces are opposite the wrong holes he tries to put the square in the triangular hole but sees his mistake and soon gets it right (Bax & Bernal, 1974).

three more complex formboards can be used and therefore in play the child begins to be able to do simple jigsaw puzzles (Fig. 4.8). This perception of shape is very important to the child in terms of later activities such as learning to read. Perception of shape comes before the ability to produce it. Thus a three-year-old can distinguish between a cross and the letter 'x' but he will fail to copy the letter 'x', making a vertical and horizontal line to form a cross. However, if asked he can point out which is right and which is wrong.

An early stage of infant development has been described previously, that of the recognition of permanence of objects. The toddler is able to remember situations and begins to be able to think about the immediate future. He can't really think conceptually at these early ages so that he learns by experience but not by working out 'what would happen if'. He finds out how hard it is to run into a wall by running into it, each new activity adds to his reservoir of intuitive knowledge, but he is not able to generalize to rules at this stage. According to Piaget the child doesn't reach the stage of being able to think of people operationally until he is around seven.

Another aspect of development which relates closely to intelligence is moral development and the knowledge of right and wrong. Clearly the attributes of conscience, guilt and altruism are learned, but the enhancement of the child's moral sense relates very much to his intelligence. It is possibly concerned too with the developing notion of self as opposed to being simply part of a family group, which is probably occurring after the age of six or seven months. The child begins to understand 'no' when firmly uttered during the second year of life and he will often respond to moral pressure 'you can't do that' with anger and frustration. It is only as language develops between two and three that he can discuss the reason why he should be prevented from doing one thing and not another. In moulding behaviour of the child both punishment and reward are effective but reward, that is, encouraging the child to do things for positive reasons, is in the long term more effective than punishment. Punishment simply teaches him that the world is controlled by a rule system with ultimate penalty if the rules are broken, rather than by an altruistic system which allows him to develop positive ideas about things he can do.

Ways of testing the child's intellectual development

The aim of an intelligence test is to get a measure of the child's intelligence by spending a fairly brief time with him. Traditional intelligence scales in adults such as the Wechsler and the Stanford–

Binet provide a score, with most of the population falling somewhere between 80 and 130 and a standardized average round about 100. There are now many intelligence tests that go down to age three. In the UK the British Ability Scales[1] are becoming more widely used. In America the Wechsler Intelligence Scales (with their scales for young children) are probably the commonest intelligence tests used. However, these tests do not really produce a score which can be used with younger children and the two best-known tests which can be used at this age are the Bayley Developmental Scales and the Griffiths Mental Development Scale. The Griffiths Scale is probably most widely used in the UK and the Bayley in America, but both have many items in common. The Griffiths has six scales: locomotor, personal social, hearing and speech, eye—hand co-ordination, performance and practical reasoning. It can be used from one month of age right through to eight years. The scores achieved by these tests are called *developmental quotients*. Prediction from developmental quotients to adult intelligence scores are not very good. However, at the lower end of the scale children who perform badly on the test are much more likely to be slow children. The great value of such tests is that they put some sort of measure on the child's present functioning, and therefore allow assessment of change over a period of time, or after some amelioration or possibly treatment. It is very useful in following up a child who has had some procedure such as the phenylalanine-free diet for phenylketonuria to see that he is staying within the range of normal development.

Clinicians often prefer to give age equivalents for children's function and say 'he's functioning at around an 18-month or a two-year-old level' without applying a score, particularly under the age of five.

There are tests also for specific aspects of function. Particularly commonly used are tests which look at speech and language function in the preschool child separately from tests of overall development. The most commonly used language test in the UK is the Reynell test (1969) which looks at both expressive and receptive language in the young child. Many of the items in the test are similar to those used in the clinic. Some of these tests (like the Reynell) have the disadvantage that they were developed with one social/cultural group and test items may not be suitable for children from a different social/cultural background.

Another group of developmental tests used by clinicians includes the test devised by the late Dr Mary Sheridan called the Stycar test[1] and, in America, the Denver Developmental Screening Test (1969).

[1] Available from NFER, Nelson, Danville House, 2 Oxford Road East, Windsor, Berks.

Again, many of the items are very similar to those which are described later in this chapter as used during the clinical examination of the child. The Denver has the disadvantage that very often key items at certain ages can be accepted by report and it does not make a clear distinction, which we feel is important, between the history — the report of the child's performance — and the observations of the child's performance by the examining physician. We favour doctors knowing about development and making their own developmental assessment as outlined but, if they want to score, going for a more formal test such as the Griffiths, the Bayley or, in the case of a speech and language problem, the Reynell Developmental Scales. These tests take time to administer whereas a developmental assessment can be done in 10 or 15 minutes.

Examination at two, three and four-and-a-half years

Technique of the examination

While it is possible to carry out a physical examination of a child without his co-operation, it is much easier if he is not crying or disturbed. It is impossible to carry out an assessment of his functions unless some degree of co-operation is being achieved. It is therefore important to organize the consultation in such a way that the child is likely to co-operate. We have discussed this in more detail elsewhere (Bax *et al.*, 1980).

First the arrangement of the room requires some attention. Many clinical rooms are set up with a desk or a table across which the doctor sits from the parents and child. Consequently when he wants to look more closely at the child, he must stand up and is then seen as an imposing figure in a white coat striding round to assault the infant. Of course it is not only the child whose co-operation and friendship are necessary; the mother and father too should be relaxed and at ease for if they are anxious this may well communicate itself to the child (Fig. 4.9a).

The doctor should therefore sit with his desk against the wall, turning round to write on it. The parents sit facing him on the same side of the desk. The young child under the age of eighteen months would sit initially on the mother's knee and we would place small toys near him on the edge of the desk to attract his attention initially. When the child is a little older he'll be standing at his mother's knee, and we find a low table beside him is useful. Initially this can be pulled round so that it is between him and the examiner, and this may make him feel safer (Fig. 4.9b). After the age of six months the examiner

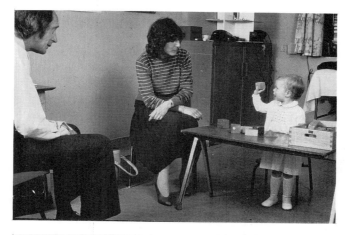

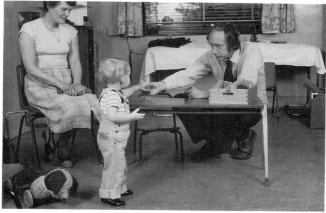

Fig. 4.9 Doctor, mother and child at the start of an assessment.

should not approach the child too rapidly, as this may distress him, and much of the developmental examination can be carried out from a distance. Those items in the examination which do not require a close approach should therefore be done first.

Some objects should be placed on the low table to attract attention, but with the older child too many should not be put out to start with, to allow observation of how he handles specific toys offered to him. Thus we usually have a box of rather nondescript blocks beside him but early in the examination, if he seems friendly, we might offer him a car or a doll which we would then ask him if he'd like to look at.

When the examiner does approach the child, he should be at child level, squatting or kneeling and not bending down. Once the child is playing at the table and perhaps looking at a book, the examiner can come up fairly close behind him and start talking to him, and then perhaps point something out to him before gently coming closer to him and actually participating in his activities. (Of course some children who are not at all shy and nervous make the examiner's life quite easy.)

In terms of equipment the Stycar boxes, apart from containing specific materials for testing hearing and vision, include a number of toys. We also have a number of toys of our own which from personal experience we have found are useful. In London the 'bus puzzle'[1] has been a very good toy but this is only suitable for children who are familiar with a London street scene. Various picture-books are helpful and many people use Ladybird Books, which are quite likely to be familiar to the child. Kitchen objects are a good stand-by with children who are not English-speaking, as are items of clothing and furniture.

It has been shown recently that the child responds less to direct questioning than to conversation. The examiner's problem is that he wishes to assess the child as rapidly as possible, and the quickest way to do this may indeed be to ask him to name specific objects. However, if the child is at all reluctant, it is much better to start talking about the material and then slip in a question almost as a conversational aside.

For the physical examination it is seldom necessary to lay the older child on a couch. Usually his abdomen and his chest are examined with him standing by his mother's knee or sitting on her lap. For the young baby, a baby table (as specified in Egan *et al.*, 1979) is extremely useful and the classic medical couch is handy too with the six-month-old, although a mat on the floor does as well and obviates the risk of the child falling off (although it would be a clumsy examiner who allowed this to happen!).

History-taking

As the child gets older it is important to know how accurate the mother's recall is about her child's health and developmental history. Parent-held records, where some of this information may have been accurately recorded, are, we believe, the best solution, but quite often earlier notes are not available. In general practice of course this information should be available but in urban areas about one-third of parents with babies under two move, so the doctor is often confronted

---

[1] Obtainable from The Test Agency Cournswood House, Northdean, High Wycombe, Bucks.

with a toddler he has not seen before. We therefore carried out some studies to see how accurate mothers' memories were of particular events in the child's life which we had recorded round about the time they had occurred. In general we found that for most developmental milestones the parents tended to record them as occurring rather earlier than they did, with one notable exception, that is, the age of the first smile. Often a mother whose baby had actually been smiling by six weeks said to us that the child didn't smile until three months. As late smiling is associated with delayed mental development, this particular piece of information is of some importance. As the child gets older parents' memories of early development may also lead one astray. Many parents of five-year-olds whom we saw in our school study reported to us that their children were talking in sentences by 18 months, although most of them were probably not doing so at that age. Parents do usually remember the birthweight of their babies accurately.

In terms of medical history parents will often remember episodes of admission to hospital but details of the child's symptoms are not so accurately recalled. This is particularly true of the neonatal period when parents are often inadequately informed of what exactly is hap-pening to their baby in the special-care baby unit. However, they will usually remember how long the child was in hospital. As the child gets older and the history of things like respiratory infections becomes more important, the doctor is again confronted with the problem of what others told the parents. We quite commonly saw mothers who told us that a doctor had said that the child had a chest infection and had given him an antibiotic, but then admitted that the doctor had not actually put a stethoscope on the chest. The rattle of clearing phlegm from the larynx and pharynx is often described as a 'chesty' cough and therefore to direct questioning — 'did he have a chest infection?' — the parents will often answer 'yes'. The doctor of course is interested in infection of the lower respiratory tract — bronchitis and pneumonia. Assessment of past ear infections is often very difficult. Earache can be obstructive in origin and the older toddler complaining of earache is not therefore a sure sign ear infection. Some doctors will give antibiotics to a mother who thinks her child has an ear infection because he seems to have a temperature and has been pulling and poking at the ear. Clearly evidence that the ear was properly examined is required to decide that there was an ear infection, and even then the examiner has difficulties deciding what a pink ear-drum means.

Physical history and examination

Essentially the history and examination are the same at two, three and four and a half years. The child's early medical history is reviewed especially for any problem in the pre- or perinatal period. Subsequent significant illnesses are noted with specific enquiry about upper respiratory tract, chest and ear infections, as these are so common. An impression is formed of how frequent these infections are, and open-ended questions are asked to identify any other illnesses the child may have had. Ask about bowel and bladder function, not only in relationship to training (see under behaviour), but also in relationship to any evidence of disease. Onset of wetting after continence has been achieved may (particularly in a little girl) indicate a urinary tract infection.

Physical examination is usually carried out at the end of the developmental assessment. Inspect the mouth and fauces and review the dentition; inspect the ear-drums and palpate the cervical lymph nodes; observe eye movements in all directions; auscultate the heart and the chest; inspect and palpate the abdomen; inspect the genitalia in both boys and girls; palpate the testes in a boy and gently part the labia majora in girls. During walking observe the position of the lower legs, looking out for any minor abnormalities of gait or bony architecture which may need further examination. Their significance will need discussing with the parents.

Developmental assessment

In assessing all functions in the young child the results of the examination are scored as 'normal', 'possibly abnormal', or 'abnormal'. Any single test used in assessing a function may be 'failed', e.g. the child may not build a tower of six bricks but the examiner decides that nevertheless fine motor function is normal. Obviously if there is no response to a high-pitched rattle hearing cannot be recorded as normal, but based on parental history and physical examination of the ear-drum the child's hearing may be considered as probably normal and therefore scored in the 'possibly abnormal' category. The child is being assessed, not the test.

Developmental history-taking at two years

Review gross motor function. Ask about walking. By two years walking should have been achieved and if it has not one needs to know why. By two the gait to a casual observer looks nearly normal. The arms now swing from the sides. If the child is not walking questions about the earlier forms of locomotion are asked: whether the child crawled, bottom shuffled or used some other method of locomotion. Look for any other obvious abnormalities in movement; ask the parents if they have noted any weakness and look for objective evidence of this.

FINE MOTOR MOVEMENTS

Ask what the child is playing with; whether he uses a spoon yet. By this age he ought to be spooning food into his mouth, although at 18 months it may still be a pretty messy procedure. Ask whether he scribbles and if he turns the pages in a book. Initially this is done two or three pages at a time, but by two years he ought to be able to turn over reasonably thick pages. Ask if the parents have felt at any time that he had a hearing problem and ask whether they have ever thought he has had any visual problems and particularly if they've noted a squint.

SPEECH AND LANGUAGE

Ask what the child is saying. By two years the child ought to have a vocabulary of 50+ words excluding naming words such as 'mum' and 'dad'. Ask both about words he says and the words he understands — does he go and get his shoes, coat, etc.; does he point at things like a teddy bear if asked to; will he carry out a simple instruction? By two one expects to hear the news that the child has begun to put words together. Distinguish between words which are genuinely being put together to create sentences, e.g. 'daddy's car', 'daddy's hat', as opposed to two words that are used as one, e.g. pick up. On average 40% of utterances at two may take the form of a sentence.

VISION AND HEARING

Ask whether the parents have any worries about the child's eyes and vision. Similarly do they feel that the child hears well.

BEHAVIOUR

Ask how he is relating to both his mother and father and any other close members of the family. Is he happy? Does he have temper tantrums? Ask whether it is a full-blown tantrum with him lying screaming and kicking on the floor or just some minor frustration which is common around this age; ask about his feeding — whether he eats adequately and whether he is faddy; ask about his sleeping: is he easy to settle? does he sleep through the night? Ask about his toileting behaviour. Sometime between eighteen months and two years many children will start being dry by day and, while it is not a particular concern if they are not at two, it may be something the parents will want to discuss with you.

Developmental examination at two years

Watch the child walk as he comes into the room. You would expect to see him pick things up and carry them about if he is walking, get up and sit down easily, bend over to pick something up from the floor and squat. All these observations of gross motor function take place normally during the course of the examination.

FINE MOTOR FUNCTION

Offer him some one-inch bricks. At 18 months he will build up three or four of them and by two he should do half a dozen. Observe the quality of the movements as he places a brick on the tower and notice that between 18 months and two the ability to use eye–hand co-ordination is improved and the placement will be more exact. Give him a pencil or a crayon and observe his scribbling. Often the crayon is held with the hand over it. Dabbing movements may be made at 18 months but around two some more coherent scribble will usually have emerged. Watch him push toy cars around and watch him when asked to feed a doll, moving the spoon appropriately and fairly accurately towards the mouth. If there is any doubt about the acquisition of a pincer grip, offer him a small object such as a Smartie to pick up between forefinger and thumb. Note also laterality, which is usually established by this age.

VISION TESTING

At two the child will cooperate with naming small objects at a distance and the Sheridan Stycar test is based on this. The child is asked to name or match a small toy which the examiner holds up. The small toys usually used are a doll's chair, a toy car, a doll, a brick, a spoon, a knife and a fork. A duplicate set of objects are placed in front of the child and he is trained to pick up the same object as the examiner shows him. Thus the examiner holds up a car and says 'show me your car'. The child may call out 'car', which makes the test quicker and easier to do. The examiner then retreats to 10 feet away from the child and shows his objects in turn. The problem with the test is that the child may not make a good distinction between a spoon and a fork at this age and consistently call both of them 'spoons', without minding which he picks up. The spoon, the fork and the knife are the smallest objects and it has been suggested that the child who fails this test has vision worse than 6/12, but we know of no good evidence to support this. Clinically, however, the test does demonstrate reasonable vision and furthermore it is a useful test for older children who are slow for one reason or another.

HEARING

By the time the child is around two it is often possible to use a spoken language test with him and get him to identify or pick up toys which are presented to him on the table. The seven-toy test involves putting out the seven familiar objects including a doll, a chair and a car and the doctor whispers the name of the object and the child picks it up. Picture materials can be used and the child can be asked to point at an array of pictures. We have used the Stycar and the Reed test material but others are available.

In our own studies of the two-year-olds we tested, just over half were able to carry out a seven-toy test for us and in the remainder we were forced to fall back on distraction testing as used with the 18-month-old child. In order to do this it is best to have the child sitting or standing at a table with something which interests him moderately and place an observer across the table from him some 10 feet away so that the child is not distracted by the observer. Then make a range of sounds to left and right and observe the child turning to the sound. The Nuffield and Manchester rattles can be used as well as other sound-making equipment. In fact, a free-field audiometer can be used which delivers a known sound level at the ear when used at an appropriate distance, but not many primary-care physicians have this available.

SPEECH AND LANGUAGE

Allow the child to play with and name some common toys. He may start talking during the course of the examination and he can then be engaged in conversation about the toy. Suggest he puts the doll to bed and ask him what he is doing. Try and engage in conversation rather than asking him specific questions. Providing the child relates it is usually possible to show him either objects or pictures and get him to name them. According to his culture he will name different objects. In London a big red bus is a good stand-by as the first object, but dogs and cats, and household objects, clothes, brushes and combs are usually seen by children every day and can readily be named. In our own studies at two years we heard 86% of the children name many objects and 68% say a two- or three-word sentence. The problem remains in deciding whether the non-responders have a problem or are simply non-cooperative at the time of the assessment.

Following the examination review the child's behaviour, i.e. did he settle easily, did he talk freely, was he very shy, etc? Relate these observations to the behavioural history.

Developmental and behavioural history at three and four-and-a-half

The history inevitably is an expansion of that described for the two-year-old. It will probably be immediately apparent that the child can walk and run about as he comes into the room but the mother can be asked about walking and running and perhaps whether the child is using a small front-wheel cycle. In terms of fine motor activity ask whether the child is scribbling and drawing. Ask if there are any concerns about vision and hearing and whether the child has any sign of squint. Ask about his communication — can he talk well in sentences, is he understood by the family and other adults? Ask about his eating and sleeping and his toilet training. Most children will be dry by day now, but in our study at age three two-thirds of children were dry at night. About 6 or 7% were still wetting during the day. At four and a half while 75% were dry every night rather more than 10% were still wetting most nights. Some 4 or 5% had occasional daytime problems. Bowel control is of more concern. We found that about 5% were still having problems at the age of three but by four and a half this had fallen to 3%.

Ask about temper tantrums — how often they occurred during the day, what time they occurred, how long they lasted and how many days a week they occurred. We found that at three years over 10% were still having temper tantrums every day and a further 5% had very frequent temper tantrums. By four and a half rates had fallen somewhat and only 2–3% of children had regular temper tantrums at this age. Particularly in the child who is presenting with behaviour problems, it is worth enquiring about his activity level and his attention span. Children who are regarded as over-active by their parents at three have a high chance of manifesting difficult behaviour later in school.

Ask how the child relates to his parents, other adults and other children. Find out if he is in any preschool nursery and how that is going. As with development the doctor should sum up in his mind the behavioural history and decide whether he thinks the child has a problem or not and also consider how far this relates to the child himself and how far it is a familial problem. In Chapter 9 we have discussed the relationship between depression in the mother and the child's behaviour and it is obviously important to review this in relation to any behaviour problems arising in a child.

Developmental examination at three

GROSS MOTOR DEVELOPMENT

Watch the child walk into the room. He should now have a relaxed gait with his arms swinging comfortably at his sides. Ask him to stand on one leg. At three nearly a third of children don't want to do this and a quarter don't succeed in doing it but 38% hold one or other leg up for a few seconds (it has been stated in the literature that they will do this for as long as 30 seconds at three). We have seen a child hop well at three but this is rare.

FINE MOTOR FUNCTION

Ask the child to build a tower and then make him copy a 'train' which the examiner makes in front of him. The train consists of five bricks laid horizontally with a funnel on the front brick. Ask the child to draw and examine his grip. By this time laterality should be established and can be scored. Ask the child to copy a vertical line, a circle and a cross. The results of fine motor testing in our study are given at the end of the chapter.

VISION TESTING

Many children will now do a letter-matching task. The Sheridan–Gardiner sets[1] include a five-letter card or a seven-letter card and the child is asked in that test to identify a letter shown him in a book at 10 feet. The letters in the book are presented singly in the centre of a white page. It has been shown recently that this task is simpler than identifying an embedded letter such as one on a row on a Snellen chart and new tests are being developed with a central letter surrounded by other letters which the child has to identify. It is possible to test the child at 20 feet in a suitably adapted room, but it is harder to hold the

[1] Obtainable from Keeler Instruments Ltd, 21–27 Marylebone Lane, London W1M 6DS.

child's attention at this distance. In the ordinary cluttered clinical room (it is often not 20 feet long) the tradition is to test the child at 10 feet and get him to identify a 6/3 letter, i.e. half the size of the 6/6 letter on the standard Snellen chart. At three it is often difficult to get the child to accept occlusion for long enough to test both eyes monocularly (there are some arguments for doing a vision screen at three and a half by which time it is easier) and obviously if the child resists occlusion it is better to get a binocular reading than nothing at all. There are a very few children who will have monocular loss of visual acuity and do not have a squint; assessment of full eye movements and looking at the light reflexes are important parts of the examination of vision. Data indicate that children's vision is still improving at three and a score of 6/9 or 6/12 monocularly in each eye does not need immediate referral but the child may be regularly observed. If the child has a family history of myopia he should be referred early. It will be found in 3–4% of children at this age.

HEARING

By three the child should co-operate with a spoken-word hearing test. There are several available, all basically using the same principle of matched words with rather similar sounds which require the child to make discriminations to identify. Either they involve showing the child pictures and asking him to indicate which is the correct picture or they involve toys. The picture tests best known are the Reed test (obtainable from the Royal National Institute for the Deaf) using a standing card containing four pictures, the child being asked to point at one whose name is whispered from 10 feet away, and the Stycar test, which has similar pictures but with a larger choice of pictures. In the Kendal toy test the child is asked to choose from a set of toys. It is best always to carry out a hearing test with an observer sitting opposite the child while the examiner speaks the word quietly from six feet away. It is always good to have a sound-level meter available so that the examiner can verify what sorts of levels of sounds he is making, and some would say this is essential.

It may be possible to get the child himself to occlude one ear but preferably the mother sits behind him and does this, although some children resist; if they do, one simply hopes that not too much sound will get round to the other ear. A common problem for the examiner is the high level of ambient noise in the room. It would be desirable always to work in properly sound-damped rooms, but these are not generally available. The examiner therefore must be very careful not to raise his voice because of the ambient noise and this is where a sound-level meter is very helpful. If a response is obtained to the quietly spoken word at appropriate levels of 20 to 30 dB, given that there is a lot of distracting noise going on, it can be accepted that the child is hearing well, but sometimes the environment is such that responses are variable and it is necessary to refer the child elsewhere. There will be a few children at three who will still fail to co-operate in any of these tests and in these instances distraction testing may be all that is possible. The same applies to a child who speaks a language with which the examiner is not familiar, although the parents may be trained to whisper the words. It is sometimes difficult to control this situation.

SPEECH AND LANGUAGE

For speech and language the child should have a conversation with the examiner and 75% of children in our studies did this. We specifically asked them to name a number of objects or pictures and to point at the arms, nose and mouth and other objects if necessary. The pictures chosen are the common objects like cars, kitchen utensils and toys. Avoid odd animals and always check with the parents that the child is familiar with the object. Delay in speech and language development is the commonest problem at this age and we recorded something like 7% as having a definite abnormality. Of those in our group that didn't talk with us, some 10% were considered socially inhibited and perhaps shy but, on further assessment by a health visitor visiting the home, we were reassured that their language was normal.

Developmental examination at four-and-a-half to five

At this age the child in the UK is just about to enter or has entered school and a rather more extensive examination should be undertaken. We have reported on the results of our infant examination and there is no question that a competently carried out neurodevelopmental examination at this age can identify children who are likely to have immediate difficulties and so they should be discussed with their teachers. They also have a likelihood of going on having difficulties throughout their school years (Bax & Whitmore, 1987).

GROSS MOTOR FUNCTION

Apart from watching the child walk as previously described, we can get the child to hop and heel—toe walk. From the results of our examinations it seems that at four and a half when the examination was performed, many children failed to hop. By five the figures are slightly different and we give those that we obtained in our school study (Bax & Whitmore, 1987).

FINE MOTOR FUNCTION

Ask the child to draw a circle, square and triangle. Carry out a finger—nose test and ask the child to pat repetitively with one hand on another. We report our results of these tests in the table on p. 145. If there are grounds for concern about the child, there are various ways of extending the testing, including looking for associated movements. The easiest way to do this is to ask the child to carry out the familiar medical test of pronation and supination of the wrist (diadochokinesia) and watch the extent of associated movements on the other side.

VISION AND HEARING TESTING

The principles of vision and hearing testing are the same at four and a half as they are at three, but the testing is very much easier and one should manage to occlude the eyes so that monocular testing is carried out. Many children will identify letters on a modified Snellen chart, which is better than using the simple letters in the Sheridan—Gardiner books.

It should be possible to occlude the ear and therefore to be certain that each ear is tested separately. At school entry all children should be tested with pure-tone audiometry (this may be carried out by a technician but is now more often done by a nurse). The audiometer delivers a pure tone at selected frequencies and sound intensities to each ear separately. Some children find the ear muffs frightening and others seem to lose concentration and do not signal a response to the quieter sounds. Clinical review of a child who has failed the pure-tone test is mandatory.

SPEECH AND LANGUAGE

By this age the child should have a large vocabulary and be able to speak in sentences. We used pictures or toys to get the child to name a number of objects and while we did this we listened to certain consonantal sounds. Commonly late-acquired or substituted consonants include 'r', 'sh', 'th', 'l' and 'k' and it is useful to listen for these. If the child has more than three substitutions or omissions it is likely that his comprehensibility will be reduced and referral for assessment of his speech development is appropriate. In terms of language where the child does not initiate sentences we use pictures from the Renfrew Developmental Language Test to initiate sentences. The pictures in this set require the child to say more than a single word. One picture, for example, shows a child who has fallen downstairs and his glasses have fallen off and broken, another picture shows a child climbing a ladder to the roof of the house where there is a cat, and a third shows a girl picking up a little boy to post a letter. Mostly children will talk to the doctor without material but it is handy to have something to use systematically which will elicit a sentence.

SOME PERCEPTUAL TESTING

Drawing the circle, square and triangle gives some idea of the child's ability to copy and understand shapes at this stage. Another set of tests, which have been standardized, are the Berges—Lezine tests of imitation of gestures (Berges & Lezine, 1965). The child is simply asked to copy the gestures the examiner makes. These are easy to carry out with children and again give some information about children who are having difficulties. The norms at three and four and a half for the items we used are given on pp. 142—5.

Behavioural assessment at three and four-and-a-half

As on every occasion it is important to think about the way the child is responding to the examiner, but given the time available there is not very good evidence on a short visit that a complete assessment of a child's social and emotional problems can be obtained. Obviously if there are parental concern and reports of temper tantrums and aggressive, difficult or withdrawn behaviour one is going to observe how the child responds to an unfamiliar adult. Occasionally extremely shy or withdrawn behaviour may be noted in the 15 or 20 minutes spent with the child doing an assessment but most children who are shy and frightened at the start of school (they may not have been to a nursery school) resolve their shyness over the first few months and it is not a significant finding. In general therefore if there is evidence of a behaviour problem it will be necessary to spend longer with the child and observe him or her in a variety of different settings.

Research findings at two years

Gross motor function

By the age of two in our sample all our children, except one who had a severe chromosome anomaly, were walking, although in larger samples normal children may not yet be walking. We noted in 6% of the children that we didn't observe running — some of them because they were too shy to move away from their mothers, but some whose gait was possibly slightly slower to develop.

Fine motor function

71% of children built a tower of six bricks or more by this age. Less successful builders may have been less co-operative rather than less effective with their hand movements. This finding emphasizes the need to make a judgement about the child's hand function (see summary of development, p. 403).

Hearing and response to hearing tests

Note that in rather more than half the sample we felt it was possible to do a seven-toy test, although in a proportion we scored them as refusing having embarked on it. In 132 children the test was not carried out. In a proportion we did distraction tests as well before deciding whether the child would carry out the seven-toy test. Results are set out below:

Hearing

Hearing	Pass		Fail		Refused	Not
	n	%	*n*	%	*n*	*n*
7-toy test	147	98	3	2	16	132
Stycar at 3 feet						
HF rattle L	158	96	6	4	13	124
HF rattle R	157	96	6	4	13	125
LF rattle L	151	98	3	2	14	128
LF rattle R	151	98	3	2	14	128
Voice 'ss' L	158	99	2	1	11	129
Voice 'ss' R	159	99	1	1	11	129
Voice 'ooo' L	152	99	1	1	14	131
Voice 'ooo' R	151	99	1	1	14	132
Bell or cup L	145	98	3	2	17	133
Bell or cup R	165	98	3	2	18	114

Localizes 45° L	165	98	3	2	18	114
Localizes 45° R	165	98	3	2	18	114

Hearing	Yes		No	
	n	%	n	%
Responds to instructions	267	97	23	3

Speech and language

	Yes		No		Refused
	n	%	n	%	n
Names many objects	234	86	45	16	15
Two- or three-word phrases heard	186	68	87	32	19

Behaviour (total $n = 303$)

		n	%
Appetite	Good	213	68
	Sometimes poor	68	12.5
	Always poor	32	12.5
Food fads	Not faddy	231	74.5
	Few fads	33	14.4
	Very faddy	29	11
Settling to sleep	Easy	247	82
	Difficult 2 or 3 nights a week	20	6
	Difficult most nights	36	12.5
Night waking	Hardly ever	244	81
	2 or 3 nights a week	18	6.5
	4 or more nights a week	41	12.5
Management	Easy to manage	203	68
	Sometimes difficult	81	27
	Frequently very difficult	14	5
Dependency	Independent	189	64
	Sometimes demands a lot of attention	79	26.5
	Demands too much attention	29	9.5

		n	%
Temper tantrums	Hardly ever	148	49
	1–4 per week	93	31
	Nearly every day	38	13
	3 or more a day	18	7
Daytime wetting	Never/hardly ever	134	43
	1 or 2 days a week	21	7
	Most days	24	9
	In nappies	123	41
Night wetting	Never/hardly ever	71	23
	1 or 2 nights a week	9	3
	Most nights	4	1
	In nappies	218	73
Soiling	Hardly ever	163	53
	1 or 2 times a week	17	5.5
	Most days	11	4.5
	In nappies	108	37
Problem to mother	No problem	269	88.5
	Problem	34	11.5
Problem to doctor	None	268	89
	Mild	23	8
	Moderate	9	3
	Severe	0	0

Summary of abnormal findings

	Normal		Possibly abnormal		Definitely abnormal		Total
	n	%	*n*	%	*n*	%	*n*
Gross motor	289	98	4	1.4	2	0.7	295
Fine motor	277	94	14	5	4	1.4	295
Vision	293	99	—	—	3	1	296
Hearing	285	97	7	2	2	1	295
Speech	234	79	50	17	14	5	298

Summary of research at three years

Fine motor tasks

Tower building

Bricks	0	1–4	5	6	7	8–	9–	10+
Nos of children	5	15	10	20	23	57	29	151
%	1.5	4.3	3.0	6.0	6.9	17.2	8.8	45.6

Copies train	Yes	No		Refused
Nos of children	225	52		41
%	68.4	15.8		12.5
Pencil grip	Normal	Awkward	Fisted	Refused
Nos of children	225	86	16	10
%	65.3	26.4	4.9	3.1
Laterality	Left	Right		Ambidextrous
Nos of children	50	249		−21
%	15.2	75.9		6.4

Copying	Yes	No	Refused
Vertical line	270 (82%)	27 (8.2%)	29 (8.8%)
Circle	220 (67%)	84 (25%)	26 (7.9%)
Cross	118 (35.8%)	178 (53.9%)	29 (8.8%)

Standing on one leg — 29% of children would not do this, 25% tried and failed, 38% succeeded

Behaviour (total $n = 331$)

		n	%
Appetite	Good	223	66.5
	Sometimes poor	56	15.5
	Always poor	52	18
Food fads	Not faddy	231	70.5
	Few fads	60	16.5
	Very faddy	40	13
Settling to sleep	Easy	270	82
	Difficult 2 or 3 nights a week	25	6.5
	Difficult most nights	26	11.5
Night waking	Hardly ever	270	82
	2 or 3 nights a week	25	6.5
	4 or more nights a week	26	11.5
Management	Easy to manage	209	64
	Sometimes difficult	92	28
	Frequently very difficult	16	8
Dependency	Independent	216	66.5
	Sometimes demands a lot of attention	83	25.5
	Demands too much attention	28	8

		n	%
Temper tantrums	Hardly ever	178	55
	1–4 per week	92	27.5
	Nearly every day	44	5.5
	3 or more a day	18	7
Daytime wetting	Never/hardly ever	284	85.5
	1 or 2 days a week	15	7.5
	Most days	17	6.0
	In nappies	5	1
Night wetting	Never/hardly ever	204	62.5
	1 or 2 nights a week	28	8
	Most nights	26	7.5
	In nappies	73	22
Soiling	Hardly ever	308	93.5
	1 or 2 times a week	10	3
	Most days	14	3
	In nappies	9	2
Problem to mother	No problem	279	86.5
	Problem	48	13.5
Problem to doctor	None	272	84
	Mild	41	12.5
	Moderate	13	3
	Severe	1	0.5

Summary of abnormal findings

	Normal		Possibly abnormal		Definitely abnormal		Total
	n	%	n	%	n	%	n
Gross motor	324	99.4	2	0.6	—	—	326
Fine motor	296	90	28	8.5	4	1.2	328
Vision	291	82.4	29	8.8	9	2.7	329
Hearing	299	91.2	22	6.7	7	2.1	326
Speech	268	81	39	11.8	23	6.9	330

Research findings at four-and-a-half years

Gross and fine motor testing

	Steady		Unsteady		Cannot		Refused
	n	%	n	%	n	%	n
Heel—toe walk	99	42.5	102	44	32	14	32
Hops L	133	55	66	27	42	17	29
Hops R	136	56	77	32	28	12	29

FINE MOTOR

	Right		Left		Both		Refused
	n	%	n	%	n	%	n
Hand preference	235	86	30	11	8	3	2

	Normal		Awkward		Fisted		Refused
	n	%	n	%	n	%	n
Grip	247	83	26	9	3	1	—

	Yes		No		Refused
	n	%	n	%	n
Draws circle	263	97	9	3	3
Draws square	168	63	99	37	6
Draws triangle	86	32.5	179	67.5	7

HAND PAT

L pat R				R pat L				
Regular		Irregular		Regular		Irregular		Refused
n	%	n	%	n	%	n	%	n
236	94	15	6	241	97	8	3	19
12 in 5 sec		12 in 5 sec		12 in 5 sec		127 in 5 sec		Refused
n	%	n	%	n	%	n	%	n
233	94	16	6	237	96	11	4	19

DIADOCHOKINESIS

	Can n	Can %	Irregular n	Irregular %	Cannot n	Cannot %	Refused n
L	179	80	41	18	3	1	31
R	173	78	43	19.5	5	2	31
L & R	164	76	50	23	3	1	34

ASSOCIATED MOVEMENTS

	Nil n	Nil %	Left n	Left %	Right n	Right %	Both n	Both %
L	53	24	56	25.5	46	21	65	29.5
R	71	32	30	14	56	25	64	29
Both	91	42.5	4	2	5	2	114	53

BERGES — LEZINE

	Pass n	Pass %	Fail n	Fail %	Refused n
5	258	98	6	2	10
6	254	96	10	4	10
7	159	61	102	39	13
8	134	52	124	48	14

FINGER — NOSE TEST

Steady n	Steady %	Unsteady n	Unsteady %	Refused n
245	98	6	2	19

Behaviour (total $n = 278$)

		n	%
Appetite	Good	180	67
	Sometimes poor	78	21
	Always poor	26	12
Food fads	Not faddy	185	68.5
	Few fads	65	22
	Very faddy	25	9.5
Settling to sleep	Easy	230	85
	Difficult 2 or 3 nights a week	22	7.5
	Difficult most nights	22	7.5
Night waking	Hardly ever	229	85
	2 or 3 nights a week	16	5
	4 or more nights a week	27	10
Management	Easy to manage	188	68
	Sometimes difficult	69	25.5
	Frequently very difficult	18	6.5
Dependency	Independent	216	66
	Sometimes demands a lot of attention	65	28
	Demands too much attention	16	6
Temper tantrums	Hardly ever	184	67.5
	1–4 per week	60	21.5
	Nearly every day	24	8
	3 or more a day	6	3
Daytime wetting	Never/hardly ever	261	93
	1 or 2 days a week	10	3
	Most days	4	2
	In nappies	10	2
Night wetting	Never/hardly ever	213	76.5
	1 or 2 nights a week	26	9.5
	Most nights	26	9.5
	In nappies	8	4.5
Soiling	Hardly ever	268	96.5
	1 or 2 times a week	3	1.5
	Most days	2	1
	In nappies	2	1
Problem to mother	No problem	265	89
	Problem	35	11
Problem to doctor	None	241	89.5
	Mild	21	6.5
	Moderate	10	3.5
	Severe	2	0.5

Summary of abnormal findings

	Normal		Possibly abnormal		Definitely abnormal		
	n	%	n	%	n	%	n
Gross motor	265	96	9	3	1	0.5	275
Fine motor	256	93	14	5	4	1.5	274
Vision	251	91	12	4	12	4	275
Hearing	256	93	10	4	8	3	274
Speech	238	88	1	7	1	5	270

References

Bax, M. & Bernal, J. (1974) *Your Child's First Five Years*. Heinemann, London.

Bax, M. & Whitmore, K. (1987) The medical examination of children on entry to school. The results and use of developmental assessment. *Developmental Medicine and Child Neurology*, **29**, 40−55.

Bax, M., Hart, H. & Jenkins, S. (1980) Assessment of speech and language development in the young child. *Pediatrics*, **66**, 350−4.

Berges, J. & Lezine, I. (1965) *The Imitation of Gestures*, trans. Parmelee, A.H. Spastics Society Medical Education and Information Unit in association with William Heinemann (Medical) Books Ltd, London.

Dunn, J. & Kendrick, C. (1982) *Siblings: Love, Envy and Understanding*. Grant McIntyre, London.

Egan, D.F., Illingworth R.S. & Mac Keith, R.C. (1979) *Developmental Screening 0−5 Years*. Spastic International Medical Publications: William Heinemann, London.

Huizinga, N. (1974) *Homo Ludens*, trans. Howe, R.F.C. Routledge & Kegan Paul, London.

Ingram, T.T.S. (1969) Developmental disorders in speech. In: *Handbook of Clinical Neurology*, Vol. 4, *Disorders of Speech, Perception and Symbolic Behaviour* (eds Vinken, P.J. & Bruyn, G.W.), p. 430. Wiley, New York.

Kalverboer, A.F. (1977) Measurement of play: clinical applications. In *Biology of Play* (eds Tizard, B. & Harvey, D.). Mac Keith Press: Blackwell Scientific Publications, Oxford.

Rosenbloom, L. & Morton, M.E. (1971) The maturation of fine prehension in young children. *Developmental Medicine and Child Neurology*, **13**, 3−8.

Sheridan, M.D. & Gardiner, P.D. (1970) Sheridan−Gardiner Test for visual acuity. *British Medical Journal*, **2**, 108−9.

Sutherland, D.H., Olshen, R.A., Biden, E.N. & Wyatt, M.P. (1988) *The development of mature walking*. Clinics in Developmental Medicine 104/105, Mac Keith Press: Blackwell Scientific Publications, Oxford.

Tizard, B. & Harvey, D. (eds) (1977) *Biology of Play*. Mac Keith Press.

Touwem, B.C.L. (1979) *Examination of the Child with Minor Neurological Dysfunction*. Spastics International Medical Publications: William Heinemann, London.

5   Social and Environmental Factors

THERE ARE many factors in the material and social environment of the child which have the potential to affect, in some cases profoundly, that child's health and welfare. A child can never be viewed in isolation from his family and environment; in this chapter we consider available evidence on some of the important social and environmental factors and how they relate to child health and development.

Because of the relatively small size of the sample followed in the Coram study, it was not possible to look in any detail at such background variables as family demography and social class effects; hence the data discussed in this chapter are taken from other available research evidence.

Since early this century statements have been made, and studies have confirmed, that poverty, overcrowding and associated disadvantages are prejudicial to health, particularly in childhood. This remains all too true in 1988. Recent reports continue to show the inverse relationship between social class and perinatal and neonatal mortality rates and later childhood morbidity and mortality rates. A similar pattern emerges whether social position is measured by occupational class, by employment status, or by assets such as house ownership (Fig. 5.1). Although with increasing standards of living the mortality rates overall have fallen over the years it is depressing that the gradient in fetal and neonatal mortality rates with respect to social class remains as steep as ever. There has, however, been a reduction of the social class gradient in respect to postneonatal death-rates.

Social class, of course, is based on the Registrar-General's classification of men's occupations, and we are still waiting for a satisfactory classification based on women's occupations. This could well be more relevant when it comes to correlating social class data with aspects of childhood morbidity or mortality. The proportion of all births included in the Registrar-General's analysis by social class has been steadily declining over recent years because of a steady increase in proportion of births to single mothers; hence some workers prefer to use women's educational experience in place of social class.

The term 'social class' while relating specifically to occupation en-

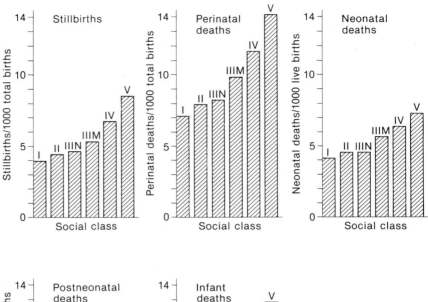

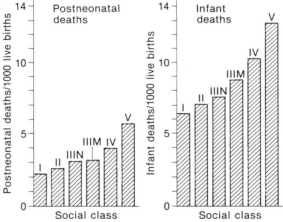

Fig. 5.1 Outcome of pregnancy by social class of father, England and Wales, 1984. Stillbirths: fetal deaths after 28 completed weeks of gestation. Perinatal deaths: stillbirths and deaths in the first week of life. Neonatal deaths: deaths in the first 28 days of life. Postneonatal deaths: deaths at ages over 28 days and under one year. Infant deaths: deaths at all ages under one year. (Source: *OPCS Mortality Statistics, Perinatal and Infant*, 1984.)

compasses many other aspects of living and reflects income, education, housing and environment as well as more subtle areas such as access to services. While it is a useful concept in that it groups together segments of the population sharing broadly similar types and levels of resources, with broadly similar styles of living, it also conceals enormous individual variations. So it is a useful concept when looking at trends in populations or large samples of children, but not such a useful concept in understanding any one family's functioning.

When grappling with historical data on populations it may help to remember that shifts in classification of occupation have been made by the various registrar-generals since Stevenson's initial classification in 1911. For instance in 1960 aircraft pilots and navigators were changed from social class III to II, whereas postmen went from III to IV and lorry drivers' mates from IV to V! Details of perinatal and neonatal mortality in relation to social class were recently reviewed in the Short report (1984), and another important and informative report, *Inequalities in Health* (the Black report), was published in 1980. More recently a report from the Health Education Authority confirms that social class differences in mortality and morbidity persist, and there is depressingly no evidence of the gap narrowing (Whitehead, 1987). The data are convincing, and the recommendations of the Black report were far-reaching. The government, however, having commissioned the report, did not feel able to support the recommendations, and there is no commitment to pursue any of the report's proposals. The Black and Short report data show that rates of stillbirth, perinatal death, neonatal death and postneonatal death are still considerably higher among babies born to manual workers than among babies of professional workers, and these class differences persist in the mortality statistics for older children. A male child of an unskilled worker is four times as likely to die before his first birthday as the son of a professional worker; he is 10 times more likely to die before he is 14 from an accident involving fire, a fall or drowning, and 7 times more likely to be killed in a road accident.

Morbidity statistics too reflect a social class bias, and are available from a number of cohort and population studies. Low birthweight (and its association with poorer neurodevelopmental outcome) is more prevalent in lower social classes; higher rates of chronic illness, respiratory infections, accidents and hearing loss have also been found associated with low social class. Social class differences have not, however, been found in most studies of children with behaviour problems.

Child development is also correlated with socioeconomic status, and data from various longitudinal studies of pre- and perinatal complications have yet to produce a single variable predictive of outcome more potent than the socioeconomic and familial characteristics of the child's environment (Neligan *et al.*, 1976; Siegel, 1982). While certain clusters of adverse perinatal events may be associated with severe handicap (without a class bias), when total outcome of a population is considered then perinatal events alone are thought to have an almost negligible effect on later development and educational achievement (Caputo *et al.*, 1981). This has, however, recently been questioned; a large follow-up study of children born in Dundee found low social class to be associated with mental retardation, global delay, speech delay and behaviour disorder, but not with cerebral palsy or motor disorder (Taylor *et al.*, 1985). However, pregnancy pathology was also found by these authors to be powerfully correlated with neurodevelopmental outcome even after controlling for social class. The children in this study were identified as having neurodevelopmental disability at the age of three, and it will be interesting to see whether social class or pregnancy events are more strongly correlated with their later educational outcome.

In understanding the nature of the associations discussed above, we need to look more closely at the resources available to families, particularly economic resources, and at how these resources are available within families. It is also necessary to look at the health care that families receive, the quality and accessibility of health services, and how they are used. It may then be possible to understand how some of the social and economic deprivations associated with social class have an adverse effect on child health.

In this chapter we shall be discussing the environment in which the child lives, the family circumstances in which children are raised and the various ways these can affect children's health and development.

Research in the field of child development has until relatively recently focused on the 'normal' child, who is often assumed to be white and living with two natural parents. Only in the last decade or so have researchers moved away from this model, and it is quite clear that many children do not fit the above description. It is becoming increasingly difficult (and increasingly undesirable) to define what is meant by a 'normal' family — more and more children are living either in single-parent families or stepfamilies or extended families; some move in and out of different family situations during their childhood years; in some cultures children are raised by multiple mothers. Should we then be labelling families and looking for differences, or should we rather be looking at the strengths and positive assets of different family situations?

The strengths of the stable nuclear family are many, and there are advantages for children in this situation. Child-rearing is very much easier where there are two parents to share the tasks, to support each other emotionally as well as in material provision for the family, and to give the child not only love and affection but two positive role models of parenting.

A family environment that provides this sort of security and stability during childhood is undoubtedly beneficial, provided the parents themselves have a good relationship. A rich network of extended family used very often to exist, with two sets of concerned grandparents and very often aunts and uncles, with the possibility within this network of important and close relationships for the child. In many cultures this kinship network still exists — but in the UK the role of the extended family has considerably diminished in recent years due to increasing mobility of the labour force and the need for young parents to move away from areas where they were themselves brought up. For some this is advantageous; for others and particularly the women, it can mean they are quite isolated from any social and supportive network during the early years when they are bringing up their children. Grandparents are still very important both as confidants and as substitute caretakers. For many children the stable nuclear family is not a reality and in this chapter we look at some of the other situations in which children are brought up and consider how these and other environmental factors can affect child development.

As in so much research, the focus has often been on the deficits and problems encountered in different situations and hence much of the evidence in this chapter reports on negative findings. However, it should be stressed that, for the majority of children, from whatever family type, affection and warmth and security are given generously, and for both child and parents the preschool years and beyond are a source of much joy, excitement and fulfilment. The pleasures and delights in the world of childhood with its unfolding of individual personality and skills are shared by all families, whatever their composition.

One-parent families

Bringing up young children brings many joys, but is also hard work in any family. The stresses on both parent and child are increased in single-parent families, and many single parents are critical of the health workers they encounter, feeling that their particular difficulties are often not sufficiently appreciated.

One-parent families are formed in a number of different ways — through single motherhood, divorce, separation or death of a partner. Obviously circumstances will vary accordingly, and for some families it is a transitional stage before finding another partner.

The number of one-parent families in the UK has been steadily rising in the past few years with the number of children in one-parent families rising by 62% between 1971 and 1981, from 1 to 1.6 million. Around one in eight families with children is now a one-parent family; 88% of these families are headed by women and 12% by men.

A large number of single parents and their children live for long periods of time at or near the poverty line, and over 60% depend wholly or partly on supplementary benefit. The 1983 Family Expenditure Survey revealed that one-parent families were the one social group whose average income had fallen in real terms over the previous few years. This clearly has implications for health. Similarly these families are more likely than two-parent families to have housing difficulties — they are more likely to live in run-down inner city areas, to occupy poor-quality housing, to share accommodation with relatives or friends, and to become homeless. Half of all the families housed under the 1977 Housing (Homeless Persons) Act are from single-parent families, and they are increasingly being placed in quite unsuitable bed-and-breakfast accommodation in hotels with severe health consequences for both mothers and children.

Becoming a one-parent family involves a time of emotional stress, even if it means relief from a difficult or damaging relationship. Practical and legal difficulties can make the situation worse, and after the initial crisis there are likely to be long periods of isolation and depression. Having sole responsibility for the care of children and having to make all decisions alone is for many parents a chronic stress, and the incidence of maternal depression among single mothers is high (Osborn *et al.*, 1984). The majority of lone parents would rather work than live on state benefits, but for many this is not possible due to the lack or high cost of suitable day-care provision for their children. There are, of course, great individual differences between 'one-parent family' situations, with some single parents being quite well supported by their extended family or friends, and others being almost totally unsupported.

The chronic stress and practical problems experienced by parents in this situation are reflected in the statistics for children in care, where it is estimated that over half the total children in care are from one-parent families.

Our society remains centred around the two-parent family, and the majority of the recommendations of the Finer report in 1974 (on the needs of one-parent families) remain unimplemented. It is clearly less easy for the needs of the child to be met in this situation, whether for love and security, a safe home, a nutritious diet, adequate warm clothing or a stimulating environment where children can reach full potential.

The Child Health and Education Study (CHES) reporting on a cohort follow-up at age five found increased rates of behaviour problems and lower abilities on test scores among children of single parents compared with those from two-parent families (Osborn *et al.*, 1984). The authors consider that this can be seen as a consequence of the poorer socioeconomic circumstances of these families compared with 'intact' families, but also conclude that 'the loss of a parent reduced the opportunity for adult−child contact with detrimental consequences for the child's general ability and vocabulary'.

Health workers will often be involved. They need to be sensitive to the pressures on single parents, and understand the increased vulnerability of their children and the health needs of both parent and child. A knowledge of rights and benefits and local self-help groups (for example, Gingerbread) is also essential, and may be what a family most needs; ongoing support by a sympathetic health visitor can also be a lifeline. Information packs, 'Caring for health', are available from the National Council for One-Parent Families.

Divorce

Divorce or separation has become reasonably commonplace in our society with dramatic increases in the past 20 years, yet insufficient attention has been paid to the effects on the children involved and the majority of families do not receive help from any health professional.

The effects of a disrupted parental relationship on a child are in fact serious and often long-lasting, and have been graphically described by Wallerstein & Kelly (1980), who conducted a longitudinal study in California on the effects of divorce on children and their parents. Further studies in the UK have been undertaken by Richards, who reviewed the topic recently (Richards, 1984).

The reactions of children vary with their age, their individual personality, their relationships with their parents before the disruption, and their previous life experiences. Whatever the age of the child, the time of parental separation is usually the most stressful period of their life, with ongoing consequences for years rather than months.

Apart from the emotional turmoil surrounding separation, many practical changes are likely to occur in the child's day-to-day life, which frequently add to the child's sense of insecurity. Perhaps the most striking of these is the economic change; the majority of families are worse off financially following a divorce or separation, and in many cases this necessitates the mother going out to work if she is not already doing so, or changing from a part-time to a full-time job. This often means changes in child care for the children involved, and for younger children maybe their first experience of full-time nursery or child-minding arrangements. So at a time when children most need their mother's presence and support, she is least likely to be available to them. Worries about money may preoccupy the parent and legal wrangling over maintenance may occur; even quite young children detect these anxieties, and discussions frequently go on in the presence of the children. As Wallerstein & Kelly (1980) state, 'certainly one of the most pressing dilemmas for the single parent is the difficulty in balancing financial and psychological needs of parent and child in the wake of the separation'.

It is common for families to move within a few months of separation, either to be further away from their spouse or to less expensive housing. This may mean a change of neighbourhood, change of school for the child and possible loss of friends, and the period preceding the move (which may take months) engenders much anxiety and a sense of insecurity. Although for some parents there may be a profound sense of relief at the divorce, the more likely reactions are anger and bitterness; depression is also a common reaction and is thought to occur in about one-third of both men and women following separation. For the children, however, relief at their parent's separation is rare (probably less than 10%) and is only likely to occur in older children and where there has been a long violent relationship between the parents. The majority of children are intensely distressed and may react with anger or sadness, but perhaps the overwhelming feeling is of fear and insecurity. It is after all logical to a child that, if a father and mother's relationship can dissolve, so too could a parent–child relationship; hence the fear, not always expressed, of 'who will take care of me?' Fear of abandonment, of coming home to an empty house, or being placed in a foster home, are common among preschool and primary school-age children.

Because parents at this time are so bound up in their own sadness and anxieties they may not be aware of their children's distress, or if aware may not have the emotional reserves to give their children what they need. The children's needs in any case are hard to meet, since their overwhelming wish is for reconciliation, and for both parents to be back at home together living harmoniously and caring for the children. Children have a limited capacity to identify with their parents' need and wish to escape from an unhappy marriage, and although there is now a commonly held belief that it is better for children to experience a broken home than to stay within an unhappy marriage there is very limited evidence for this. While it is certainly true for the parents, for the children involved both situations are stressful, and unless there is overt violence children tend to be more secure and happy within a stable partnership or marriage.

Following a separation, in the Californian study (Wallerstein & Kelly, 1980) over one-third of children felt that their mother (who was in nearly all cases the caretaker of the children) was entirely unaware of their distress. Correspondingly, within a few months of the separation around a third of the mothers were less available to their children physically as well as emotionally, as they both increased their hours of work and became occupied with new social relationships.

Children show their distress at this time in a number of ways, and this relates to their age and developmental level. Anger is manifested as temper tantrums in the younger children, or outbursts of aggression directed towards siblings or other children at playgroup; overall the children generally become much more difficult to manage. Older children's anger may be more verbal, often with intense hostility towards the custodial parent, who is blamed for the loss of the other parent. Fear and anxiety are usually manifested in younger children by an increase in clinginess, reluctance to be left at nursery or other people's houses, and often difficulties with separation at bedtime, and an increase in night-waking and nightmares. Psychosomatic symptoms are also common. Previously acquired developmental skills are sometimes lost and the child again wets the bed or rediscovers the discarded security blanket or bottle. Vivid fantasies of reconciliation are common and may be acted out in play or talked of openly with trusted adults. It is the younger children who may feel in some way responsible for the parental separation, although in recent studies this was not found to be a common anxiety. The demonstration of intense emotional need has also been described, with apparently random hunger for affection and physical contact (for instance with a nursery schoolteacher). These effects are all maximal in the early period following the separation, and may have resolved by a year or so later. However, outbursts of anger may occur for years, and certainly the resulting insecurity can persist for a very long time.

How the child copes with this distress both immediately and in the long term is largely dependent on how the parents behave, and there are certainly mitigating factors. For some children, parental separation may mean losing all contact with one parent, and Richards found this to be true of half the families he studied. Clearly this represents an enormous loss to the child which can never be adequately compensated for. On the other hand some non-custodial parents develop a closer and warmer relationship with their child than they had prior to the separation.

Where parents continue to direct anger and hostilities to each other, and particularly where the children are encouraged to take part in these, the outlook for the child's emotional future is more bleak than when both parents behave responsibly, avoiding voicing the criticism they may feel and being sensitive to the needs and feelings of the child. Parents should be encouraged to communicate directly with each other, and avoid using the child as message-bearer.

A warm ongoing relationship with both separated parents appears to be in the best interest of the child, although the legal process does not always encourage this. Certainly both children and their parents need a lot of support and opportunity to talk about their feelings both during the crisis and for some time afterwards, and an understanding of the children's needs and fears is important for all professionals who may become involved. General practitioners and health visitors are very likely to see these families at crisis point and afterwards, and are in an ideal position to offer ongoing support and counselling.

Stepfamilies

For the majority of young children their mother's remarriage and the creation of a stepfamily is a positive step, bringing a greater sense of security, which is welcomed.

Making a new relationship with a stepfather or mother is easier for younger children than for older, who are more likely to be resentful and cool or outright angry at the new man in their mother's life. There is always a period of observation and weighing up, with initial with-holding of affection, but providing the child is reassured that this new adult is not being presented as a substitute for their absent parent then a warm and loving relationship is very likely to develop, and is gratifying to both adult and child.

The emotional development of the child within a stepfamily will to a considerable extent be determined by that child's previous experience and how the initial disruption of the family was handled. Children who are likely to be unsettled within the reconstituted family are those who are asked to renounce their love and loyalty to the absent parent, and where hostilities and criticisms continue to abound. Many parents are considerably happier when they remarry, and, provided they are not bound up in their new relationship to the neglect of the child's needs, this is clearly beneficial to the child. Other factors may be in-fluential, as remarriage often involves additional readjustments such as moving house and neighbourhood, changing schools, and coping with a step-parent who perhaps has different values and culture and ways of child-rearing from the absent parent. Often too there will be stepsiblings — a bonus for many children, but for others a source of anxiety and a resulting feeling of needing to compete for parental attention and affection. Where the stepsiblings are older, many demands may be made on the mother, and maternal depression was found to be a greater risk in stepfamilies where there are two or more older children. The Child Health and Development Study found that on some tests of ability at five years children in stepfamilies did less well than children in both 'natural' two-parent families and one-parent families, but the main differences were in the children's behaviour (Osborn *et al.*, 1984). The mean scores for antisocial behaviour were significantly higher for children in stepfamilies than for children with both natural parents, and this was felt to represent the prolonged effects of the previous disruption of the family.

The most successful outcomes in terms of the children's emotional well-being are where the child continues to have a close and respected relationship with the non-custodial parent, as well as a positive and enriching relationship with the new step-parent within the reconstituted family.

Adoption

The practice of adoption is deeply rooted in history, and is known to have been practised in ancient Greece and Rome, as well as in many more primitive cultures. The original purpose of adoption was for the continuation of the family line, particularly in cultures where a male heir or successor was considered essential; adoption was also a common method of acquiring additional labour. The needs and rights of the parent were then paramount, and it is really only in the past century that there has been some control of adoption practices, with concern being focused on the best interests of the child.

In the UK the proportion of children who are adopted is around 1%; in the USA it is nearer 2%, possibly due to the higher incidence of 'trans-country' adoption of, for instance, Vietnamese children.

Although there are fewer children available for adoption than previously due to easier access both to effective contraception and to legal abortion, children who might otherwise have spent their lives in children's homes are increasingly being offered for adoption as it is now recognized that this offers the best chance of a secure and affectionate home. These children include those who are in care, and have special needs, including many severely handicapped children who are increasingly being found homes despite being 'hard to place'.

Complex psychological adjustments have to be made by adoptive parents, and also by children if they are beyond infancy. Pre-adoptive counselling is essential, and this should ideally be an ongoing process, as for many parents there continue to be difficulties as their adopted child grows up. They are faced with trying to accept the child as their own, yet having to tell the child he is adopted, and increasingly encouraging the child to know of (and possibly later to meet) his natural parents. Adoptive parents are mainly highly committed and concerned individuals and the majority of adopted children do very well, making a normal adjustment to family life.

Clearly the age of the child is relevant, and it is easier for all concerned to make bonds with a baby than an older child, particularly one who has had several caretakers and is likely to be suspicious and insecure and acting out. However, with careful selection and support the outcome can be very successful even for older children (Tizard, 1977). The most successful adoptions are, however, the early ones and unnecessary delays are to be avoided. The incidence of behaviour problems in adopted children is somewhat higher than in the general population, particularly in boys, and this is likely to reflect their different life experiences rather than their biological background. It is a further reason for ongoing support and counselling being available to adoptive parents. It is also worth noting that rates of behaviour problems amongst adopted children are considerably lower than for children in one-parent families or in residential care.

Paediatric examination of the child and careful appraisal of the family medical and social background is an essential prerequisite to adoption, and most social services or private agencies have specialist advisers in this field. It is clearly essential that the implications of any medical problem are adequately explained to the prospective parents, who must have a realistic understanding of how these might affect the child's future health and development.

The medical aspects of adoption, including a discussion of psychiatric assessment of adoptive parents can be found in Wolkind (1979). The needs of the child are those of any child in a 'natural' family; in addition he needs to be told truthfully of his adoption from the earliest age, by his parents not others, and with an ongoing discussion about the facts, which will need to be retold and reinterpreted according to the child's age and maturation.

The father's role

For the past two decades fathers have been encouraged to be present at the birth of their child, and it is now fairly unusual for a father not to participate in some way at the birth. The feelings fathers describe at this time, of elation, relief and pride, are much the same as those of mothers. Most fathers comment that they feel closer to their baby as a result of this experience; they are also likely to be more supportive of their partner than if they had not shared the initial experience of birth. The increasing role of fathers in caring for their young children is partly a reflection of the women's movement and partly reflecting a social movement in which men feel free to demonstrate the emotional and caring aspects of their natures, without being deemed 'unmanly', something which was far less easy for the previous generation.

So there is now the possibility of sharing the caretaking aspects of bringing up a family, although in reality the majority of child-rearing tasks are still being carried out by women.

Professionals have perhaps been rather slow to recognize the importance of the father's role in the development and health of the young child, and often it is only in the context of the child with special needs that the father's role is fully recognized. It is now accepted good practice that both parents be seen together when a paediatrician has to break the news of perhaps a major congenital abnormality in a baby, but it is relatively less common for both parents to attend out-patients with their unwell child, or for both parents to be invited to a developmental check-up. The reasoning has always been that the fathers are at work — and clearly this may be true — but perhaps we have not given sufficient thought to the importance of their involvement with their children. By not acknowledging this we unconsciously undermine their role.

The research on father–infant interaction (mainly from the States) has shown that fathers are sensitive to the cues of their infants and that complex relationships often develop soon after birth. When studying the social interactions between fathers and infants from two weeks to six months of age, Yogman (1984) found that fathers were as sensitive and communicative as mothers with their infants, responding to cues and skilfully adapting to their infant's behavioural rhythms. Other studies have shown that by eight months infants in normal home environments are attached to both their mother and father, and prefer either parent to a stranger (Lamb, 1977). It has also been shown that an infant can develop a secure attachment with the father even if there is an insecure attachment with the mother. Research has found that in nearly a third of cases the young child's main attachment is to her father, and fathers may well be the child's preferred person.

Although the great majority of fathers spend less time with young children than their mothers, that time is more likely to be spent playing rather than on other caretaking tasks (such as feeding or changing nappies). Father-play is generally much more physical than mother-play, with much vigorous stimulation and games involving rough-and-tumble, throwing and catching, swinging, tickling and so on. Most of these games are mutually enjoyed and highly arousing to the child, who responds with chuckles and laughter, and, when older, cries of 'more'. Mother-play on the other hand tends to include more verbal and visual stimulation but is generally calmer. Both types of play are thought to be necessary for the infant's optimal development, and it is fascinating that similar findings are reproduced from studies in many different cultural and social groups. It seems likely that there is a biological basis for these differences in play styles, although the argument about biological versus social determinants continues. A further aspect to consider is the father's indirect influence on child development via his support (or lack of it) for the child's mother.

In the Thomas Coram Study, where the father was reported as actively involved and helping in the first six weeks (on health visitor assessment), we found that babies were more likely to be reported as settled, waking less at night, and having fewer feeding difficulties. In addition, where fathers were helpful, the mothers were more confident in their caretaking role and were more likely to be enjoying motherhood.

A supportive relationship with the spouse is a good mitigating factor for maternal depression, and where a mother has a warm caring relationship with the man she lives with she is more likely to be successful and confident in her mothering role.

The studies of the effects of fathering on child development and child behaviour are still in their infancy, but the implications for health professionals are fairly clear. There is a need to include fathers far more than is routine at present when seeing children, and certainly when problems are apparent (whether physical, developmental or emotional) there is a need to understand the father's role in the family. Both parents should be involved in discussions about any proposed intervention, and the outcome for managing, for example, a child with a behaviour problem is far more likely to be successful when both father and mother are agreed on a course of action. This may mean flexibility of clinic times with the opportunity for fathers to attend to fit in with working hours.

Family size

Several studies have looked at the effect of birth order and family size on children's abilities and attributes, and some interesting findings have emerged. Perhaps the most striking finding, replicated in many large cohort studies as well as smaller studies, is that to be born into a family of five or more siblings puts a child at a disadvantage compared with his peers in smaller families. In 1973 the National Children's Bureau's report, *Born to Fail*, was published, and the authors cited three main factors as constituting disadvantage, one of them being large family size (Wedge & Prosser, 1973). These and other authors have shown significant differences in abilities and attainments between children according to family size, with children from large families consistently achieving less than their peers. Workers involved in the Child Health and Education Study (Osborn *et al.*, 1984), reporting on the social life of Britain's five-year-olds, attempted to discover which family and social factors were most strongly associated with differences in children's abilities and behaviour at the beginning of their school career. Again, family size was a significant factor; children with no siblings were considerably ahead on tests of general ability and conceptual maturity as well as on language tests at age five, compared with children from large families. The differences in achievement tend to become even more marked as children progress through their school careers.

There are, of course, many reasons for this apart from simply the number of brothers and sisters in a family. Large family size is very often associated with lower socio-economic status, poorer housing, fewer material resources, and an increased risk of the mother becoming depressed. What resources there are available are spread more thinly, and this applies to parental time and attention devoted to individual children as well as to there being fewer outings and almost certainly a poorer diet. It may be the latter which partially explains the decrease in height in later-born children of large families compared with those in small families. Behaviour problems are more common in children from large families, and parenting styles will be different; some writers have emphasized the more authoritarian role and increased use of physical punishment by parents of five or more children, presumably in an effort to retain control. In smaller families more individual attention is possible, and each child's individual personality is more likely to be taken into account in child-rearing.

Only children in contrast are more likely to be high achievers, displaying greater creativity and motivation, and are reportedly likely to be upwardly socially mobile. They are likely to have greater parental pressures on them to achieve, but also spend more time in adult company and in interactive vocalization, with often quite mature language development for their age. However, they are also more likely to display neurotic behaviours, and an increased incidence of psychosomatic disorders is reported in first-borns and only children, compared with later-born siblings.

Second and third children are sometimes described as more socially active and gregarious, and less conforming, as well as less highly achieving. These are, of course, generalizations and everyone will be familiar with families in whom none of these remarks apply. Parenting styles vary enormously, and also importantly children's temperaments are individual and different regardless of their birth order. Parents are understandably less confident with their first-born and more anxious both about physical care and about their own abilities in parenting; attitudes may well be more relaxed by the time the second or third child is born, but we need to recognize that the child's personality greatly influences the style of parenting.

Birth spacing too plays a part. Where children are closely spaced there is less opportunity for individual attention, and, where two children are born less than 18 months apart, one study found that mothers tended to talk to the children as a unit, and at the level of the youngest child. Children may also be dressed the same, and closely spaced siblings, like twins, may suffer later identity problems.

In some communities, and particularly where weaning the child from the breast depends on the birth of a subsequent child, birth spacing is of crucial importance to a child's physical and emotional development, and health workers try to encourage a minimum of two years between pregnancies.

Teenage parents

Many studies have pointed out the disadvantages of being born to a teenage mother, and indeed the increased risk to the mother of child-bearing in her teens.

Almost one child in 10 in 1982 was born to a teenage mother, and around 50% of teenage mothers are unmarried (compared with around 12% of older mothers). The total number of teenage births in England and Wales for 1984 was 59 900. The total number (and proportion) of births to teenage parents has declined in the past decade, probably reflecting easier access to contraceptive services and improvements in sex education for schoolchildren (Table 5.1).

Children of younger mothers have been shown to do less well than children born to older mothers in a variety of ways, perhaps the most striking being the higher fetal, perinatal and infant mortality rates, as well as higher risks of maternal mortality. Unmarried teenage mothers are now more likely to keep their babies than decide to have them adopted, and parenthood may be seen as a preferable alternative to unemployment or a low-paid job.

Many of these young mothers will have lacked adequate parenting

Table 5.1 Conception rates in teenage girls, 1974 and 1984, England and Wales.

Age (years)	Conception rates per thousand	
	1974	1984
13–15	8.5	8.6
16	47.6	41.9
17	73.8	61.4
18	94.8	77.9
19	110.7	89.3
Rates for all girls under 20	69.7	59.9

Source: OPCS (1986) *Birth Statistics 1985, England and Wales*, FMI no. 12.

themselves, and lack confidence in their own parenting skills. Isolation and depression are common, exacerbated by the frequent lack of support from a stable partnership or family. There are now fewer residential mother-and-baby homes than a decade or two ago, when a facility run by a religious or voluntary organization would offer a home and support for several months. Many young mothers now find themselves placed in bed-and-breakfast accommodation, a poor environment which many people believe constitutes a health risk to mother and child (Conway, 1988).

The Child Health and Education Study (Osborn *et al.*, 1984) (follow-up of a cohort of births from one week in April 1970) reported on just over a thousand children born to teenage mothers. They found that at five years these children performed less well on some educational tests, particularly of vocabulary, and also exhibited more behaviour disturbance than children of older mothers. They were also on average shorter at age five, and had smaller head circumferences. It was notable that the younger mothers appeared to suffer more from depression (with higher *malaise* scores) than the older mothers, and this was strongly correlated with the reporting of child behaviour problems. During the pregnancies there were higher rates of smoking, and the birthweights of children of younger mothers were lower than the comparison group.

Other studies have reported high rates of physical illness, hospital admissions, and accidents among children of teenage mothers, and there is also a higher incidence of sudden infant death syndrome. Teenage parenthood is one characteristic often associated with child abuse, and Lynch & Roberts (1978) found that half the abusing mothers in their study were under 20 years at the time of birth of their first child, compared with 16% in a control group.

It is difficult to sort out issues of causality among these associations, as in all the studies it is striking that teenage mothering is associated with lower socioeconomic status, unemployment, and poor housing and social environment, which all represent the comparative poverty of many of these families. A recent paper on this topic (Wadsworth *et al.*, 1984) supported the belief that low maternal age adversely affects children's health and development not through some biological effect, but through disadvantage which frequently accompanies teenage mothering. Hence the outlook is not always bleak but clearly depends on the amount of support, both social and financial, available to the young mother.

Rates of teenage pregnancy vary enormously from one country to another. A study of 36 western nations found the highest rate in the USA (96 per 1000) and among culturally comparable countries the lowest rate (14 per 1000) was found in the Netherlands. It seems likely that an enlightened attitude towards sex (as in the Netherlands) together with formal and informal sex education and readily accessible contraceptive services for young people predispose towards much lower rates of teenage pregnancy and abortion.

Unemployment and children

While there are several descriptive studies of the effects of unemployment on family life, there is remarkably little research relating to the effects on children of having an unemployed parent. Figures from 1983 indicated that around 1.2 million children in Britain were growing up in families where the main earner was unemployed and the numbers must now be considerably higher since 13.8% of the work-force were registered unemployed in October 1985. What literature there is relating to children was well reviewed by Madge in 1983, who makes the valid point that the meaning of unemployment and the type of men likely to be affected depends considerably on the social context and the current level of joblessness (Madge, 1983).

A considerable amount is known, however, about the effects of unemployment in adults, and Smith has written several excellent reviews on various aspects of this, which were published in the *British Medical Journal* at the end of 1985. There is evidence that unemployment in adults causes additional and premature deaths; there are also strong correlations between unemployment and ill health, and the best evidence suggests that unemployment causes extra physical illness (Smith, 1985b). Certainly the unemployed are less healthy than the employed, although part of this association is due to the unhealthy having a higher chance of becoming unemployed. There is evidence too that unemployment leads to a deterioration in mental health and many good accounts of this have been written (e.g. Jahoda, 1982). Both suicide and parasuicide rates are higher among unemployed men and some of the association is thought to be causal (Smith, 1985a). Poverty is known to be extremely common in unemployed families.

In view of this it would be surprising if there were no observable effects on the wives and children of unemployed men, and the literature and research that is available suggests that unemployment in a family can be seriously damaging to children (Smith, 1985c). The chronic stress, misery and low self-esteem of the unemployed lead to a deterioration in mental health of an individual, and can be destructive to family relationships. In addition to financial hardship the family are also on top of each other in the home each day, very often generating tensions or arguments. In these circumstances marital breakdown is common, and for all age groups the divorce rate of the unemployed is twice that of the national average, with obvious consequences for the children. Physical violence at home is reported more commonly when the main breadwinner is unemployed, and two studies of women seeking help because of wife-battering found that in almost half the cases the man concerned was unemployed.

Child abuse too has been reported to be associated with unemployment, and the rates of both have risen dramatically in the past five years. Many cases of child abuse are registered with the National Society for the Prevention of Cruelty to Children, and in the five years to the end of 1982 over six thousand children were registered; the most common factors cited as precipitating the abuse were unemployment, marital discord, financial problems and lack of self-esteem (Creighton, 1984). Another study of abused children in Scotland found that almost one-third of their fathers were out of work (Cater & Easton, 1980). A more recent study of abused children from Sheffield, however, did not find a higher than expected level of unemployment among their parents (Taitz et al., 1987). Related to child abuse and neglect is the issue of taking children into the care of the local authority; again unsurprisingly the proportion of parents of children taken into care who are unemployed is extremely high.

Ethnic minority groups

Despite the fact that over the last few generations Britain has become a multiracial society, there is inadequate training of both doctors and nurses concerning the health needs of minority groups. A lack of understanding of culture, religion and custom, together with poor appreciation of the difficulties faced by many families in adapting to life in Britain, often results in stereotyping of individuals by health professionals and others. Communication difficulties may arise in attempting to deliver health care, and the family may be blamed for not speaking English or an older child or relative inappropriately used as an interpreter.

In a few districts, teams of multi-ethnic health workers have been appointed to act as advocates (note not simply interpreters) for families from different ethnic groups, with consequent improvements in service delivery. The DHSS in the mid-1980s supported the Asian mother-and-baby campaign, with the appointment of link-workers in many health districts; health professionals valued this service greatly and some districts have continued to fund these posts.

Rates of certain illnesses are higher in certain groups, such as sickle-cell disease in the Afro-Caribbean population, β-thalassaemia in people from Mediterranean countries and India, and sensorineural deafness in certain Asian groups. In districts where a high proportion of the population are at risk from these diseases, counselling services are available, and antenatal (for thalassaemia) or postnatal (for sickle-cell) screening may be offered.

Social and environmental factors may contribute to poorer health; immigrant families (even second or third generation) in general tend to live in worse accommodation, often in poorer run-down council estates, and adults in employment are often working for long hours in poorly paid employment (for example, the catering and hotel business).

Studies in pregnancy outcome have consistently shown higher infant mortality rates among babies and mothers born outside the UK and this is particularly true for mothers originating from Pakistan and Bangladesh (Fig. 5.2). Risk factors have been thought to include low maternal height, high parity, anaemia, poor antenatal attendance, and consanguinity (Whitehead, 1987).

A particular concern in the field of child health is the programme of child health surveillance. All of the screening and assessment tools in common use (for example, Denver, Stycar, Griffiths) were standardized on white Caucasian populations (predominantly middle class) and are often inappropriate to a child from a different cultural background. This is particularly true of language assessment tools, and so far only limited attempts have been made to overcome this. A speech screening test along the lines of the Kendall toy test had been devised for Bengali children (S. Bellman, personal communication) and work is being done on measures of early language development in Asian populations

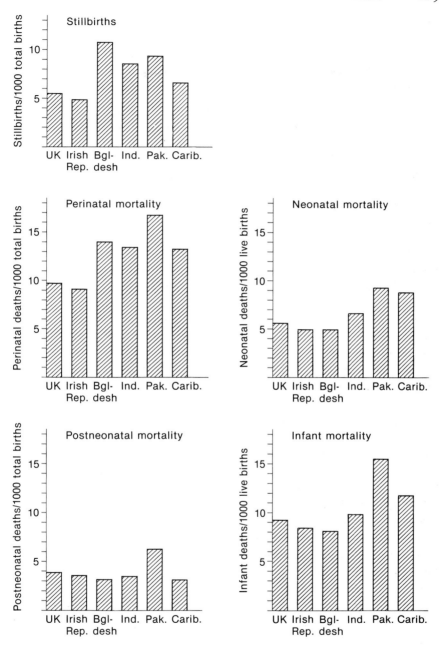

Fig. 5.2 Outcome of pregnancy by mother's country of birth, England and Wales, 1984. UK: United Kingdom. Irish Rep.: Irish Republic. B'dsh: Bangladesh. Ind.: India. Pak.: Pakistan. Carib.: Caribbean Commonwealth.

in East London, but these are still at the level of preliminary research.

Clearly, when presented with a child from a non-English-speaking background, in attempting to assess speech and language (and indeed other aspects of development) one can often only hazard an inaccurate guess as to the child's level of attainment. The parent is of course a major source of information and expertise, but if there appears to be any concern then it is mandatory to arrange for a further assessment with a suitably trained interpreter present.

Another area of major concern is the advice and support offered to ethnic minority families where there is a child with a disability or handicap. Many of these families feel isolated and unsupported with inadequate understanding of the services available and how to use them, and often no attempt is made by the health service to address these issues. Studies in Tower Hamlets have shown how effective trained counsellors from similar cultural backgrounds can be in support-ing such families. The effectiveness of a parent-adviser scheme has been shown to be impressive, with improvements noted in many measures of both child and family health and function (Davis, 1987).

It has to be said, though, that much more thought and effort need to be made to improve accessibility and acceptability of health services for families of ethnic minorities, and a lot more input is needed on these aspects of health care in both medical and nursing training.

Mortality, morbidity and unemployment

Perinatal and infant mortality rates have been gradually declining, and this was true even for the period of the depression in the 1930s. There is a positive association between death rates of children zero−four years and unemployment, low socio-economic status, and inadequate or overcrowded housing, and, although these are all interrelated the unemployment rate seems to have an effect independent of class (data from 1971 census). Latest figures from Scotland show a small increase in perinatal mortality, and this may lend weight to conclusions from studies which suggest an association between unemployment and perinatal mortality. However, in unemployed families all other risk factors are likely to be high, so both large numbers and sophisticated studies are necessary to examine the associations accurately.

More convincing are the morbidity data, although research in this area is again sparse. A large-population-based study in Glasgow found strong associations between admission rates of children to hospital and unemployment, as well as with overcrowding and other deprivation variables (Maclure & Stewart, 1984). Children living in deprived areas of Glasgow were on average nine times more likely to be admitted to hospital for any reason than children in non-deprived districts. Some districts had very low rates of admission, and these districts had low rates of unemployment (6%) and overcrowding (1%). At the other extreme unemployment affected 33% and overcrowding 30% of households, and it was from these districts that the admission rates of children were highest.

Again from Glasgow a study of 655 babies found a lower mean birthweight by 150 g among those whose fathers were unemployed compared with those with employed fathers, and also some growth deficit in the first year (Cole *et al.*, 1983). National studies of child growth have shown that children of the unemployed tend to be shorter than those whose fathers are working, and the effect is most marked for children of the long-term unemployed. Some evidence from the same study suggests there may be an effect on developmental status also; at the age of two the children of the unemployed did significantly less well on developmental tests, despite no differences in groups being apparent at one year of age (Chinnock *et al.*, 1984). Others have written about the relationship between childhood accidents and unemployment, and increased rates of physical illness, behaviour problems, and feeding and sleep disturbances. Many writers have reported on the psychological impact concluding that children can become emotionally unstable and suffer from anxiety and depression (particularly older children) and that even young children can feel embarrassment. Just as parents may feel ashamed and embarrassed to be out of work, so too may their children, and one can speculate that 'my dad's unemployed' does not benefit one's peer group image in the nursery or infant school as much as 'my dad's a fireman'. It is likely though that the stigma of unemployment is lessened when rates of unemployment are high, as in the mid-1980s, and this may possibly be the only positive spin-off from a dismal situation.

A further possible spin-off could be that unemployed men spend more time in positive aspects of child care, and hence are more involved with their children in recreational and other activities. However, where people have studied this it only appears true in a minority of families, with most men not adopting a greater child-rearing role.

Physical environment

Because the physical environment of the country or small country town appears far more attractive and less stressful than an inner city environment it is sometimes assumed that the latter is detrimental to child development. However, the evidence in support of this is not straightforward, and although studies have shown increased rates of antisocial behaviour and behaviour problems in children living in urban environments compared with rural environments (e.g. Rutter *et al.*, 1975; Osborn *et al.*, 1984) there are other factors which have to be considered. There is often a clustering of adverse factors which affect children in inner cities: rates of poor housing, overcrowding, and larger family size are all more common and are associated with lower socioeconomic status, with poorer academic achievement and with increased rates of behaviour problems. But children of middle-class families in inner cities are less likely to be adversely affected, and clearly cultural and child-rearing patterns, as well as material resources, are influential.

There are certainly clear risk factors associated with city dwelling. There is likely to be lack of safe, supervised play space for children, and it is known that parents in overcrowded conditions are more likely to allow or encourage their children to play outside the home. Thus, there is a greater risk of accidents, and of course the large numbers of cars, vans and lorries in cities increase the risk of road accidents. Environmental toxins are mostly higher in cities, and lead from petrol fumes and other sources is one health hazard which has received a lot of attention in recent years (Smith *et al.*, 1983).

Some environments do seem to encourage violence and vandalism (certain estates and high-rise blocks) and the design has been implicated in causing this; the characteristics of the residents may also be a determining factor. Another factor in inner urban environments is that social support systems may be less defined and strong — families may be housed far from their relatives, and forming new social networks is less easy in urban than village environments. Disruption of social networks is known to be associated with maternal depression and is likely to have other, more direct effects on children, with fewer close adult relatives to share in aspects of child-rearing.

While the idyll of country life remains the aspiration of many city dwellers, the reality is that family influences and material resources are probably most important in determining the quality of a child's life, and exchanging urban poverty for rural poverty may not bring many advantages.

Preconceptual and antenatal factors

The influence of many factors which potentially affect child health and development is already operating in the preconceptual and early perinatal period.

As improvements in obstetric and neonatal care continue to reduce the numbers of babies handicapped as a consequence of adverse perinatal events, attention is increasingly focused on the prenatal and indeed preconception period as a target for prevention of handicaps. About one-third of handicap is thought to originate in the first trimester of pregnancy; in children with severe mental handicap where the cause can be ascertained with certainly 55% of cases are found to originate from prenatal causes (Mackay, 1982). The causes are not just genetically determined disorders (which can increasingly be diagnosed in the antenatal period) but adverse environmental events affecting the fetus.

Factors known to affect the fetus with varying degrees of severity include irradiation, maternal nutrition, ingestion of drugs and alcohol, and cigarette-smoking, as well as pesticides and other less common toxins.

Nutrition

It has long been recognized that an adequate diet both before and during pregnancy is important for optimal growth and health of the baby. Much research has focused on maternal nutrition, and a great deal of health educational material has been generated. The majority of mothers receive some sort of dietary advice when they attend antenatal clinics, and many hospitals provide diet sheets. While the average diet in this country meets the energy and nutritional levels recommended by the DHSS, a significant minority have an intake, particularly of minerals and vitamins, which falls short of this. The most at-risk groups are those on low incomes, particularly pregnant women in families on supplementary benefit, and single parents. Because nutritional status tends to improve with higher income, it is possible that some of the social class differences in low birthweight and perinatal mortality may be explainable by differences in maternal diet, both preconception and during pregnancy (Wynn & Wynn, 1979). This hypothesis is supported by more recent evidence from a study of maternal diet amongst pregnant women in Hackney and Hampstead; the former were predominantly of lower social class and low income, whereas the latter were mainly from social class I and II. The rates of low birthweight were strikingly higher among the Hackney mothers and analysis of their diet revealed caloric intake below recommended levels, as well as other nutritional deficiencies (Crawford et al., 1986).

Central nervous system malformations such as spina bifida are particularly thought to be related to deficiencies of vitamins and folic acid (Smithells et al., 1976). Preconceptual nutritional status is of crucial importance here due to the rapid growth of the nervous system in the first four weeks after conception (the neural tube is normally completely closed by 28 days) before many women recognize that they are pregnant, and long before any antenatal dietary advice is likely to be given. The effects of acute malnutrition in previously well-nourished populations have been reported, from the siege of Leningrad in 1941–1943 and the period of acute famine during the winter of 1944–1945 in Holland (Smith, 1947). In both groups of pregnant women mean birthweight was significantly reduced (by 550 g in Leningrad and 300 g in Holland) but an increase in congenital malformations was not reported.

In reality women are unlikely to change their diet significantly during pregnancy without practical help, and insufficient attention has been paid to cultural and economic factors that influence what pregnant women eat. A recent study by the Maternity Alliance (Durward, 1984) costed an adequate diet for a pregnant mother, and measured this as a proportion of income. The average cost of the diet which met DHSS recommended levels of nutrients and accorded with antenatal clinic advice was £13.87 per week (in 1984). While this worked out at 14% of the income of a couple whose income was £100 a week, the situation is far worse for a couple dependent on supplementary benefit. For them, the cost of the diet to feed one person was 32% of the total income excluding housing costs (based on rates in February 1984), leaving only £31.50 for all other essentials including the man's diet, fuel, clothing, transport and so on. Hence health education alone without practical economic subsidy can have only limited effectiveness.

Lack of money is a major factor restricting food choice, as well as limiting the quantity of food consumed. One study of families on supplementary benefit found that some parents themselves went without food in order to provide enough for their children, and this was borne out by Graham's study (1976) in Milton Keynes, where 51% of lone parents with preschool children, and 30% of low-income parents in two-parent families were cutting down on food consumption for financial reasons.

Many studies have found social class differences in consumption of fresh fruit and vegetables, and, despite increased consumption of wholemeal bread and high-fibre foods and decreased sugar consumption in the past decade among all social classes, the richest income group continues to have a healthier diet than poorer groups. Lack of money is frequently cited for the lack of fresh fruit and vegetables among poor families.

Cigarette-smoking

The association of maternal smoking with adverse outcome of pregnancy has been described now for over 25 years. Many studies have demonstrated an increased perinatal mortality rate among offspring of mothers who smoke, and intra-uterine growth deficiency, with the infants being significantly lighter than infants of non-smokers. The effects of smoking on birthweight still hold after controlling for social class.

The effects persist after birth (in most cases so too does the smoking); a significantly greater mortality has been reported up to the age of five years, and children of smoking mothers are admitted to hospital more often than children of non-smoking controls. The Child Health and Development Study reported shorter stature and long-term behavioural effects with poor reading ability at the age of 11 years among the children of smokers (Butler & Goldstein, 1973). There are of course likely to be other characteristics of women who smoke which may account for some of the adverse outcomes noted, and these cannot always be accurately assessed and controlled for. For instance heavy-smoking women tend to be in a lower socio-economic group, and their housing conditions are often poorer; they are also more likely to be exposed to stressful circumstances. These factors, circuitously, may partly explain their need to smoke. Many mothers do stop smoking in pregnancy, others find it impossible despite knowing that it may be harmful, and they should not be regarded as irresponsible. Some mothers temper the advice given with their own experience, which is more powerful, of having smoked in a previous pregnancy and given birth to a large healthy baby. Data from a study by Graham (1976) suggest that for many low-income mothers smoking is a response to a particular situation, and provides one way of coping with day-to-day responsibilities and stresses. Hence entreating women to give up smoking is unlikely to be successful without acknowledgement of their particular circumstances and suggestions of alternative strategies for reducing stress.

Drug effects

A number of drugs are known to be teratogenic in the developing fetus, and thalidomide is probably the best-known example of this. Drugs can have harmful effects on the fetus at any time during pregnancy, but the period of greatest risk of producing congenital malformations is from the third to the eleventh week of pregnancy. Drugs given during the second and third trimester may affect fetal growth or have toxic effects on fetal tissue; those given shortly before term may have an adverse effect on the newborn baby after delivery.

The safest policy is for no drugs to be taken during pregnancy unless necessary to the mother's health. While there is a small risk of congenital malformations from some of the anticonvulsant drugs, the benefits of controlling epilepsy during pregnancy usually outweigh the risks. Phenytoin is thought to carry the highest risk (probably around 10%) of fetal malformation, but primidone, carbamazepine, ethosuximide and sodium valproate are also suspect.

Antidepressants and anxiolytics are again somewhat suspect but no particular abnormalities are associated with them other than for lithium which is known to be associated particularly with congenital heart defects.

Alcohol is a known teratogen, and if any of the above drugs are habitually taken in conjunction with alcohol the risk of adverse effects to the fetus is enhanced.

Many antibiotics are safe during pregnancy. However, the amino-glycosides (particularly streptomycin and kanamycin) can cause eighth-nerve damage resulting in deafness. Tetracyclines cause yellow discoloration of deciduous teeth, and enamel hypoplasia. The sul-phonamides and dapsone may cause neonatal haemolysis, and most antimalarials are contra-indicated. The safest antibiotic during preg-nancy is probably penicillin.

A full list of drugs which should be either avoided or used with caution during pregnancy can be found in the British National Formulary.

Self-administered drugs

Although there is no convincing evidence to date that occasional use of cannabis or LSD produces adverse effects on the fetus or newborn infant, data in this area are scanty, and it is possible that both may be harmful. Chronic usage of both is associated with increased rates of spontaneous abortion, and the high tar and hydrocarbon content of cannabis-smoking is thought to have the same effect as ordinary cigarette-smoking on fetal growth rates. No teratogenic effects have been reported associated with usage of marihuana, LSD, amphetamines or cocaine, although we know of no reported controlled studies.

Heroin usage is again not associated with congenital abnormalities. However, withdrawal symptoms in the newborn may be severe, requiring prolonged treatment, and the behavioural effects are thought to be quite long-lasting. Attention deficits and learning disorders are reported in children born to heroin addicts, and there is some association with mild growth retardation. Because of the many adverse social and environmental factors that are often associated with having a parent who is a heroin addict, some of the later effects described in these children are likely to be due to environmental factors, in addition to the biological effects on the fetal nervous system.

Alcohol effects

Damage to the fetus from alcohol is stated to be the largest known teratogenic cause of mental handicap in the western world, and is preventable. The range of abnormalities caused is wide, and the effects vary from none to intra-uterine death, or severe mental retardation together with growth retardation and malformation. The full clinical effects are described as the 'fetal alcohol syndrome', and the incidence varies according to the population studied (UK one per 2500, USA and Sweden one per thousand). Until recently it has undoubtedly been under-diagnosed since women who drink excessively during pregnancy may be reluctant to volunteer this information. Clustering of cases is likely to occur in deprived inner city areas, hence descriptions in this country from paediatricians in cities such as Liverpool and Glasgow. A long list of abnormalities has been reported in the fetal alcohol syndrome, with many types of skeletal, cardiac, renal and facial abnormalities described. Cardiac abnormalities have been described in 25–50% of affected children, and are more common than renal abnormalities. The key features of the full syndrome are prenatal and/or postnatal growth retardation, neurological abnormality and developmental delay or intellectual impairment, and characteristic facial features. The dysmorphic facial features should include at least two of the following: microcephaly (head circumference < 3rd percentile), micropthalmia and/or short palpebral fissures, poorly developed phil-trum, thin upper lip and flattening of maxillary area (Poskitt, 1984). A partial fetal alcohol syndrome would be considered in children who show some of these features in addition to other significant abnormalities in cardiac, central nervous, or skeletal systems.

When women continue to drink heavily until shortly before delivery, the infant may develop withdrawal symptoms after birth, with agitated restless behaviour, hypertonia and jitteriness. Abnormal behaviour in the first few days may be a clue, or feeding difficulties in the baby and lack of early socialization may alert the clinician to early evidence of developmental delay. Poor maternal–infant interaction may be present, and can be contributed to by both the infant's neurological state and the mother's state of mind. Clearly if she continues to drink this is prejudicial to the infant's development, both physically and emotionally. Late effects described in affected children include poor attention, hyper-activity and behaviour problems.

The most important consequence of fetal alcohol syndrome is mental retardation, and this may only be manifest after the first few months of life. However, the range of IQ found in different studies has been large, varying from some children with apparently normal intelligence to those with very severe retardation, with a mean IQ estimate for affected children of 65.

One question which remains unanswered is how much alcohol it is safe to drink during pregnancy. Women are currently advised not to drink more than the equivalent of 30 ml absolute alcohol per day (equivalent to one-and-a-half glasses of wine or one-and-a-half pints of beer) but 'binge' drinking with abstinent days is considered probably more dangerous. If drugs or cigarettes are also consumed, the 'safe' dose of alcohol is likely to be even lower than this. It is thought that a reduction in alcohol intake during pregnancy will reduce the risk to the fetus, so ongoing health education as to the risks involved from alcohol is needed. As with cigarette-smoking, health education alone is insufficient to deter many women who drink for multiple social and emotional reasons. They are likely to come from deprived and stressful environments, and, until society has something positive to offer them, more than medical help is needed. Health education regarding the ill effects of both alcohol and cigarettes can perhaps most usefully be directed at schoolchildren, from primary school age upwards.

Stress and morbidity

Most people recognize an association between stress and illness even though the mechanism may be poorly understood, and in adults associations have been described between adverse life events and such disparate illness as coronary thrombosis, appendicitis and neoplastic disease, to mention just a few.

Similar associations have been reported in childhood, and the ill effects of stress in relation to pregnancy and childbirth have long been recognized. Early in this century writers linked raised levels of anxiety in pregnancy with obstetric abnormalities in labour and the rationale that lay behind some antenatal classes was that an understanding of the processes of pregnancy and labour together with relaxation tech-niques would lead to less intrapartum complications. While there is some sense in this, it was often assumed that ignorance was the cause of the anxiety experienced by many pregnant women, and it is only more recently that researchers in this field have recognized the importance of identifying and understanding the sources of stress and anxiety. For many women, of course, their anxiety results from factors external to the pregnancy itself, and once this issue is examined it appears that 'life stress' is more significantly related to obstetric complications than 'anxious disposition'.

Life stress is usually measured by a scaled score of life events which have been found to be significantly disturbing to people who experience them, and includes factors such as divorce (or separation), death of a close relative or friend, moving house, becoming unemployed, severe financial worries, a family member being arrested, serious illness in the family and so on. A recent careful study of life events in pregnancy found significant correlations between high scores for adverse life events and both low birthweight and premature birth, even after controlling for maternal smoking and socioeconomic factors (Newton & Hunt, 1984). It is apparent that traditional antenatal support is unlikely to be effective in ameliorating the effects of such issues as a marital split or unemployment, and we should be looking more at social support networks and how to increase these and render them more effective.

As Lumley & Astbury (1982) state 'if, for example, anxiety stems largely from crowded housing conditions, unemployment, marital conflict or inadequate income, it is highly unlikely to be alleviated by a course of childbirth preparation which stresses relaxation and breathing patterns in labour'. There is now considerable evidence of the value of supportive relationships, and the lack of a supportive environment in times of stress seems to be a major reason why some people respond with increased susceptibility to disease.

While stressful life events during the nine months of pregnancy are common, they are all the more so during the early years of childhood. A study in America of 500 families in New York county found that over a one-year period 42% of families had experienced the death of a near relative, and 20% had experienced divorce or the arrest of a family member. Families with high rates of life events were found to have significantly increased numbers of contacts with the medical profession, either as consultations or admissions to hospital. In another study the same researchers found an increased susceptibility to streptococcal infection in children who had suffered recent stressful events; and some mechanisms for these findings were postulated (Haggerty, 1980).

A further study in New Zealand (Beautrais, 1982) looked at the relationship between family life events and the risk of morbidity in a birth cohort of one thousand children between the ages of one and four years. Morbidity rates for most common childhood illnesses and accidents were found to increase in almost direct proportion to the number of family life events, and, specifically, children from families experiencing 12 or more life events (over the three-year period) had on average six times the risk of hospital admission compared with children from families with three or fewer life events. Higher rates of medical attendance were also reported, and in all cases the associations between life events and rates of morbidity were highly statistically significant. These authors were careful to control for other factors which might have explained the higher morbidity rates, but the findings held true after controlling for family social background (including mother's educational level) and living standards. They suggest two explanations for their findings: first that the presence of stress in the family reduces maternal coping ability with a resulting decrease in child-rearing standards and hence increase in risk of childhood morbidity; secondly that the effects of stress directly alter the child's susceptibility to illness. Probably both factors are involved, and in support of the second explanation is evidence that decreased immunoglobulin (Ig) A levels and increased catecholamine secretion can occur as a response to stress.

Maternal factors too undoubtedly play a part, since stress in families, resulting in reduced maternal vigilance, has been recognized as accounting for the persistent correlations found between childhood accidents, poisoning, burns and scalds and adverse life events.

References

Beautrais, A.L., Fergusson, D.M. & Shannon, F.T. (1982) Life events and childhood morbidity: a prospective study. *Pediatrics*, **70**(6), 935−40.

Butler, N.R. & Goldstein, H. (1973) Smoking in pregnancy and subsequent child development. *British Medical Journal*, **4**, 573−5.

Caputo, D.V., Goldstein, K.M. & Taub, H.B. (1981) Neonatal compromise and later psychological development. In *Preterm Birth and Psychological Development* (eds Friedman, S.L. & Sigman, M.) Academic Press, New York.

Cater, J. & Easton, P. (1980) Separation and other stress in child abuse. *Lancet*, i, 972−3.

Chinnock, A., Keegan, P.T., Fox, P.T. & Elston, M.D. (1984) Associations between growth patterns, social factors, morbidity and developmental delay in a longitudinal survey of preschool children. In *Human Growth and Development* (ed. Borns, J.). Plenum, London.

Cole, T.J., Donnet, M.L. & Stanfield, J.P. (1983) Unemployment, birthweight and growth in the first year. *Archives of Disease in Childhood*, **58**, 717−21.

Conway, J. (ed) (1988) *Prescription for Poor Health: The Crisis for Homeless families*. London Food Commission, Maternity Alliance, SHAC & Shelter.

Crawford, M.A., Doyle, W., Craft, I.C. & Laurance, B.M. (1986) A comparison of food intake during pregnancy and birthweight in high and low socio-economic groups. *Progress in Lipid Research*, **25**, 249−54.

Creighton, S.J. (1984) *Trends in Child Abuse*. National Society for the Prevention of Cruelty to Children, London.

Davis, H. & Ali Choudry, P. (1987) *Helping Bangladeshi Families: the Parent Adviser Scheme: Mental Handicap*.

Department of Health and Social Security (1980) *Inequalities in Health*. London, DHSS.

Durward, L. (1984) *Poverty in Pregnancy: the Cost of an Adequate Diet for Expectant Mothers*. Maternity Alliance, London.

Graham, H. (1976) Smoking in pregnancy: the attitudes of expectant mothers. *Social Science and Medicine*, **10**, 399−405.

Haggerty, R.J. (1980) Life stress, illness and social supports. *Developmental Medicine and Child Neurology*, **22**, 391−400.

House of Commons Social Services Committee. *Third Report: Perinatal and Neonatal Mortality Report 1984*. London, HMSO.

Jahoda, M. (1982) *Employment and Unemployment*. Cambridge University Press, Cambridge.

Lamb, M.E. (1977) Father−infant and mother−infant interaction in the first year of life. *Child Development*, **48**, 167−81.

Lumley, J. & Astbury, J. (1982) Advice in pregnancy: perfect remedies, imperfect science. In *Effectiveness and Satisfaction in Antenatal Care* (eds Enkin, M. & Chalmers, I.). Spastics International Medical Publications, William Heinemann, London (132−50).

Lynch, M. & Roberts, J. (1978) Early alerting signs. In *Child Abuse* (ed. Franklin, A.W.). Churchill Livingstone, Edinburgh.

Mackay, R.I. (1982) The causes of severe mental retardation. *Developmental Medicine and Child Neurology*, **24**(3), 386−8.

Maclure, A. & Stewart, G.T. (1984) Admission of children to hospitals in Glasgow: relation to unemployment and other deprivation variables. *Lancet*, **ii**, 682−5.

Madge, N. (1983) Unemployment and its effects on children. *Journal of Child Psychology and Psychiatry*, **24**(2), 311−19.

Neligan, G.A., Kolvin, I., Scott, D.McI., Garside, R.F. (1976) *Born Too Soon or Born Too Small*. Spastics International Publications, London: Heinemann Medical.

Newton, R.W. & Hunt, L.P. (1984) Psychosocial stress in pregnancy and its relation to low birth weight. *British Medical Journal*, **288**, 1191−4.

Osborn, A.F., Butler, N.R. & Morris, A.C. (1984) *The Social Life of Britain's Five-year-olds*. Routledge & Kegan Paul, London.

Poskitt, E.M.E. (1984) Fetal alcohol syndrome and fetal alcohol effects. In *Progress in Child Health*, vol. 1. (ed. Macfarlane, A.). Churchill Livingstone, Edinburgh.

Richards, M.P.M. (1984) Children and divorce. In *Progress in Child Health*, vol. 1. (ed. Macfarlane, J.A.). Churchill Livingstone, Edinburgh.

Rutter, M., Cox, A., Tupling, C., Berger, M.Y. & Yule, W. (1975) Attainment and adjustment in two geographical areas. I. Prevalence of psychiatric disorders. *British Journal of Psychiatry*, **126**, 493−509.

Siegel, L.S. (1982) Reproductive, perinatal and environmental factors as predictors of the cognitive and language development of preterm and fullterm infants. *Child Development*, **53**, 963−73.

Smith, C.A. (1947) The effect of wartime starvation in Holland upon pregnancy and its product. *American Journal of Obstetrics and Gynecology*, **53**, 599−608.

Smith, M., Delves, T., Lansdown, R., Clayton, B. & Graham, P. (1983) The effects of lead exposure on urban children: the Institute of Child Health/Southampton Study. *Developmental Medicine and Child Neurology*, suppl. 47, **25**(5).

Smith, R. (1985a) 'I couldn't stand it any more': suicide and unemployment. *British Medical Journal*, **291**, 1563−6.

Smith, R. (1985b) 'I'm just not right': the physical health of the unemployed. *British Medical Journal*, **291**, 1626–9.

Smith, R. (1985c) 'We get on each other's nerves': unemployment and the family. *British Medical Journal*, **291**, 1707–10.

Smithells, R.W., Sheppard, S. & Sclorch, C.J. (1976) Vitamin deficiencies and neural tube defects. *Archives of Disease in Childhood*, **51**, 944.

Taitz, L., King, J.M., Nicholson, J. & Kessel, M. (1987) Unemployment and child abuse. *British Medical Journal*, **294**, 1074–6.

Taylor, D.J., Howie, P.W., Davidson, J., Davidson, D. & Drillien, C.M. (1985) Do pregnancy complications contribute to neurodevelopmental disability? *Lancet*, **1**, 713–16.

Tizard, B. (1977) *Adoption: a Second Chance*. Open Books, London.

Wadsworth, J., Taylor, B., Osborn, A. & Butler, N. (1984) Teenage mothering: child development at 5 years. *Journal of Child Psychology and Psychiatry*, **25**, 305–14.

Wallerstein, J.S. & Kelly, J.B. (1980) *Surviving the Breakup*. Grant McIntyre, London.

Wedge, P. & Prosser, H. (1973) *Born to Fail*. Arrow Books in association with the National Children's Bureau, London.

Whitehead, M. (1987) *The Health Divide: Inequalities in Health in the 1980s*. Health Education Authority.

Wolkind, S. (1979) *Medical Aspects of Adoption and Foster Care*. Clinics in Developmental Medicine No. 74, Spastics International Medical Publications with Heinemann, London.

Wynn, A. & Wynn, M. (1979) *Prevention of Handicap and the Health of Women*. Routledge & Kegan Paul, London.

Yogman, M.W. (1984) Competence and performance of fathers and infants. In *Progress in Child Health*, vol. 1 (ed. Macfarlane, J.A.). Churchill Livingstone, Edinburgh.

6 Health Care — Feeding and Immunization

THE FIRST SECTION of this chapter focuses on three areas which are of major concern to parents, health visitors and doctors in the first few years of life, namely infant feeding, weight gain and problems concerning the digestive system. For many mothers feeding seems to dominate the first few months of life. Practical and realistic advice from health visitors, doctors and other mothers can provide the necessary support for mothers over this difficult period so that they can enjoy their babies.

The smaller section concerns immunization and aims to clarify the situation regarding contra-indications to immunization in order to prevent misunderstandings and to encourage more mothers to have their children fully immunized. Unfortunately rates of immunization in the UK compare poorly with those in the United States and clearly there is considerable room for improvement. Doctors and health visitors need to be informed of the latest policies and recommendations so that they can counsel parents appropriately.

Infant feeding patterns

Incidence and duration of breast-feeding

Despite mounting evidence of the advantages of breast-feeding the incidence in the UK is disappointingly low. A national survey in 1980 showed that two-thirds of mothers attempted to breast-feed but only 42% were still breast-feeding at six weeks and just over a quarter continued for as long as four months (Martin & Monk, 1980). In 1985 the proportion of mothers breast-feeding was very similar, with 65% attempting breast-feeding and 40% and 26% continuing at six weeks and four months respectively (Oppé et al., 1988).

One encouraging feature is the increase in breast-feeding rates over the period 1975–1980. In 1975, 51% attempted breast-feeding but only a quarter of mothers were breast-feeding at six weeks, falling to 13% at four months (Martin & Monk, 1980). However, the increase has levelled off since 1980. A striking feature of all three studies was the tendency for many mothers to give up breast-feeding after only a week or two.

Influence of health professionals during pregnancy

Although virtually all mothers attend antenatal clinics surprisingly few, 40%, reported having discussed infant feeding at these visits (Martin & Monk, 1980). Antenatal clinics could provide an ideal opportunity to discuss feeding, especially since many women do not attend mothercraft classes. Very often the mothers who are least likely to breast-feed are also the poorest attenders at antenatal classes.

However, lack of time in busy clinics may prevent adequate discussion of feeding and general anxieties. The health visitor can play a valuable role in antenatal care by visiting mothers at home antenatally. She is in the unique position of being able to provide continuing care from the antenatal period through to the postnatal weeks and childhood years. The effectiveness of health visitors' intervention on lactation was demonstrated in a study in two areas of London (Hart *et al.*, 1980). Higher breast-feeding rates were achieved, compared with a control group, by increasing health visitor contacts antenatally and in the first six weeks. Many mothers give up breast-feeding soon after discharge from hospital and the programme was aimed particularly at providing support at this crucial time. Often the midwives and health visitors overlapped but generally this arrangement worked well.

Since many mothers choose to bottle-feed the technique of mixing feeds and giving bottles also needs to be covered antenatally. Bottle-feeding mothers with problems need as much health visitor support in the early weeks as breast-feeding mothers. In the 1980 survey, health visitors were the most common source of advice on infant feeding.

Factors affecting the success of breast-feeding

The 1980 study highlighted some aspects of delivery and hospital practice which appear to affect the chances of successful lactation. Putting the baby to the breast within four hours of delivery, demand feeding and avoiding giving complementary bottle-feeds all enhanced the success of lactation. Not surprisingly, having a caesarean section or an ill or low-birthweight infant prejudiced the outcome of breast-feeding. The practice of rooming-in enables mother and baby to be together continuously, making demand feeding more practicable. With the increased trend towards shortened hospital stays, as in the scheme in which mothers spend only a few hours in hospital, mothers will have more opportunity to organize their own feeding schedules in relaxed surroundings. Some workers (e.g. Sosa *et al.*, 1976) stress the importance of 'skin-to-skin' contact in establishing a close bond between infant and mother and encouraging breast-feeding. Mothers need a sympathetic environment to foster this intimate relationship with their baby, which is best provided in the mother's own home.

The commonest reason given for stopping breast-feeding was 'insufficient milk'. Other reasons included painful breasts, baby would not suck, breast-feeding took too long, mother did not like breast-feeding. Clearly, some mothers are not sufficiently motivated to persevere despite some discomfort and inconvenience but in the majority an improved success rate could be achieved by offering a high level of information and support. The attitude and support of the father can greatly influence both the mother's desire to breast-feed and the likelihood of a successful outcome. Ideally antenatal discussion should involve both parents, not only concerning feeding but also in other aspects of childbirth and child development.

Breast versus bottle

Despite extensive modification of cow's milk to provide a safe substitute for human milk, increasing evidence suggests that even in the developed world breast-feeding affords numerous advantages to the infant's health. However, where breast-feeding is impossible or the mother prefers not to breast-feed, bottle-feeding well done is an adequate substitute. The advantages of breast-feeding need to be publicized by health professionals, schools and the media. Ultimately, the mother will do what she wishes and needs competent advice about her chosen method. Most mothers can breast-feed given the right circumstances but as we know many fail at an early stage. Health professionals must avoid giving the impression that bottle-feeding mothers are providing second-best care, as they may already feel disappointed at not succeeding at breast-feeding. Feeding is only one element of infant care; valuable interactions occur with both parents throughout the day. There has been a tendency to overemphasize breast-feeding as the only satisfactory method and, whilst we wholeheartedly recommend it, in clinical practice a balanced approach is needed to accommodate the wishes of all mothers.

Advantages of breast-feeding

PSYCHOLOGICAL SATISFACTION

Most mothers find suckling an infant a satisfying and enjoyable experience. Satisfaction may be derived from the feeling that the infant is being nourished from the mother's own body. 'Skin-to-skin' physical contact is pleasurable to mother and infant and cements a bond between them. Although most of us feel instinctively that breast-feeding has emotional benefits there is very little hard evidence to support this. Probably a baby who is bottle-fed in a loving and caring manner is just as likely to fare well emotionally as a breast-fed infant.

PROTECTION AGAINST ILLNESS

Infections

Breast-fed infants have a reduced risk of infections including gastro-enteritis, otitis media, respiratory illness and pneumonia. One study (Cunningham, 1977) found that no life-threatening illness occurred in 106 breast-fed infants during the first year, whereas five of the 147 bottle-fed infants developed pneumonia, one was severely ill with meningitis and one died of sudden infant death syndrome. In poorly developed countries it has been found that breast-fed babies rarely develop diarrhoea after exposure to *E. coli*, *Shigella* and *Salmonella*.

The anti-infective properties of colostrum and breast milk can be attributed to the presence of maternal antibodies (immunoglobulins), living cells — macrophages, lymphocytes, complement and interferon-producing cells — and different whey-soluble proteins. Secretory IgA limits bacterial and viral multiplication in the lumen of the gut. IgG and IgM are present in smaller quantities and have distinct antimicrobial activities. Human milk contains a growth factor for *Lactobacillus bifidus*, which facilitates colonization. The acetic and lactic acids produced increase the acidity of the intestinal contents and inhibit growth of pathogens. Whey-soluble proteins include lactoferrin and the enzyme lysozyme. Lactoferrin encourages iron absorption and lysozyme inhibits bacterial growth.

Allergies

Asthma and eczema appear to be less common in breast-fed infants though the subject is still highly controversial. Evidence suggests that it is worth while encouraging mothers with an atopic family history to breast-feed. It is thought that atopic infants have a transient IgA deficiency in the early months which allows penetration of sensitizing macromolecules such as cow's milk protein. However, sensitization to food allergies can occur in fully breast-fed infants (Warner, 1980), presumably because allergens ingested by mothers are excreted in milk.

Electrolyte balance

Breast-fed babies are less likely to develop electrolyte disturbances such as neonatal tetany, due to hypocalcaemia, idiopathic hypercalcaemia and hyperosmolar 'dehydration'. Cot death is less common in breast-fed infants, possibly because of decreased liability to electrolyte imbalance.

Optimum nutrition

Breast-feeding is the safest method of feeding in poorly developed countries but, if maternal nutrition is inadequate, supplements from local foods will probably be needed for the mother during pregnancy and lactation and for the baby from three months onwards to prevent under-nutrition. In the Third World early introduction of solids is associated with high rates of diarrhoea, largely because of unhygienic conditions for food preparation. In the developed world, where obesity is more of a problem, the breast-fed infant is less likely than the bottle-fed baby to gain weight rapidly in the early weeks and to go on to develop childhood obesity. However, recent evidence suggests that obesity is declining in this country (Taitz, 1977; Whitelaw, 1977). Furthermore the obese infant does not necessarily become an obese schoolchild. Poskitt & Cole (1977) found that only 10−20% of fat babies were still fat at five to seven years of age.

ECONOMY

Although breast-feeding involves the cost of extra food for the mother it is cheaper than the cost of artificial milk, bottles, teats and sterilizing equipment. However, the cost factor appears not to influence mothers' choice, since the least well-off mothers are least likely to breast-feed.

CONVENIENCE

Most mothers find that having breast milk available at all times is far easier than making up bottles. One disadvantage is that the father cannot take over if the mother is tired, but there are other ways in which fathers can become involved with child care to help the mother.

OTHER

Some mothers attribute tiredness to breast-feeding but this is more likely to be due to lack of sleep. Possibly, this rationalization may accompany a wish to stop breast-feeding or be a symptom of underlying anxieties or depression.

Breast-feeding confers some advantage for mothers' physical health. Suckling the baby immediately after birth encourages expulsion of the placenta and continued breast-feeding promotes involution of the uterus.

In less developed countries infertility during lactation and in some cultures abstention from intercourse during this time helps to increase the interval between pregnancies.

Reasons why some mothers prefer bottle-feeding

1 Belief that they have insufficient breast milk.
2 Previous experience of breast-feeding unsuccessful.
3 Revulsion from idea of breast-feeding.
4 Embarrassed by breast-feeding.
5 Too tying — wish to go out or go back to work.
6 Fear of cracked nipples and painful engorgement.
7 Other people can help with feeding.

Physiology of lactation

During pregnancy the secretory alveoli and lactiferous ducts of the breast develop under the influence of oestrogens, progesterone, adreno-corticosteroids and prolactin. Milk secretion is stimulated by prolactin, a hormone produced by the anterior pituitary gland. During pregnancy, milk secretion is kept at a low level as high blood oestrogen and progesterone levels suppress prolactin release. After delivery the levels fall and prolactin is released, stimulating milk production. Between feeds milk is secreted into the lumen of the alveolus. At feed time milk is ejected into the ducts where it is available to the sucking infant by the 'draught' reflex (Fig. 6.1). This neurohumoral reflex is stimulated not only by the sucking action of the infant on the richly innervated nipple but also by psychological stimuli such as hearing the infant cry and thinking about the approaching feed time. The reflex mechanism is mediated via the hypothalamus to the postpituitary where oxytocin is released, causing contraction of the myo-epithelial cells which envelop the alveoli. The sucking infant will not be able to obtain milk unless active propulsion also occurs. Tension and anxiety may inhibit the draught reflex, setting up a cycle of frustrated hunger and further worry.

The amount, vigour and frequency of sucking have a powerful effect

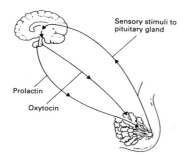

Fig. 6.1 Lactation and breast feeding. Prolactin from the anterior pituitary gland causes the lacteal glands to secrete milk. Oxytocin from the posterior pituitary acts on the myo-epithelial cells surrounding the glands and causes the milk to be secreted into the lactiferous ducts and thence to the nipple. Oxytocin also stimulates the output of more prolactin.

on milk secretion. The sucking stimulus not only promotes a good release of oxytocin but also increases the output of prolactin and hence promotes milk supply. It is useful for mothers to be aware of the link between frequent suckling and stimulation of milk production and if the baby appears to be unsatisfied more frequent feeds, up to two-hourly, encourage increased milk supply. There is no evidence that it is necessary to empty the breasts at a feed but prolonged engorgement, particularly in the early puerperium, can suppress potential lactation.

Composition of colostrum and mature milk

Colostrum is produced initially in small quantities up to 50 ml a day. It differs from mature breast milk, containing five times as much protein initially, and less fat, carbohydrate and calories. It contains more elec-trolytes, lysosyme and lactoferrin. About one-fifth of the protein is casein and four-fifths is a mixture of soluble whey proteins of which half is secretory IgA. By the third or fourth day transitional milk leads on to the production of mature milk.

Human milk has a higher fat content than cow's milk but tends to have a more watery appearance because the fat is more finely divided. Mothers may be anxious about this watery appearance giving the impression that the milk is weak and under-nutritious and it can be reassuring to explain the changes in composition of milk and its variation during feeding. At the beginning of a feed breast milk contains more protein and less fat giving a watery appearance. Towards the end the milk is creamier due to a fourfold increase in fat content. Compo-sition of milk also varies between different feeds in the day, the concentration of fat being least in the early hours of the morning. After the first month the volume of breast milk secreted and taken by the baby increases relatively little compared with the infant's rapid growth rate. Maternal milk volume averages 600 ml a day at two months rising to 900 ml at six months. As the baby grows his increased energy requirement is provided by an increase in fat content in the milk.

Initial stages of breast-feeding

Studies on demand feeding in maternity units have shown that as lactation is being established the infant's demand for feeding rises to a maximum of 10−12 times daily by the fifth day. During the first few days, before the supply of breast milk is properly established the baby has a physiological weight loss averaging 230 g (7%) due to redistribution of body fluids along with loss of water from the body. Supplementary feeds should not be given to prevent hunger and weight loss at this time as the baby's vigorous sucking is an important factor in stimulating milk production. It is not surprising therefore that adhering to a four-hour schedule in the early stages will not fulfil the baby's needs and may discourage persevering with breast-feeding. Studies of milk composition indicate that human milk is similar to that of animals who carry their young around and feed them continuously or frequently. Mothers who appreciate the need for frequent feeds are less likely to run into problems with lactation.

Outline of management of breast-feeding by the doctor, midwife and health visitor

ANTENATALLY

1   Discuss expectant mother's feeding preferences pointing out pros and cons of breast and bottle.
2   Provide basic information on physiology of lactation including the let-down reflex, and the mechanism of milk stimulation.
3   Check nipples and advise on how to draw out retracted nipples between finger and thumb.
4   Suggest that mother asks to put the baby to the breast as soon as possible after delivery, preferably in the delivery room. The infant is likely to be more alert and eager to suck immediately after birth than in the next couple of days.
5   Warn mother that her infant is likely to appear hungry for the first few days and may need feeding up to a dozen times daily initially. Complement only with boiled water.

6 Discourage using complementary milk feeds both in hospital and after discharge since the infant will spend less time sucking and milk supply will dwindle.

7 Point out that many mothers need guidance on breast-feeding technique and advise asking for help from nursing staff as soon as difficulties arise.

8 Give mother telephone number of health visitor and midwife to phone when she comes out of hospital and if she has problems. Also, the local branch of National Childbirth Trust, Lalleche League or Association of Breast-Feeding Mothers can provide help and support.

AFTER DISCHARGE

9 Visit the mother as soon as possible after discharge. Many mothers give up breast-feeding at this time.

10 Observe feeding and check that nipple is correctly inserted into baby's mouth and the breast is not obstructing the baby's nostrils.

11 Advise starting each feed on alternate breasts. Express milk only if mother feels discomfort after a feed, over-expression encourages over-production of milk and further engorgement.

12 Some babies may appear satisfied after only five minutes' feeding. Reassure that this is quite normal since babies obtain 90% of feed in the first five minutes. After a few weeks 10–15 minutes each side is average, which usually provides sufficient nourishment and sucking stimulation.

13 Discuss a sensible demand-feeding schedule. Explain that babies may sometimes need feeding every two to three hours and at others every four to five hours. Demand feeding is intended to give both mother and baby flexibility. Feeds can be brought forward or delayed for an hour or so to fit in with the mother's schedule such as when there are older children to take and collect from school.

14 Explain that if baby appears hungry increasing frequency of feeds up to two-hourly stimulates milk supply. Discuss reasons other than hunger why baby may be crying such as thirst, wet nappy, wind, demand for attention.

15 Introduce mother to other mothers who are successfully breast-feeding.

Early problems with breast-feeding

RETRACTED NIPPLES

The nipples should be examined around the sixth month of pregnancy to determine whether they protract when the areola is squeezed. About a quarter of pregnant women may have retracted nipples but if Waller's glass or plastic shields are worn in the last trimester studies have shown that all will have protractile nipples when the baby is born. Drawing the nipples out with thumb and finger, imitating the action of the baby's jaw, also helps nipples to protract.

DIFFICULTY FIXING BABY ON TO BREAST

Mothers often need help with the technique of breast-feeding initially and correct positioning is very important. The baby should take the whole of the nipple into his mouth, placing his gums round the areola so that the nipple lies between the tongue and the palate. Soreness can easily develop if the baby grasps the nipple rather than the areola. The small, sick or sleepy infant may be reluctant to suck and require patience and encouragement. If the infant is too weak to suck initially milk can be expressed manually and given by spoon, but a nasogastric tube may be necessary. The supply of breast milk can be maintained by use of a breast pump until the infant is able to suck the breast. Some babies may appear to actively resist sucking and cry with frustration. A nurse or midwife can be of great assistance for the first few feeds by holding the baby on to the breast. Poorly protractile nipples may make fixation difficult. The mother should draw her nipples out first to enable suckling to take place and the nurse or midwife can help to hold the breast in the baby's mouth so that the sucking action can draw out the nipple and enable suckling. The mother should be encouraged to draw her nipples outwards between fingers and thumb several times a day and continue to wear Waller shields.

PAINFUL NIPPLES

Sore nipples may easily develop during the early weeks due to prolonged vigorous sucking particularly on poorly protractile nipples. The problem is best avoided by treating non-protractile nipples prenatally, ensuring that the infant grasps the areola and gradually increasing feeding time from two minutes up to 10 minutes each side. The nipple is so sensitive that even a tiny erosion is exquisitely painful and may discourage continuing with feeding. Superficial erosions and petechial lesions tend to occur during the first week whereas after this time a fissure crack may appear at the side of the nipple.

Antiseptics such as Rotacept spray and local anaesthetics should be avoided in the treatment of sore nipples. A popular remedy is the application of egg white. Wearing breast pads may encourage sogginess and soreness. An alternative is to protect the nipple by the plastic mesh cut from a tea strainer. Petechial lesions and ulcers can be successfully treated with a steroid and neomycin cream (washed off before feeds). The fissure ulcer is often infected with thrush, requiring application of Nystan cream.

ENGORGEMENT

Painful engorgement of the breasts developing at about the fourth of fifth day is due to both increased blood flow and accumulation of milk. The more engorged the breast becomes, the less the nipple is protractile, creating a vicious circle of difficulties in suckling and further engorgement. Manual expression of milk after feeds just sufficient to relieve any residual feeling of fullness and discomfort prevents serious engorgement developing. If manual expression is unsuccessful a sterilized breast pump can be used. However, complete emptying of the breasts after each feed is unnecessary and may create further problems as this process will stimulate additional milk production rather than allowing the baby's demand to regulate supply.

MASTITIS

Mastitis may occur in the early stage of breast-feeding when engorgement is common but also sporadically during lactation and weaning. A nipple abrasion may provide a portal of entry for staphylococci, or infection may arise in a distended segment of breast. Superficial mastitis is infection of the skin or areola which then spreads into the breast. Treatment is with flucloxacillin 250 mg six-hourly, and occasionally incision of a local abscess is necessary. In intramammary mastitis typically a whole segment of the breast becomes distended and milk stagnates leading to secondary infection. The overlying skin is red and there is often fever, severe pain, a firm swelling and axillary lymphadenopathy. Early treatment with penicillin 500 mg and flucloxacillin 500 mg six-hourly should prevent abscess formation.

Emptying of the breast assists resolution and the continuation of feeding should be encouraged with the help of analgesics. Supplementary manual emptying of the breast may be necessary.

BREAST-MILK JAUNDICE

Breast-milk jaundice may occasionally complicate breast-feeding, usually presenting a week after birth and persisting for six to eight weeks. It arises as a result of the presence of an inhibitor to hepatic glucuronyl transferase in the mother's milk which prevents conjugation of bilirubin. Thus the infant's blood may contain up to 20 mg (per 100 ml) (340 mmol) of unconjugated, lipid-soluble bilirubin. If the infant is deeply jaundiced in the first week, breast-feeding may be interrupted for a few days but can be safely resumed when the bilirubin has come down. After the first week the blood–brain barrier is no longer permeable to bilirubin. Moderate breast-milk jaundice is not an indication for stopping breast-feeding but may make the baby sleepy.

BREAST-FEEDING AND HIV

Infection with HIV has been reported to have been transmitted from an HIV-seropositive mother to her infant by breast-feeding. It is therefore recommended that women known to be HIV antibody-positive or those at high risk who have not been serologically tested should be discourage from breast-feeding in the UK (Oppé *et al.*, 1988).

EXCRETION OF SUBSTANCES IN BREAST MILK

A wide variety of substances including alcohol and nicotine pass unchanged into breast milk. Although alcohol may make the baby sleepy no serious ill effects have been found with moderate intake. Nicotine has not been shown to have harmful effects but there are numerous other reasons, such as a higher incidence of respiratory illness, why smoking should be discouraged whatever the method of feeding.

Prescribing for the lactating as for the pregnant mother should be carefully considered and guidelines are given in the British National Formulary.

Many therapeutic substances are excreted in milk and the baby receives roughly one-tenth of the mother's dose. Methaemoglobinaemia and vitamin D deficiency have been reported with phenobarbitone and phenytoin. Phenobarbitone, diazepam, antidepressants and other psychotropic drugs can cause sedation in the infant. Therefore these drugs are best avoided completely during lactation and mothers on anti-epileptic drugs should be advised not to breast-feed. As there is a small risk of aspirin causing a bleeding tendency it is prudent to recommend paracetamol as an analgesic during lactation. Anticoagulants can also cause bleeding problems and most authorities consider that breast-feeding is contra-indicated during therapy.

Antibiotics, salicylates, barbiturates and sulphonamides may cause skin rashes in the baby. Penicillin sensitivity can be transmitted by this route and bowel flora can be disturbed. Tetracyclines are best avoided. Metronidazole may give a bitter taste to the milk.

Senna anthraquinones and phenolphthalein laxatives taken by the mother can have an aperient effect on the baby but no other laxatives do this. Bronchodilators of the sympathomimetic groups should be given by aerosol to reduce the amount reaching the baby. Theophylline is probably safe as are digoxin, propranolol and thiazides. Continuous therapy with high doses of corticosteroids (>10 mg prednisolone daily) may affect the infant's adrenal function.

The combined oral contraceptive pill is contra-indicated in lactating mothers since it suppresses milk production. On the other hand the progesterone only pill (POP) does not interfere significantly with the quantity and quality of breast milk. A very tiny amount of the hormone in the POP has been shown to get into the milk, the least being found in milk from women who use pills containing only levonorgestrel — especially Norgeston and Microval.

Stopping breast-feeding

Breast-feeding even for a few days offers advantages to the infant since he receives valuable antibodies. The ideal period for breast-feeding is probably three to six months although some mothers are happy to breast-feed for longer periods, well after the first year. Delaying weaning until after three months avoids exposing the infant to cow's milk at a time when the gastrointestinal tract is less resistant to passage of antigens. Milk production increases in quantity and protein and energy content during the early months until by six months about 900 ml (approximately one and a half pints) are produced. After four months the infant is likely to need iron from additional food sources such as eggs, vegetables and meat.

In the national survey (Martin & Monk, 1980) the proportion of mothers still breast-feeding at six weeks, four months and six months was 42%, 27% and 23% respectively.

Gradual weaning from the breast is best achieved over a four- to six-week period, replacing one feed at a time with milk formula from a bottle or cup. Stopping more rapidly entails a risk of engorgement and breast infection. Parents with a family history of allergy may be advised to use soya milk during the first year.

Mothers often get upset when their baby cries furiously when offered a bottle and refuses to suck from it, closing his lips tightly and turning away. Sometimes the bottle is accepted more readily from the father or a friend. As a rule if the bottle is offered every day the infant will eventually accept it. Reluctance and irritability at first is not surprising since the breast is strongly attractive to the infant and the bottle is a strange experience. The infant may not like the taste of cow's milk at first since it is less sweet than breast milk. Sweetening the first one or two feeds may be effective in encouraging acceptance of the bottle but this practice should not be continued for obvious reasons.

Nutritional requirement of the infant — formulae, composition of human, cow's and modified cow's milk

Providing a substitute for breast milk requires knowledge of the nutritional requirements of the average baby. The daily energy requirements for a baby on the 50th centile for weight is 110 kcal per kg of expected weight but some babies need more and some less. The calculated requirement makes allowance for basal metabolic rate, growth, activity and replacement of heat loss. If a baby is contented and thriving coaxing him to take more feed will result in laying down of extra tissue fat. The energy value of human and cow's milk is similar, around 70 kcal per 100 ml or 20 kcal per oz (Table 6.1).

WATER

The term infant requires 150–175 ml per kg of fluid per day. After the age of a year fluid requirements per unit bodyweight diminish to about 1.5 litres a day throughout childhood. The relative amounts of water and solids in human and cow's milk are about the same.

ELECTROLYTES

Cow's milk contains four times as much sodium and two and a half times as much potassium as mature breast milk. Colostrum contains a relatively high concentration of sodium, which is essential for the development of the secretory function of the mammary gland but since the volume of colostrum is small the total intake by the newborn infant is not harmful. Modified cow's milk formula contains reduced levels of sodium, chloride and phosphorus, but the levels of these solutes are still higher than in human milk. Particularly in the first three months urine-concentrating capacity is limited so that the kidneys cannot handle sodium overload without excreting large volumes of water. Hence, if fluid is restricted or lost through diarrhoea, there is a

Table 6.1 Composition of milk.

Constituent (g per litre) except where stated)	Mature human milk (mean)	Cow's milk (mean)
Energy (kcal per litre)	7·47	7·01
Protein		
Total	10·6	30·9
Casein	3·7	25·0
Lactalbumin	3·6	2·3
Lactoglobulin	2·0	2·1
Amino acids		
Total	12·8	33·0
Essential total	5·4	19·6
Fats		
Total	45·4	38·0
Carbohydrate		
Lactose	71·0	47·0
Minerals (mg per litre)		
Sodium	18·9	77·0
Potassium	55·3	143·0
Calcium	27·1	137·0
Magnesium	3·5	13·0
Iron	0·5	0·4

From *Geigy Scientific Tables* (1977) and McLaren & Blennan (1976).

danger of hypertonic, hyperosmolar dehydration. This danger is increased if mothers make feeds too strong or when a thirsty baby is given extra food instead of water. Hyperosmolality has been shown to cause permanent neurological damage and is present in some babies with sudden infant death syndrome.

PROTEIN

The protein intake of a breast-fed infant ingesting 150 mg per kg per day is 1.8–2.5 kg per day. Human milk contains less than half the amount of protein per litre (10.6 g) contained in cow's milk (30.9 g) but contains relatively more lactalbumin (whey) than caseinogen (casein). In some cow's milk formulae (group I) the protein is unmodified but reduced in amount and in others (group II) using demineralized whey the protein has been modified so that the ratio of whey protein (lactalbumin) to casein resembles human milk more closely.

CARBOHYDRATE

Of total daily calories 40—50% is derived from carbohydrate (10—15 g per kg per day) during the first year of life. Both human and cow's milk contain lactose in proportions of 6.7—7% and 4.5% respectively. Most modified milks contain additional lactose.

FAT

Fats usually provide more than 50% of calories (5—6 kg per day). Fatty acids in human milk reflect maternal diet to some extent and generally cow's milk has less polyunsaturated fat (linoleic, arachidonic) than human milk. Most modified formulae have a mixture of vegetable and animal fat substituted for butter fat resulting in a composition of fatty acids resembling human milk fat more closely than the fat in cow's milk.

MINERALS

Calcium, phosphorus, magnesium, iron, copper, zinc, sulphur, cobalt, iodine and fluorine are all required by the growing infant. Human milk contains more iron and copper than cow's milk. The levels of the other minerals are somewhat lower in human milk but are adequate for the infant's needs. The infant accumulates iron stores in the liver during the last month of pregnancy. The iron in breast milk together with stored iron are sufficient for blood formation during the first six months but after this time iron stores are almost exhausted and iron is needed in the diet. Formula milks usually contain sufficient iron for the infant's needs during the first six months. The infant of short gestation is likely to be deficient in iron stores and may require iron supplement in the form of ferrous fumarate or gluconate to prevent anaemia.

VITAMINS

Human and cow's milk both contain adequate amounts of vitamin A, thiamine, riboflavin and nicotinic acid. Cow's milk is low in vitamins C and D whereas breast milk usually contains adequate amounts provided the mother's intake is satisfactory and exposure to sunlight is sufficient. Modified milks are fortified with vitamins C and D. Vitamin D is present in concentration of about 400—440 i.u. per litre. The infant requires 400 i.u. per day. *Present-day practice in infant feeding* (Oppé *et al.*, 1988) recommends that all mothers, whether breast- or bottle-feeding, give their babies vitamin drops from the age of one month until at least two years, and until five years of age when the diet is less than optimal. Children's vitamin drops are available from child health clinics and the recommended dose of five drops daily gives the child approximately 700 i.u. of vitamin A, 300 i.u. of vitamin D and 20 mg of vitamin C.

A vitamin supplement is particularly important in certain groups of children: low-birthweight infants, those who receive household milk, children from some ethnic minorities and those who have reduced exposure to ultraviolet radiation on the skin. Only one preparation of supplementary vitamins should be used as excesses of vitamins can be harmful. A dose of vitamin D equivalent to about four to fourteen doses of children's vitamin drops given daily for several weeks has been associated with hypercalcaemia in children particularly sensitive to vitamin D. Excess vitamin A is probably only harmful in about a twentyfold dose whereas excesses of vitamin C and the B vitamins have no ill effects and are excreted in the urine.

Infant formulae based on cow's milk

GROUP I

Group I consists of skimmed milk (which contains all nutrients of cow's milk except fat and fat-soluble vitamins) with added carbo-hydrates and mixed fats. The protein is unmodified cow's milk protein, the fat is a mixture of vegetable oils and animal fats and the carbo-hydrate is lactose from skimmed milk plus either more lactose or maltodextrin and starch. Examples:
Cow and Gate Plus (added lactose).
Milumil (added maltodextrin and starch).
Ostermilk Complete Formula (added maltodextrin).
Ostermilk Two (added maltodextrin).
SMA (added lactose).

GROUP II

Group II consists of skimmed milk with demineralized whey and mixed fats. The protein is modified to contain proportionately more whey proteins (lactalbumin) and less casein. The fat is a mixture of vegetable oils and animal fats. The carbohydrate is lactose from skimmed milk and demineralized whey. The mineral content is reduced by use

of demineralized whey to approach the mineral concentration of human milk. Examples:
Cow and Gate Premium.
Osterfeed.
SMA Gold Cap.
Nan (Nestlé).

Soya-based milk substitutes

Some soya-based milks are suitable as the sole source of nourishment for young infants. Examples:
Formula S Soya Food.
Pro Sobee.
Isomil.
Wysoy.
These milks are free of lactose as well as cow's milk protein. Occasionally allergies to soya protein may develop.

Goat's milk

Like cow's milk, unmodified goat's milk is unsuitable for nutrition of infants under the age of six months. It contains an excess of protein and minerals and a deficiency of some vitamins. Boiling is necessary to reduce the risk of tuberculosis, brucellosis and other infections but this process further reduces the concentration of folic acid and heat-labile vitamins. Goat's milk may be used in infant feeding after six months but vitamins A, D, C, folic acid and B_{12} must be included in the diet or given as a supplement. Allergy to goat's milk protein may develop.

Bottle-feeding

PREPARATION OF FEED

Instructions on reconstituting dried milks should be followed accurately and hygienically. Guidance on making up feeds is needed antenatally and in the lying-in period. The bottle and teats are first washed and then sterilized either by boiling or immersion in hypochlorite solution for one and a half to three hours. Hurriedly dipping bottles in the solution does not achieve adequate sterilization. Milk can be made up directly in the bottle or in a sterilized jug. The required amount of milk powder is measured out in the scoop provided and placed in the bottle or jug. The milk should be loosely contained in the scoop rather than packed down and the top should be levelled off using a knife. Generally, 1 oz (about 30 ml) of just boiled water is added per scoop of powder though adding an extra 0.5 oz is a safeguard against over-concentrated feeds. The resulting volume of milk will be greater than the amount of water added due to the added bulk of the milk powder.

Reconstituted milk can be stored in a refrigerator for 24 hours and brought up to body temperature before using. Keeping milk warm for several hours in an insulated container is inadvisable since bacteria may be incubated.

The health visitor or midwife should observe that feeds are being made up correctly since mishaps can have serious consequences. The quantity of milk in the scoop and the amount of water added need careful checking to avoid over-strength feeds. If a baby appears hungry some mothers may be tempted to add an extra scoop of milk powder. Mixing over-strength feeds or giving a thirsty baby extra milk instead of water can lead to hypernatraemia.

TECHNIQUE, FREQUENCY AND AMOUNTS OF FEEDS

The formula is warmed so that a drop shaken on the back of the hand feels warm but not hot. The teat should have a hole which allows milk to drip readily but not too fast when the bottle is held upside down. The infant normally takes 10–20 minutes to complete a feed. Boiled water is usually given for the first 12 hours after birth and then a small milk feed of about 30 ml. Over the next few days feeds are increased to about 90–120 ml per feed given at three- to four-hourly intervals according to demand. The infant needs about 150 ml per kg per day (2½ fl. oz per lb per day). For an infant weighing 3.5 kg this means six feeds of 90 ml at the end of the first week. The amount taken at each feed may vary and it is sensible to offer the infant 20 to 30 ml more than he usually takes. As he is growing rapidly in the early weeks the amount offered will need to be increased every week or so to keep up with his increasing demand. By about three months the average infant weighing 6 kg will be taking five feeds of 180 ml (6 oz).

Bottle- and breast-fed babies should gain 110–220 g (4–8 oz) a week for the first four months of life, falling to 90–200 g (3–7 oz) in the second four months and to 60–110 g (2–4 oz) a week in the third four months.

Water and juices

Babies often get thirsty between milk feeds, particularly in hot weather. Mothers should be encouraged to offer extra drinks from the early weeks. Water is preferable initially but after four weeks the infant can have juices in the appropriate dilution. There are a number of sucrose-free juices available which have the advantage of being less harmful to the teeth.

Introduction of solid foods

AGE OF INTRODUCTION OF SOLIDS

Introduction of solid foods before the age of three months has no proven nutritional advantage and evidence suggests that it may predispose to the development of obesity and allergy and increase the risk of hypernatraemia due to high solute load. *Present-day Practice in Infant Feeding* (Oppé et al., 1988) recommends starting solids between the ages of three and six months. Nevertheless the 1980 and 1985 Infant Feeding Surveys reported that 55% of mothers had given solid food by three months and 14% by six weeks. Bottle-fed babies were likely to receive solids earlier than breast-fed infants. Cereal and rusks were the most common first foods introduced.

Despite the DHSS recommendation, many mothers clearly feel that their infant needs solid food either to satisfy hunger or to help with sleeping through the night. The advice of friends and family rather than the health visitor or doctor may be heeded. More education is needed antenatally since once a mother has started using solids it is difficult and indeed undesirable to persuade her to withdraw them.

CHEWING

Chewing is an important achievement in the development of feeding behaviour. Chewing movements begin around eight weeks and are well developed by 12−16 weeks. The ability to transfer food from the tongue to the back of the mouth in order to swallow it develops by three to four months. The infant needs to practice chewing at four to five months whilst the skill is developing or it may not be properly acquired (Illingworth & Lister, 1964). Chewing may be delayed in mentally retarded infants and the gradual introduction of lumpy foods needs to be postponed until chewing movements emerge.

Around four to five months the infant readily welcomes new flavours and textures but may be more cautious if mixed feeding is delayed until the end of the first year. Success is best achieved by offering only two or three spoonfuls of a new food at a time. Initially cereals or sieved or liquidized food are mixed to a semi-solid consistency. By five months the baby enjoys chewing a rusk, piece of bread or biscuit and at five to six months can begin to cope with small lumps in food. At this time, increasing the lumpiness of food by serving mashed or finely chopped foods allows the infant to become accustomed to meals of varying consistencies. Delay in introducing lumpy foods may lead to a child of a year or more only eating sieved foods, a situation which is difficult to remedy.

Many children do not acquire teeth until after six months, but this does not affect the introduction of lumpy foods. Most infants have some teeth by the end of the first year, by which time they can manage most family foods provided they are cut up into reasonably small pieces.

Foods from three months to one year

Cereals containing rice, oats and barley rather than wheat (to reduce exposure to gluten) are suitable first foods, mixed to a semi-solid consistency with breast milk, milk formula or boiled water according to instructions. Puréed fruits such as apples, pears or bananas, vegetables such as carrots, and plain or fruit yoghurt are also easily digested and nutritious. Egg yolk contains iron and may be added from five to six months. Babies with a family history of allergy may be advised to adopt a low-allergenic weaning programme although there is no conclusive evidence that this is beneficial. Eggs, dairy produce, fish, nuts and fruits with lots of pips are avoided for the first 6–12 months and then cautiously introduced. Advice from a dietitian is advisable if a prolonged low-allergenic diet is planned, to ensure a balanced diet.

By the age of six months the normal infant usually has three meals a day and various kinds of minced meats and fish can be introduced. It is recommended that either breast milk or milk formula should be continued until the age of one year. After six months the infant needs at least 500 ml (1 pint) of breast or milk formula. Once the infant is eating three meals a day fruit juice can be substituted for one or more of the meal-time milk feeds. In view of the risk of obesity and dental caries, added sugar (sucrose) should be kept to a minimum and additional salt should be avoided. The infant's food may taste bland to an adult's palate but there is sufficient natural sugar and salt in fresh foods for nutritional needs. Some prepared baby foods have especially low salt contents and no added sugar or artificial colourings or flavourings.

From six months onwards the baby gradually adopts the family feeding pattern. He will be able to finger-feed from about six months and start to hold a spoon at nine months. Efficient self-feeding with a spoon is achieved around 15 months and it is advisable to allow the infant to practise this skill despite the messiness and time involved.

Vitamin A, D and C supplements are advisable at least during the first two years and until the age of five where the diet is less than optimal.

Diet from one to five years

By the end of the first year the child's protein and calorie requirements per unit bodyweight are beginning to fall along with a corresponding deceleration of weight gain. The infant requires 110 kcal per kg per day falling to 60 kcal per kg per day by the age of 10 years. The drop in calorie requirement and weight gain may lead to parental anxiety over adequacy of nutrition. Plotting the child's weight on a percentile chart will demonstrate to parents that their child is behaving in the same way as others of his age. It is difficult to specify an exact diet for any child since requirements and energy output vary widely. A simple guide to a balanced diet would include daily:

> 600 ml (1 pint) of milk.
> One portion of meat, fish, poultry or pulses.
> One egg.
> Vegetables.
> Fruit, preferably citrus.
> Staples such as bread, cereals, pasta and potatoes to fill the energy gap.

With the mounting evidence of the influence of diet on obesity and on a wide variety of diseases in adulthood such as ischaemic heart disease, vascular disease, hypertension, diabetes, appendicitis, diverticulitis, hiatus hernia, and cancers such as bowel cancer, it seems logical to bring children up with eating habits which are least likely to impair their future health. Intake of high-fibre foods, such as wholemeal bread, bran, pulses and vegetables such as peas and sweet-corn, should be encouraged. Refined carbohydrates (i.e. sugary foods) and fatty foods should be kept to a minimum. Potato chips, crisps, sweetened fizzy drinks, sweets, biscuits and chocolate are particularly undesirable as they satisfy the appetite but have excessive amounts of calories, fat and refined carbohydrates.

Vegetarian diets

An increasing number of young children are receiving vegetarian diets because of parental preference for religious, health, social or cultural reasons, or dislike of meat products. Vegetarian diets can supply all necessary nutrients provided vegetables are selected from different classes. Vegetables are high in fibre content, vitamins and minerals. Pulses can contain up to 40% protein. Vegetarians usually have faster gastrointestinal transfer times, bulkier stools and lower serum cholesterol levels. Vegetarians who exclude eggs and milk are known as vegans and may develop vitamin B_{12} deficiency and deficiency of trace elements such as zinc due to the high-fibre intake. Vegan children and pregnant vegan mothers need vitamin B_{12} and mineral supplements. After breast-feeding has ceased the growing vegetarian child requires a suitable milk substitute to maintain adequate nutrition. Soya milks are usually acceptable to vegans.

Common feeding problems in infancy

POOR SUCKING AND SLOW FEEDING

The infant who sucks weakly, who tires easily or who refuses the bottle or breast before a reasonable amount is consumed causes great concern to his mother. Some disorders such as oral thrush may be easy to detect and remedy but often the problem is complex and requires patient history-taking by the health visitor and doctor and ideally observation of feeding. When an infant presents with a history of poor feeding it is essential to measure weight gain, preferably based on repeated weighings since birth. This not only gives an indication of the seriousness of the problem but also pin-points the onset.

Sucking is the young infant's most exhausting activity and not surprisingly small or ill infants tire easily. The mother of the small or preterm infant should be encouraged to offer small quantities of milk of 30–60 ml (1–2 oz) every two to three hours in the early stages rather than spend longer periods trying to complete a larger feed.

Underlying infection may be the root of failure to suck adequately. Oral thrush, ear infection, skin or umbilical sepsis, pneumonia or urinary tract infection should all be considered. Upper respiratory infection resulting in temporary nasal obstruction commonly affects feeding and can be alleviated by saline, 0.05% xylometazoline or 0.5% ephedrine nose drops given for a few days only together with advice to offer smaller, more frequent feeds.

Cardiac or respiratory disorders associated with rapid breathing

may interfere with sucking. Jaundiced infants and infants with neurological damage may also suck poorly. Congenital abnormalities such as
cleft palate and choanal atresia are other causes of feeding difficulty.

Poor feeding technique may result in the infant consuming too
little milk or taking excessively long at feed time. In the breast-fed
infant the most frequent difficulties arise from incorrect insertion of
the nipple into the infant's mouth, obstruction of the nose by the
breast and failure to appreciate that frequent, short feeds promote
more successful lactation than prolonged feeds at four-hourly intervals.

In the bottle-fed infant the hole in the teat should be checked and
the bottle should be tilted so that no air enters the teat. Some artificially
fed infants fare better on smaller more frequent feeds along the lines of
breast-feeding schedules.

Frequently feeding problems reflect a mother's inexperience or lack
of confidence. Occasionally the root of the problem lies in a disturbed
mother–child interaction. Perhaps a mother who is impatient in temperament finds she cannot cope with a slow, reflective feeder. Another
possibility is that a mother who is not 'in love' with her baby or who
is depressed, tense or anxious because of her own problems may not
hold her baby in a relaxing and comforting position and may not
recognize the baby's signals of hunger, wind or satisfaction. A mother
who is at a low emotional ebb herself may not be able to respond to
her infant's exhausting demands. This may generate a cycle of dissatis-
faction in which the infant becomes tired and lethargic due to crying
and lack of comfort and is then disinclined to suck at feed time. These
more subtle clues may take some time to identify and the health
visitor is ideally placed to do this in the mother's own home. Since
feeding occupies a large part of the day in the early weeks it is not
surprising that successful feeding together with a satisfactory weight
gain is a sensitive index to the well-being of mother and child. Of
course, the father and other members of the family may be involved in
feeding and their behaviour and interactions must also be considered
when assessing a feeding problem.

REGURGITATION AND VOMITING

Regurgitation of a mouthful of food often occurs soon after a feed
when the baby is being winded. It is common in hungry, lusty feeders
who consume more milk rapidly and also in the slow, difficult feeder,
who probably takes in excessive air which encourages regurgitation of
milk on winding.

The hole in the teat should be checked, as too large a hole allows gulping of milk and air, leading to regurgitation. Provided that the baby is not being overfed and is thriving, parents can be reassured that some regurgitation is no cause for concern.

The term vomiting is applied to return of stomach contents rather forcefully in large amounts, often after an interval following a feed. Vomiting (and diarrhoea) may occur with any infective condition such as gastroenteritis, otitis media, respiratory or urinary tract infection or meningitis. Projectile vomiting is characteristic of pyloric stenosis and is associated with weight loss, visible peristalsis and a palpable pyloric 'tumour' felt during a feed.

A fairly common cause of regurgitation and vomiting in the infant is gastro-oesophageal reflux due to an incompetent lower oesophageal sphincter. In mild cases weight gain is not affected and the vomiting diminishes if the infant is propped up for an hour after feeds and the feed is thickened with a thickening agent such as Carobel, Nestargel (containing carob seed) or Benger Food (containing wheat flour). A considerable proportion of infants with gastro-oesophageal reflux suffer from chronic cough. Aspiration pneumonia is a possible complication to watch out for. Infants with respiratory symptoms and poor weight gain with signs of oesophagitis such as haematemesis need referral for further assessment and more intensive treatment. These symptoms may be associated with hiatus hernia in which the upper part of the stomach lies in the thorax. Most infants with hiatus hernia improve with propping up after feeds, thickened feeds and the use of antacids between feeds. Surgery is rarely necessary. In simple reflux, symptoms diminish during the second six months as the oesophageal sphincter becomes more competent.

Rumination is a form of chronic regurgitation either associated with gastro-oesophageal reflux or self-induced by the infant. The infant may produce this by vigorously moving the abdomen or occasionally may actively gag himself with the tongue or fingers. It may occur as a habit in the under-stimulated, emotionally deprived infant and is an indication to look closely at the mother−child relationship.

WIND AND COLIC

The infant always swallows some air with the feed and will take in large gulps when crying. Commonly wind starts to build up due to crying, but the ensuing discomfort causes still more crying and further air swallowing. Most babies bring up wind easily when held in the upright position either in the middle or after a feed. The infant continues to bring up wind whilst lying in the cot preferably on the abdomen.

A hungry baby who sucks ravenously may take in large amounts of air which causes him to stop sucking midway through the feed.

Sometimes a little warm boiled water given before the feed may help. At the start of a breast feed, milk may enter the baby's mouth too fast as a result of the let-down reflex and the baby may gulp and take in air. This may be prevented by expressing the initial rush of milk. In the bottle-fed infant the hole in the teat should allow milk to drip readily when the bottle is held upside down. Too large a hole will lead to excessively rapid intake of milk and air.

The term colic describes paroxysmal abdominal pain often associated with screaming attacks. Typically the problem occurs in infants under three months, often at one particular time of day, usually the evening. Parents usually describe bouts of screaming associated with drawing up of the knees, distended abdomen, flushed face and clenched fists. The infant does not respond to usual methods of comforting such as feeding, dummies or cuddling and parents may resort to taking the child out in the pram or car, often without success. The bout may be relieved if the infant passes a bowel motion or flatus or may continue until the infant is exhausted and eventually falls asleep.

In our study about half the mothers of six-week-old babies reported that their baby suffered from excessive wind and colic two or three days a week, and half of these reported it occurring most days. Clearly wind and colic occur so commonly that they must be regarded as part of the pattern of normal infant development. However, in a few infants the problem is such that it dominates a large part of the baby's waking hours and can strain parent–child relationships to breaking point. Fortunately, as our study showed, virtually all colicky infants are happy and contented at six months.

Colic has recently been linked to cow's milk protein. One study (Jakobsson & Lindberg, 1983) found that, in half of a group of breast-fed babies with colic, the problem disappeared when mothers were put on a diet free from cow's milk. It may be worth trying cow's milk avoidance in severe cases of colic but the problem is so common that such measures would not be appropriate for the majority of babies.

Dicyclomine, an antispasmodic, is effective in relieving colic but should not be prescribed for infants under six months. Certain commercial antacid mixtures are formulated for infants and may help alleviate symptoms. Herbal teas such as camomile and fennel are increasingly popular although as yet there are no studies to support their efficacy. Carrying the baby around in a baby sling, particularly if this is started from birth, has been shown to reduce colicky crying (Hunziker & Barr, 1986).

Other behavioural and physical conditions may be interpreted by parents as being wind or colic. Underfeeding and overfeeding may both result in crying and excessive wind. Mothers may be tempted to offer more feed to a crying infant but the infant may be thirsty rather than hungry and settle better with a drink of boiled water. It is important to rule out other painful conditions such as strangulated hernia, otitis media or intussusception. Crying may be thought to be due to colic when it is actually a signal for more attention. Some very young infants require and demand an enormous amount of attention. Some mothers may be anxious not to 'spoil' their baby by picking him up too often, but it is doubtful that very young babies can be 'spoiled' in this way. Babies like a consistent response which is gauged to their individual needs.

There is no doubt that the symptom of colic occurring most days is wearing to even the most patient and loving parent. Despite the fact that little can be done in the way of treatment the complaint should always be taken seriously. In our experience sympathy and support from the health visitor and doctor are by far the most important aspects of the management of colic until the condition resolves spontaneously, usually by three months.

TEETHING

Teething probably causes a variety of short-lived minor symptoms such as crying at night, irritability and loose stools, but the diagnosis should only be made when other more serious causes have been excluded. Parents may attribute these health problems to teething over a matter of weeks or even months but another reason should be sought for any symptoms lasting more than a week or two. Paracetamol syrup is probably as effective as any treatment for teething but again it should not be administered for longer than a few days.

Common variations in infants' stools — normal and abnormal

The colour, consistency and frequency of normal infant stools vary widely and commonly give rise to maternal anxiety.

The breast-fed baby's stools may be yellow or green and vary in consistency from almost liquid to a soft paste. The average breast-fed baby passes a motion after each feed but may have as many as eight motions a day and continue to thrive. Conversely the interval between bowel actions may be as long as 10 days without adversely affecting the baby. Mothers may worry that this represents constipation but can be reassured that provided the baby is contented and the stools remain soft, there is no need to alter feeding patterns. The underfed breast-fed baby may pass frequent, small, dark green motions. The greedy, demanding baby may be taking more breast milk than he requires, which leads to the passage of frequent stools in large amounts.

The artificially fed infant usually has paler, firmer stools with a more offensive smell. Green soft stools occur as a result of increased transit time through the gut and are normal in an otherwise healthy infant. They may occur during the recovery phase after an attack of gastroenteritis. Small, hard green stools are more characteristic of underfeeding.

Bowel action in the bottle-fed infant is on average one to four times a day, usually after feeds as a result of the gastrocolic reflex. Constipation is more common in the bottle-fed baby and the passage of hard stools may lead to anal abrasion with bleeding. Mothers may interpret straining as being due to constipation but it does not necessarily mean that the baby is in discomfort or having difficulty with defaecation; if the stools remain soft mothers can be reassured that this represents the normal effort involved in defaecation. Underfeeding may lead to the infrequent passage of hard stools and increasing the amount of feed may give more frequent stools. Some healthy babies absorb more water from the colon than others do, leading to hard stools. Where milk intake seems adequate, increasing the water intake either as boiled water or dilute fruit juice helps soften stools. Addition of a teaspoon of brown sugar to the formula acts as a mild aperient but should be restricted to once or twice a day for a week or two only as the baby will receive unnecessary calories, and excessive sugar intake can lead to an osmotic diuresis. After the age of three months aperient foods such as sieved prunes and vegetables can be effective in managing constipation but a few infants may require other measures.

A painful anal fissure may need application of xylocaine ointment and occasionally glycerine suppositories are indicated to ease stubborn constipation. Some babies over three months may require a non-absorbed bulk-forming agent such as sodium docusate, which is useful to alleviate the cycle of constipation and pain on defaecation. The child who 'holds back' the act of defaecation either because of a painful anal fissure or sometimes as a result of over-enthusiastic toilet training may develop stubborn constipation, typically associated with overflow of liquid stools around the hard faecal mass. Early treatment of constipation along with encouragement for mothers of toddlers to adopt a relaxed attitude towards toilet training should prevent severe constipation. In older children it may occasionally be necessary to use an aperient such as Senokot syrup and rarely hospital admission for enemas is needed. Hirschsprung's disease, which should be recognized in the neonatal period, is a rare cause of persistent constipation with abdominal distension. Stools are pellets or ribbon-like due to the narrowed aganglionic segment of the rectum and colon. The diagnosis is likely where rectal examination reveals a narrow, undilated, empty rectum.

Frequent, copious stools occur with overfeeding and may be accompanied by excessive weight gain, wind, colic and regurgitation. Crying at the end of a feed may be interpreted as hunger and one occasionally meets the infant who consumes two full bottles of milk at a feed. Convincing a mother that her infant is overfed can be exceedingly difficult. Chronic diarrhoea is discussed in the following section.

Acute gastroenteritis

Acute gastroenteritis is the syndrome of vomiting and/or diarrhoea of acute onset due to infection of the gastrointestinal tract. A similar syndrome also occurs when infection is present elsewhere such as in the respiratory or urinary tracts.

Bacterial pathogens are isolated in only about 10% of children with gastroenteritis admitted to hospital. They are usually enteropathogenic strains of *E. coli, Salmonella, Shigella* and *Campylobacter*. Rotavirus may be identified in up to 50% of children with gastroenteritis in the winter months when this type of infection has a peak incidence. The pathogen may not be identified in a large proportion of children and when viruses are isolated their exact causative role remains uncertain.

A careful history is needed to determine the exact frequency, nature and amount of diarrhoea and vomiting. The child may also have constitutional symptoms such as fever, irritability and colicky abdominal pain. Examination includes looking for other signs of infection, such as otitis media, abdominal examination to detect a surgical lesion and assessment of the state of hydration. In mild dehydration (2−3%) the child will be unduly thirsty and mildly oliguric. At approximately 5% dehydration there will be alteration in skin tone, slightly sunken eyes, thirst, oliguria and sunken fontanelle in infants. Children with this level of dehydration or more will need intravenous fluids.

In the initial stages of gastroenteritis with no dehydration or mild dehydration normal feeds should be replaced by a water−electrolyte mixture either as a commercially available glucose/electrolyte powder such as Dioralyte or as a home-made mixture containing one dessertspoon of sugar and half a teaspoon of salt to one pint of boiled water. It is of the utmost importance not to exceed the recommended salt and sugar levels. Excessive sodium can lead to hypernatraemic dehydration and excess sugar also promotes an osmotic diuresis exacerbating dehydration.

The mixture should be given in frequent small amounts and after 24 hours half-strength milk can be reintroduced. If vomiting or diarrhoea returns, the mixture can be reintroduced for a further 24 hours but return of diarrhoea each time milk is given raises the possibilities of lactose or cow's milk intolerance. These two conditions are discussed on p. 213—14.

Antibiotics have little place in the management of gastroenteritis. An exception is the use of erythromycin for the treatment of severe *Campylobacter* infections with systemic disturbance and the rare occasions when toxicity occurs in severe *Shigella* and *Salmonella* infections. Anti-emetics and drugs such as kaolin preparations and loperamide have no place in the routine management of gastroenteritis in young children.

Chronic diarrhoea in children under five

Chronic diarrhoea is diagnosed when a child passes several loose stools a day for two or more weeks.

HISTORY

A detailed history from the mother will often reveal the cause of chronic diarrhoea in the child. The history should include timing of onset of diarrhoea, particularly in relation to acute gastroenteritis, and introduction of new foods into the diet. The frequency, consistency, colour and odour of stools are all important. General symptoms may be present, notably poor appetite, weight loss and abdominal pain, and the child may demonstrate behavioural disturbances such as difficulty in management, miserable mood and poor sleeping.

PHYSICAL EXAMINATION

The child's weight, height and head circumference should be measured and plotted on a chart with previous measurements. Observations of the child's appearance may reveal lack of subcutaneous fat and this clinical impression of his nutritional status should be viewed in conjunction with the pattern on the growth chart. Abdominal distension, wasted buttocks, muscular hypotonia, pallor and persistent nappy rash may also be observed.

INVESTIGATIONS

Initial investigations

Weight, height, head circumference
Stools
    Culture
    Microscopy for ova, parasites, fat globules, reducing substances
Full blood count and differential white cell count

Further tests

Immunoglobulins especially IgA and IgE
Skin test
Specific radio-allergosorbent test (RAST)
Sweat test
Jejunal biopsy
Barium studies

CONDITIONS CAUSING CHRONIC DIARRHOEA

Infection

Diarrhoea may persist after acute infection by viruses and bacteria due
to delayed recovery of the intestinal mucosa or secondary lactose
intolerance or cow's milk sensitivity. Chronic infective diarrhoea may
be associated with failure to thrive. Stool culture may reveal infection
with organisms such as *Campylobacter*, which responds to treatment
with erythromycin. Parasites such as *Giardia lamblia* can cause chronic
diarrhoea, often with abdominal distension, wind and the passage of
pale offensive stools. Treatment with metronidazole is effective.

Carbohydrate intolerance

Disaccharide and rarely monosaccharide deficiency may occur as a rare
primary inborn condition or develop due to intestinal mucosal damage
as a result of gastroenteritis. If either condition persists weight gain
will be affected. In the more common secondary conditions the infant
develops diarrhoea when milk is reintroduced after gastroenteritis.
The stools are watery, due to the osmotic action of the sugars remaining
in the bowel, and acidic, often causing persistent nappy rash. The
diagnosis is made by demonstrating reducing substances in the stools.
The condition may last days, weeks or months and is easily managed

by using minimal-lactose milks, such as Pregestimil or Nutramigen, or soya-based milks. To determine whether intolerance has resolved, cow's milk can be introduced at monthly intervals. Return of diarrhoea indicates that the reintroduction of cow's milk should be delayed for at least another month.

Testing for reducing substances in stool. The stool is collected using a plastic lining to the nappy. A small part of the fluid stool is placed in a test-tube with an equal part of water. Fourteen drops of this mixture is placed in another tube and a Clinitest tablet added. More than 0.5% reducing substances is evidence of sugar intolerance.

Cow's milk protein intolerance (cow's milk allergy)

Intolerance to cow's milk is a well-recognized clinical syndrome which may involve several systems of the body in infancy and childhood. Allergy to the protein component of cow's milk, primarily to lacto-globulin, is thought to occur due to sensitization by protein molecules entering the intestinal mucosa. One theory postulates that transiently low levels of IgA, usually around the age of three months, reduce protection to the intestinal mucosa and allow passage of antigens. In some cases sensitization occurs following mucosal damage caused by gastroenteritis. Lactose intolerance may coexist either as a result of gastroenteritis or as a secondary result of allergic gut damage caused by milk intolerance.

The clinical picture of milk intolerance varies widely and can include severe anaphylactic reactions, wheezing, urticaria, chronic diarrhoea and steatorrhoea, failure to thrive, vomiting and abdominal pain, protein-losing enteropathy and eczema. The infants may present with diarrhoea, abdominal distension, fatty stools and occasionally blood in the stools. Children with any of the above symptoms may also suffer from behavioural symptoms such as miserable mood, excessive crying, wind, colic, poor sleeping and difficulty in management. However, milk allergy is probably over-diagnosed as a cause of vague behavioural symptoms and there is no justification for eliminating cow's milk unless there is chronic diarrhoea or definite exacerbation of behaviour problems, or of eczema or asthma.

The diagnosis of cow's milk intolerance rests largely on the clinical history and the response to milk withdrawal. Infants with failure to thrive, malabsorption and protein-losing enteropathy will need fuller investigations, in some cases involving jejunal biopsy.

Cow's milk intolerance is usually a self-limiting disorder and tends to clear up in the second year of life. Management involves replacing cow's milk with a milk containing protein hydrolysates (e.g. Nutramigen and Pregestimil) or soya milk. Soya protein can also cause signs of gastrointestinal intolerance and many paediatricians recommend that proven cow's milk intolerance should be treated with formula containing protein hydrolysates.

There is conflicting evidence on whether soy formula feeding reduces the incidence of allergy in infants predisposed to atopy. In view of possible benefits to these infants, avoidance of cow's milk for the first six months or preferably a year is usually recommended.

A wide variety of vague signs and symptoms may be attributed to cow's milk intolerance and on the whole the condition tends to be over-diagnosed. In view of the possibility of soya milk intolerance the widespread substitution of soya for cow's milk should be avoided.

Intolerance to other foods

Certain other foods may cause sensitivity reactions involving several systems. Egg white, nuts, seafood, tartrazine dyes and some fruit are the most common allergens and may produce a variety of effects including local mouth symptoms such as lip swelling, tingling in the mouth or throat and vomiting. Diarrhoea, bloating and steatorrhoea can occur as well as remote symptoms including urticaria, asthma, headaches and joint pains.

Cystic fibrosis

Cystic fibrosis occurs in 1 : 2000 children and is recessively inherited. It involves abnormality in secretory glands producing unusually tenacious mucus which accumulates and produces local obstruction.

It may present in the neonatal period as bowel obstruction due to meconium ileus. From the early months of life onwards infants may develop recurrent pulmonary infections, wheezing as a result of sticky mucus blocking the bronchi and bronchioles. Gastrointestinal involvement may present from early infancy onwards. There is absence of pancreatic enzymes, resulting in poor digestion of protein and fat. Typically the infant presents with chronic cough, pallor, abdominal distension, pale, loose, offensive stools and failure to thrive. Unlike in coeliac disease the infant is usually cheerful and may have a voracious appetite.

Diagnosis is established by demonstrating an increased concentration of sodium chloride in sweat and saliva.

Coeliac disease

The incidence of coeliac disease ranges from 1:300 (in the west of Ireland) to 1:2000 in other areas. It is characterized by a lifelong intolerance of gluten and is thought to be inherited as a Mendelian dominant with incomplete penetrance.

Symptoms may occur any time after cereals are introduced. The onset may be obviously related to starting cereals but the condition may begin insidiously and not be diagnosed until later in childhood. Typically the infant suffers from diarrhoea, which may be intermittent. Stools are frequent, large, pale and offensive. Failure to thrive, muscle wasting, pallor and abdominal distension are common. Anaemia and rickets may eventually develop if the condition is unrecognized. Characteristically the infant is miserable and has a poor appetite in contrast to cystic fibrosis.

Diagnosis involves jejunal biopsy which demonstrates an abnormal intestinal mucosa. Clinical improvement occurs on a gluten-free diet, which must be continued for life.

Toddler diarrhoea

Toddler diarrhoea is the commonest form of chronic diarrhoea seen in children aged one to four but the diagnosis can only be considered when the child is thriving and in good general health. If failure to thrive or poor health is present, then other causes should be sought.

Toddler diarrhoea is thought to be a form of irritable bowel syndrome in childhood. Evidence suggests that small intestinal motility is affected so that propulsive activity remains high after meals resulting in a shortened intestinal transit time. Diarrhoea is thought to be exacerbated by sugary foods and drinks as these stimulate propulsion and also cause some osmotic diarrhoea. There is some evidence that increasing fat in the diet may help slow down propulsive activity.

Children usually present with chronic diarrhoea, which may be intermittent and interspersed with periods of constipation and is frequently associated with abdominal pains. The stools may be profuse and watery or simply loose and frequent. A severe nappy rash may be present. Mothers may be anxious because they notice remnants of food, resulting in the nickname 'peas and carrots' syndrome. Although the condition has been thought to be self-limiting, evidence suggests that a small proportion of children will continue to have symptoms resembling the irritable bowel syndrome seen in adults.

Management largely consists of strong reassurance to parents that their child is healthy and growing well and will probably grow out of the problem. Reducing intake of sugary foods and drinks may help alleviate symptoms. Toilet training may present a problem if the child is prone to sudden diarrhoea and this may lead to delay in starting nursery school. The use of anti-diarrhoea drugs in children is generally inadvisable but loperamide may be occasionally justified to help control symptoms in the older toddler who is having diarrhoea which interferes with leading a normal life at nursery school.

Immunization

The immunization schedule (Table 6.2)

The immunization schedule in the UK begins at the age of three months, at which age there is evidence that the infant is capable of producing a satisfactory immunological response and will therefore benefit from early protection against infection. Measles immunization was formerly given at 15 months but has been brought forward to 13 months to increase protection of younger babies. During 1988 a combined measles, mumps and rubella vaccine was introduced in the UK in line with policy in the USA.

Interval between doses and interrupted immunization

An interval of six to eight weeks between the first and second doses of diphtheria/tetanus/whooping-cough and polio vaccine gives the optimum immunological response. An even longer interval of four to six months between the second and third doses obtains the most durable immunity.

Commonly infants may miss doses due to illness or, for various reasons such as travel, parents may request immunization at other

Table 6.2 The immunization schedule.

Primary	
Birth	BCG for at-risk groups and those in contact with tuberculosis
3 months	Polio plus diphtheria/tetanus/whooping-cough
5 months	Polio plus diphtheria/tetanus/whooping-cough
10 months	Polio plus diphtheria/tetanus/whooping-cough
13 months	Measles/mumps/rubella
Secondary	
4–6 years	Polio plus diphtheria/tetanus

than scheduled times. It is necessary to observe a minimum of three weeks between first and second doses to allow secondary responsiveness to develop. There is no maximum interval between doses as immunological memory is long-lasting; hence the immunization course can be completed later in the preschool period instead of starting all over again. Children or adults who have not had pertussis immunization along with diphtheria/tetanus can be immunized at any age with three doses of pertussis vaccine at monthly intervals. Measles or measles/mumps/rubella vaccine may be given at any age after one year. More than one live vaccine can be given simultaneously at different sites. However, if not given together administration of live virus vaccines should be separated by an interval of at least three weeks. A three-week period should also be allowed between giving a live virus and BCG.

Administration

Diphtheria/tetanus/whooping-cough and measles vaccine are normally given intramuscularly or deep subcutaneously into the upper arm, thigh or upper outer quadrant of the buttock. Recently the British Paediatric Association and the DHSS have recommended that in young babies immunization should be given in the anterolateral aspect of the upper thigh to minimize trauma of underlying bone and nerves. In older children the upper arm is a suitable site. Three drops of oral polio vaccine can be given directly into the mouth. A sterile 1 ml syringe and adrenaline injection BP (1 : 1000 adrenaline) should be ready for use in case of an anaphylactic reaction. Such a reaction is characterized by collapse, pallor, apnoea, limpness, sweating, tachycardia or bradycardia stridor and is very rare.

The dose (Table 6.3) of 1 : 1000 adrenaline should be given by deep

Table 6.3 Adrenaline for anaphylactic reaction.

Age	Dose of 1 : 1000 adrenaline (1 mg per ml)
Less than 1 year	0.05 ml
1 year	0.1 ml
2 year	0.2 ml
3–4 year	0.3 ml
5 year	0.4 ml
6–10 year	0.5 ml

intramuscular injection unless there is a strong central pulse and the patient's condition is good. The patient should be placed in the left lateral position and if unconscious an airway inserted. Oxygen should be given by face mask and cardiopulmonary resuscitation begun if appropriate. If there is no improvement in 10 minutes the dose of adrenaline may be repeated up to a maximum of three doses. Hydrocortisone 100 mg and/or chlorpheniramine (Piriton) 2.5−5 mg may be given intravenously.

All cases should be admitted to hospital for observation and the reaction reported to the Committee on Safety of Medicine.

General contra-indications to immunization

It is advisable to postpone immunization if the child is suffering from an acute febrile illness, particularly respiratory. Minor infections without systemic upset are not a contra-indication; this is particularly true for babies who are always snuffly.

Live vaccines (Table 6.4) should not be given to children who may have a poor immune response such as those with leukaemia or lymphoma and other cancers affecting the reticulo-endothelial system and those receiving treatment with high-dose corticosteroids and immunosuppressive drugs.

IMMUNIZATION OF HIV-POSITIVE CHILDREN

HIV-positive individuals with or without symptoms may receive measles, mumps, rubella, polio/whooping-cough, diphtheria, tetanus, typhoid, cholera and hepatitis B vaccines. BCG vaccine is contra-indicated as there have been reports of dissemination and there is as yet insufficient evidence for the safety of use of yellow fever vaccine.

Table 6.4 Types of vaccine.

Live attenuated virus	Inactivated bacteria of virus	Toxoid (inactivated bacterial toxin)
Oral polio	Whooping-cough	Tetanus
Measles	Typhoid	Diphtheria
Rubella	Inactivated polio	
Mumps		
BCG		

Whooping-cough

Immunization against whooping-cough has been promoted in the UK since 1957. However, the incidence of the disease has been declining since the beginning of this century. At the start of the century the death-rate from whooping-cough was one per 1000 among children under 15 years of age. In 1945 the number of annual deaths in England and Wales was 749, falling to 90 in 1955–1956, and 14 in 1982. It has been argued that this decline was predictable, irrespective of the introduction of mass vaccination. Other factors such as medical management of the illness and its complications also affect mortality figures. Despite the evidence that a wide variety of social and economic factors affect the incidence of pertussis there is no doubt that variations in uptake of pertussis vaccine have resulted in a corresponding variation in the incidence of the disease. Following the decline in acceptance rates of the vaccine by parents in 1974–1976, an epidemic occurred in 1977–1979 resulting in 27 deaths and 17 children with brain damage in England and Wales.

Morbidity associated with whooping-cough is also an important criterion for assessing the value of preventive measures. In the 1977 epidemic 102 500 children in the UK were notified as having pertussis, of whom 5 000 children in England and Wales were hospitalized. Fifty required admission to intensive-care units, 200 developed pneumonia, 83 experienced convulsions and 17 were left brain-damaged (Office of Health Economics, 1984) Long-term respiratory sequelae have also been reported in children following whooping-cough (Swansea, 1981).

Because of parental anxiety about adverse effects, acceptance of pertussis immunization fell to 30% in 1975 and was this followed by the epidemics of 1977–1978 and 1981–1983. More recently, public confidence has increased and acceptance had risen to 64% in 1985.

The protective efficacy of pertussis vaccine has been estimated as about 80%. Thus a proportion of vaccinated children will develop the disease but they are likely to suffer from a milder illness and are less likely to need hospital admission.

ADVERSE REACTIONS TO PERTUSSIS IMMUNIZATION

Mild reaction

About 15% of babies have a mild reaction in the first 48 hours after injection. Slight fever, mild irritability, crying and some local swelling are typical and are not a contra-indication to future pertussis immunization. Likewise, a skin rash without systemic disturbance is not a bar to further injections.

Severe reactions

Severe reactions occur rarely after immunization. The baby may have a severe local reaction with a very swollen red injection site. A severe systemic reaction may occur with extreme irritability or excessive screaming. Neurological reactions range in severity from an episode of excessive screaming to convulsions and severe encephalopathy resulting in permanent brain damage. Fortunately these complications are extremely rare and their relationship to pertussis vaccine has been the subject of intense controversy. Concern about the lack of sound scientific evidence led to the setting up of the National Childhood Encephalopathy Study (NCEP). The study concluded that there does appear to be a very small risk of serious neurological reaction within seven days of DTP immunization.

The size of this risk was estimated at approximately 1 : 110 000 injections but most of the children experiencing neurological episodes appear to recover (DHSS, 1981). The risk of permanent neurological sequelae is estimated at 1 : 310 000 immunizations equivalent to approximately 1 : 100 000 children receiving the full recommended course of three injections. On the basis of these findings the Joint Committee on Vaccination and Immunization concluded that 'the benefits of vaccination greatly outweigh the very small risk of serious neurological reactions which may arise in relation to pertussis vaccine'.

CONTRA-INDICATIONS TO WHOOPING-COUGH IMMUNIZATION

Apart from the general contra-indications to immunization, contra-indications can be considered under two groups.

Definite contra-indications

Definite contra-indications exist when there is a history of a severe local or general reaction to a preceding dose:
1   A local reaction can be regarded as severe if there is an extensive area of redness and swelling which becomes indurated and involves the greater part of the anterolateral surface of the thigh or major part of the upper arm.
2   A severe general reaction is one which includes one or more of the

following signs and symptoms: fever of 39.5 °C or more within 48 hours of vaccine; anaphylaxis; bronchospasm; laryngeal oedema; collapse, prolonged unresponsiveness or screaming; convulsion occurring within 72 hours.

Children with problem histories

There are some children whose own or family history may predispose them to a slightly higher risk from vaccine. However, the effects of whooping-cough disease could be more severe and the risks and benefits should be assessed in each case. These groups are:

1 Children with a documented history of cerebral damage in the neonatal period.
2 Children with a personal history of convulsions.
3 Children whose parents or siblings have a history of idiopathic epilepsy. In such children there may be a risk of developing a similar condition irrespective of vaccine.

Measles

Measles is a highly contagious viral disease which has a death rate of 1:5000 cases and a complication rate of 10%. Otitis media (45% of all complications) or respiratory conditions (40%) are the most common complications but neurological sequelae occur in 7:100 cases (6%). There is no evidence that the disease is becoming less dangerous over time and since the national acceptance rate is disappointingly low (50–60%) measles epidemics continue to occur.

Reasons why children are not immunized range from a belief that measles is a trivial illness or that the child has had measles in the first year of life, to avoidance because of apparent contra-indications. In fact, only 5% of children would be excluded because of contra-indications. Eradication of measles would require an uptake rate of 96% but, in contrast to the United States where legislation ensures almost universal uptake, such uptake levels are unlikely to be achieved in Britain. In 1986 acceptance of measles vaccine ranged from 29% to 89% in different districts in England and Wales, with an average of 71%.

Since the introduction of measles vaccine in 1968 the number of notifications in England and Wales has declined from about 500 000 in 1967 to about 100 000 in 1982. Mortality from measles has been declining since the beginning of the century, falling from 12 000 a year in 1900, to 100 in 1940 and to 90 in 1968 (England and Wales). Since 1968 deaths have continued to decline to a level of 13 a year in England and Wales.

Children should be immunized at the age of 13 months, regardless of a history of 'measles'. The vaccine is now usually given together with mumps and rubella vaccine (MMR). Older unprotected children can be immunized at any age and develop a more rapid antibody response to the vaccine than to natural measles. Therefore immunization of an unprotected contact can protect against disease if administered within three days of contact.

ADVERSE REACTION TO MEASLES IMMUNIZATION

Side-effects of measles vaccine are very few compared with those associated with natural measles. In about 15% of children a subclinical infection of measles occurs, resulting in malaise and fever with or without a rash occurring 5 to 10 days after vaccination. This illness seldom lasts more than 24 to 48 hours and is not transmitted to contacts.

Neurological complications occur in only one in every million doses and can take the form of encephalitis or subacute sclerosing panencephalitis (SSPE). These sequelae are about one-tenth as common after immunization as with natural measles.

CONTRA-INDICATIONS

The general contra-indications to immunization, particularly those involving live virus, apply.

The specific contraindications are:

1 Hypersensitivity to neomycin or kanamycin (very rare in children).
2 Allergy to hens' eggs is no longer considered to be a contra-indication except in children with severe reaction such as anaphylactoid type reactions (generalized urticaria, swelling of the mouth and throat, difficulty in breathing, shock).
3 The vaccine should be avoided where there is a history of anaphylaxis due to any cause.

Measles/mumps/rubella vaccine

Measles/mumps/rubella vaccine (MMR) is now recommended for all children at the age of 13 months. This has been introduced with the aim of *eliminating* rubella, congenital rubella syndrome, measles and mumps. To achieve this an uptake of 90% must be achieved. In other countries, such as the USA, in which it has been introduced it has proved popular and has increased the uptake of measles vaccine.

Rubella is most common amongst children aged four to nine, who present a risk of infection to non-immune women. Despite immunization of prepubertal girls, in 1986 and 1987 there were 362 laboratory-confirmed cases of rubella in pregnancy in England and Wales. Many of these pregnancies were terminated but on average 20 cases of congenital rubella syndrome are notified annually.

Mumps vaccine is recommended because of the morbidity associated with mumps. In the under-15s it is the most common cause of viral meningitis and may cause permanent deafness.

MMR vaccine may be given to children of any age after one year whose parents request it, regardless of a history of one of the illnesses.

ADVERSE REACTIONS TO MMR VACCINE

As with measles vaccine, malaise, fever and/or a rash may occur, most commonly about a week after vaccination and lasting about two to three days. Parotid swelling occasionally occurs, usually in the third week.

CONTRA-INDICATIONS

The general contra-indications to immunization apply, particularly those which apply to live vaccines.

Children with allergy to neomycin and kanamycin or those with a history of an anaphylactic reaction to eggs or to anything else should not receive MMR.

Common queries about immunizations

Child has a history of fits

In most cases the effects of whooping-cough disease are likely to be higher than risk from vaccine. The balance of risk and benefit should be discussed with parents and if in doubt advice should be sought from a paediatrician with special experience.

The child may have measles vaccine or MMR. Simultaneous immunoglobulin is no longer recommended to be given with measles vaccine and is contra-indicated with MMR as it reduces efficacy.

Parents should be given clear instruction on prevention and control of fever, using paracetamol and tepid sponging.

Parents or siblings have had fits

It is worth while pointing out that a child with such a family history may run an increased risk of developing fits irrespective of immunization. The balance between the harmful effects of increased risk from vaccine need to be discussed with parents before reaching a decision but generally whooping-cough vaccine is recommended. The child may have measles vaccine or MMR.

Advice on prevention and treatment of fever should be given.

Relatives other than parents or siblings have had fits

All immunizations may be given.

Perinatal problems

The child with a documented history of cerebral damage in the neonatal period may have a higher risk from vaccine but the risk of serious effects of whooping-cough disease may be higher still. If there is no evidence of progressive brain damage pertussis immunization is usually recommended. *Progressive* neurological conditions are a contra-indication to pertussis vaccine. The neonatal unit will usually make recommendations on the advisability of immunization against pertussis.

Babies with a history of jitteriness or fits due to hypocalcaemia, hypoglycaemia or anoxia or of apnoeic attacks can receive pertussis immunization.

All children with the above histories can receive measles or MMR vaccine.

Severe developmental delay

Children with a developmental delay due to a non-progressive condition are at risk from the effects of whooping-cough and should receive the vaccine. It is advisable to document the child's developmental level at the time of immunization in case subsequent poor progress is attributed to the effects of vaccine.

Measles and MMR can be given.

Asthma or eczema

All immunizations can be given.

Recent illness/antibiotic treatment

Provided the baby is well all immunizations can be given. Immunizations work perfectly well in children on antibiotics.

Small or preterm baby

Start immunization at three months after birth no matter how immature or how small the baby is. The small preterm baby runs a high risk of complication if he catches whooping-cough.

Child is reported to have had measles

Immunize against measles.

Child has been in contact with measles

Immunize against measles.

Child has been in contact with other infectious disease

All immunization can be given providing the child is well.

Child has cystic fibrosis, congenital malformation of the heart, spina bifida

All immunizations can be given.

Child has hydrocephalus, cerebral palsy, Down's syndrome

These are static conditions and all immunizations may be given.

Diphtheria

Diphtheria immunization began in 1940 and has resulted in a dramatic fall in the number of cases from 46 281 in 1940 to 37 in 1957. In the last five years there have been 14 cases notified and only one death in England and Wales.

REACTIONS AND CONTRA-INDICATIONS

Mild reactions may occur such as fever, headache, malaise and small nodules at the injection site. Severe neurological reactions and anaphylaxis are extremely rare.

There are no contra-indications apart from general considerations such as a child who is unwell.

Tetanus

Routine immunization against tetanus was introduced in 1961. Since then there has been a steep decline in cases notified, particularly in those aged under 20 years with no recorded cases in this age group in 1978—1979.

REACTIONS AND CONTRA-INDICATIONS

Nodules may arise at the injection site but general reactions such as headache, fever and malaise are uncommon. Acute anaphylaxis and urticaria may occasionally occur. Severe reactions are a contra-indication to further immunization but there are no other specific contra-indications.

Poliomyelitis

Inactivated poliomyelitis vaccine (Salk) was introduced in 1956 and was replaced by attenuated live oral vaccine (Sabin) in 1962. Since their introduction notifications of paralytic poliomyelitis have dropped from nearly 4000 in 1955 to 257 in 1960 and to only five cases during 1974—1978 in England and Wales. The oral vaccines contain strains of three polio virus types and the full basic course of three doses produces a long-lasting immunity to all three polio virus types. The vaccine may lose its potency if not stored at 0—4°C and when the containers are opened.

REACTIONS AND CONTRA-INDICATIONS

There is a small risk — about one in three million doses — of vaccine-induced poliomyelitis, but this risk is considered too small to restrict the vaccination programme.

Apart from general considerations there are no specific contra-indications. Breast-fed infants respond satisfactorily to the vaccine.

Parents who are unimmunized should be given polio vaccine at the same time as their children. Faecal excretion of vaccine virus can lead to infection of unimmunized contacts. Parents born before 1958 and recent immigrants from countries such as Asia are more likely not to have been immunized.

Note

The immunization policies outlined here are based on DHSS policies published in 1988; they may be modified in the future and current guidelines should be available for consultation.

References

Blaikley, J. *et al.* (1953) Breast feeding: factors affecting success. Report of the trial of Woolwich methods in a group of primiparae. *Journal of Obstetrics and Gynaecology of the British Empire*, **60**, 657.

Cunningham, A. (1977) Morbidity in breast-fed and artificially fed infants. *Journal of Pediatrics*, **90** (5), 726—9.

DHSS (1981) *Whooping Cough: Report from the Committee on Safety of Medicines and the Joint Committee on Vaccination and Immunization*. HMSO, London.

DHSS (1988) *Immunization against Infectious Disease*. HMSO, London. *Geigy Scientific Tables*, 8th edn (1977).

Hart, H., Bax, M. & Jenkins, S. (1980) Community influences on breast feeding. *Child Care, Health and Development*, **6**, 175—87.

Hunziker, U.A. & Barr, R.G. (1986) Increased carrying reduces infant crying: a randomized control trial. *Pediatrics*, **77**, 641—8.

Illingworth, R.S. & Lister, J. (1964) The critical and sensitive period, with special reference to certain feeding problems in infants and young children. *Journal of Pediatrics*, **65**, 839.

Jakobsson, I. & Lindberg, T. (1983) Cow's milk proteins cause infantile colic in breast-fed infants: a double blind crossover study. *Pediatrics*, **71** (2), 268—71.

Martin, J. & Monk, J. (1980) *Infant Feeding*. OPCS: London.

Office of Health Economics (1984) *Childhood Vaccination — Current Controversies*. Office of Health Economics, London.

Oppé *et al.* (1980) *Present-day Practice in Infant Feeding*. HMSO, London. Practical Guide to Immunization in Children. Supplement to Immunization against Infectious Disease. DHSS: London.

Oppé *et al.* (1988) *Present-day Practice in Infant Feeding*. HMSO, London. Practical Guide to Immunization in Children. Supplement to Immunization against Infectious Disease. DHSS: London.

Poskitt, E.M.E. & Cole, J.T. (1977) Do fat babies stay fat? *British Medical Journal*, **1**, 7—9.

Sosa, R., Kennell, J.H., Klaus, M. & Urrutio, J.J. (1976) The effect of early mother—infant contact on breast feeding, infection and growth. In *Breast Feeding and the Mother*, pp. 179—88. CIBA Foundation Symposium 45 (new series), Elsevier, Amsterdam.

Swansea Research Unit of the Royal College of General Practitioners (1981) *British Medical Journal*, **1**, 23—6.

Taitz, L.S. (1977) Infantile obesity. *Paediatric Clinics of North America*, **24**, 107—15.

Warner, J.O. (1980) Food allergy in fully breast-fed infants. *Clinical Allergy*, **10**, 133—6.

Whitelaw, A. (1977) Infant feeding and subcutaneous fat at birth and at one year. *Lancet*, **ii**, 1089—99.

7   Developmental Disorders

THE TERM 'developmental disorder' simply describes any condition which interferes with the child's normal course of development. Development may either be delayed, so that for example, the child is late walking but eventually walks normally, or it can be disturbed, so that the child with cerebral palsy not only walks late but, when he does walk, has an abnormal gait. Similarly one child may be slow at talking but eventually talk quite normally, while another may have abnormalities of speech and language development. Where there is clear-cut evidence of impaired cerebral function we can talk about a *neuro*developmental disorder. Often there is significant delay but no evidence of any central pathology and here we describe the child as having a developmental disorder. Developmental disorders are frequently associated with congenital disorders — literally disorders present from birth — and this may be due to genetic effects or some interference with the child during the nine months of intra-uterine life.

There are many hundreds of genetic diseases and while not all are associated with disturbed development many of them are. The problem for the primary care physician is that he cannot possibly know about all of them, and he has therefore to devise some way of understanding the problems of the children and families despite his restricted knowledge of any particular condition. Very often referral will be necessary for appropriate diagnostic help and assessment, but the primary clinician will want to play his part in providing a service to the child and the family. He is able to do this by focusing on the child's functional disorder rather than on the specifics related to the disease, although with any particular child he will try and supplement his knowledge as quickly as possible.

The WHO has attempted to clarify some of the words used to discuss the problems of children with developmental disorders. Thus the term *impairment* is used to describe the actual pathology or lesion the child has (this might be certified brain damage on CT scan); the *disability* describes the functional effect of that impairment (which might be hemiplegia) and *handicap* describes the practical consequences of the impairment or the disability. A *handicap* is thus a social phenom-

229

enon. A child with a severe port-wine naevus over the face may be so overwhelmed by his disfigurement that he is shy and retiring and perhaps as an adult will be unable to go out except at night. Such a person could be described as handicapped. If on the other hand the individual's personality was such that he was able to come to terms with his disfigurement and lead a perfectly normal social life he would not be considered as handicapped. In an illiterate society, illiteracy is not handicapping, but in most developed countries now inability to read is socially restricting and makes ordinary life impossible. Handicap, too, is very much in the eye of the beholder. Thus a man in a wheelchair said to me that he did not regard himself as handicapped; later, however, he reported spending some time waiting at the bottom of a lift (elevator) because he was unable to reach the buttons. He regarded himself as being unhandicapped; we would say he was handicapped. Obviously the young child is unaware of the consequences of his impairment or disability and his parents and those professionals around him make the judgement that he is handicapped. As he gets older, he realizes the social consequences of his impairment or disability.

Terminology used in 'learning difficulties'

The terminology used in dealing with people with handicaps has to be chosen with care. Words tend to become derogatory over time so that nobody would now like to be called an idiot. The word spastic is sometimes used as a term of abuse (particularly in the USA). In this country 'mental handicap' is not liked by some (because of remarks like 'you are mental') and some prefer to talk of children with learning difficulties when referring to children with mental handicap. We certainly want to avoid giving our patients and their families offence but equally we try to avoid euphemisms. Reality must be faced. It is better to talk of a child with a handicap than a handicapped child, but the latter is shorter and we have not always avoided it in this text written for the professional.

Normal or abnormal

One problem is in deciding whether a child's development is normal or abnormally delayed. Development shows wide variations and inevitably some members of the population are going to be in the bottom 3% for a particular norm for their age. Thus most children whose heights or weights lie below the 3rd percentile will prove to be 'normal' (often they will have short parents) whereas a small proportion will have an organic or emotional disorder which requires investigation and treatment. Most children who do not walk until 18 months will prove to have no dysfunction or impairment, but a significant proportion will have a disorder such as cerebral palsy or Duchenne muscular dystrophy. The clinician faced with a child whose speech and language are delayed has to decide whether he falls within the limits of normality or whether his delay represents pathology. Sometimes this distinction is academic. Thus the child who is not talking at three is, by this time, in a world where his peers and adults around him expect him to talk and he will be at a disadvantage. Therefore, even if his delay comes within the range of biologically normal, it seems reasonable to try and help him. If the clinician discovers evidence of some impairment such as a genetic disorder, the developmental delay may be coincidental but more commonly it is associated with or caused by the condition which has been identified.

Meeting the needs of the child with a developmental disorder

The child needs:

1 *Diagnosis*. The aim of the diagnosis is to identify the cause of the impairment or delay. A full diagnosis allows one to state something about the cause of the condition, the pathological process and the likely prognosis. It may have implications for treatment (e.g. response to dietary restriction in phenylketonuria) or prevention (thus the identification of a child with Duchenne muscular dystrophy can lead to genetic counselling and the prevention of the birth of a second handicapped child). The parents, reasonably, wish to know why their child is handicapped and the implication of that knowledge may have consequences which will affect their behaviour towards the child.

2 *Assessment*. Diagnosis rarely gives one clear information about the child's functioning. To plan a management programme, one needs to know what the child is actually doing and able to do. Thus children with Down's syndrome show as much variation in their range of functioning as normal children, but their mean achievement scores are considerably lower. The clinician therefore reviews the child's ability in terms of gross and fine motor function, vision, hearing, speech and language, perceptual, intellectual and social development. Assessment needs to be repeated at regular intervals.

3 *Treatment*. To the lay person (and to the doctor) treatment implies a promise of cure. The aim is to provide a specific remedy for an ill. For most developmental disorders there is not the possibility of cure,

particularly when the basic impairment involves damage to the central nervous system. One of the first essentials therefore is to make sure that the family understand this. Many parents have been told that the doctor will arrange treatment for their child with cerebral palsy and have gone away thinking he will be cured. For some conditions there are treatments which imply cure, such as the dietary treatment of phenylketonuria or the use of glasses to correct a fault in visual acuity. However, the glasses correct the dysfunction but don't cure the impairment. It is also worth remembering that many developmental disorders show a changing symptomatology with age. Thus a child who does not talk at three may achieve low but near-normal speech and language scores by five, only to have problems with reading when he is eight or nine.

4 *Management.* Management aims to alleviate what cannot be cured and to prevent secondary deficits and problems from developing. Good management helps the family look after their child. Based on the assessment, the clinician tries to ensure that the child functions optimally within his capacities, however limited.

5 *Care and counselling.* Families of children with handicaps need advice, counselling and comfort as they try and accept their child's disability and understand the way in which his functioning is limited. The parents of a child with severe handicap may go through a process not unlike mourning, which may involve periods of denial and rejection of the abnormality (and of the doctor). They often seek help from others and this wish should be respected. A good description of the reaction of the family to a handicapped child is given by Mac Keith (1973) (a classic account of the problem, which we print as an appendix).

As the handicapped child grows, however limited his development may be, he needs to be able to discuss his disabilities and adjust to his handicap as far as possible. From the toddler age the clinician should inform the child what is happening to him and why it is happening. He should not talk over the child's head at the parents.

6 *Periodic diagnostic review and periodic reassessment.* Parents sometimes complain that they keep seeing new doctors who ask the same questions again and again. This is undoubtedly true, but at the same time a clinician who sees a handicapped child who was first assessed some time ago may realize that a much better attempt at understanding the child's impairment can now be made, e.g. because developments in diagnostic procedure may have occurred (a good example is the introduction of CT scans). And while unnecessary investigations should not be undertaken, particularly when these are unpleasant for the child, the family are often grateful for the further information about their child that now becomes available.

Assessment needs repeating as the child's chronological age increases and new functions emerge or should be emerging whose presence or absence need to be documented. Periodic assessment also monitors the efficacy of treatment and management.

Treatment and management should be reviewed regularly. Goals should be set for the time by which a management tactic should have achieved success; for example, if a programme is initiated to help a motor handicapped child to walk, a time-scale should be set by which walking should be achieved. Whether it is achieved or not the situation should be reviewed at the end of that time. It is not uncommon to find handicapped children continuing with 'treatment' initiated years previously, for example, children put on drugs for epilepsy may have the same prescription unchanged for long periods of time. They should of course be reviewed very regularly and change (or withdrawal) of drugs considered at least on a two-yearly basis.

The application of these principles will be described as individual conditions are discussed. Cerebral palsy is primarily a motor disorder but frequently has so many other components that it is a good model on which to base an account of general management. The causes of impairment and developmental delay are considered under each of the main headings of neurodevelopmental disorder.

Disorders of motor development

The commonest causes of delayed motor development are cerebral palsy, muscular dystrophy and spina bifida (the last is currently much less common than it was). Approximately two per thousand children have cerebral palsy. In the 1960s the rate of spina bifida was somewhat similar but is now under one per thousand. The next most common physical handicap, Duchene muscular dystrophy, occurs in about one in three thousand boys. The diagnosis of muscular dystrophy will often be made in the preschool period, while the difficulties of management become more complex as the child gets older.

Cerebral palsy

Cerebral palsy is a disorder of movement and posture due to a non-progressive lesion occurring in the early years of life. While the lesion is non-progressive, the cerebral palsy shows a changing pattern with time. While most cases are of pre- or perinatal origin, a small proportion of children have cerebral palsy due to postnatal causes, including infections, trauma and strokes. Cerebral palsy is a syndrome, not a disease state but the result of damage to areas of the brain which are involved in controlling movement in the child. It is classically divided into three main types of disorders: spastic, athetoid and ataxic cerebral palsy.

In spastic cerebral palsy the child has increased muscle tone with brisk reflexes but is also paradoxically weak. Approximately one-third of cerebral palsy sufferers have a spastic hemiplegia, with the arm being more severely affected than the leg. A third of cases of hemiplegia are postnatally caused, usually due to 'stroke', and these have the 'purest' form of hemiplegia. Others are due to birth anoxia or vascular occlusion occurring at or around the time of birth and may actually involve damage to other areas of the brain; a careful examination may reveal that, while the child has a predominantly right- or left-sided palsy there are also signs on the other side.

In spastic diplegia, which affects about 40% of cerebral palsy patients, the child is affected in all four limbs, with the legs more severely affected than the arms. This condition is often associated with early birth. Milder cases where the arms are barely affected are sometimes referred to as spastic paraplegia but the term should be avoided in relationship to cerebral palsy and reserved for true paraplegics where the neurological function in the upper limbs is normal.

In spastic quadriplegia where more severe damage has occurred the child has severe spasticity and weakness in all four limbs, more or less evenly distributed. These are the most severe cases of cerebral palsy and are frequently associated with profound mental retardation. Some are associated with intraventricular haemorrhage occurring in the immediate postnatal period.

All the above types of cerebral palsy predominantly feature weakness and spasticity or stiffness in the limbs. There are two other types of cerebral palsy which are much less common, representing perhaps 5 to 10% of the population of cerebral-palsied young people. Choreoathetoid cerebral palsy is characterized by unwanted movements which overwhelm purposeful movement. Usually the condition involves all four limbs but it may involve only a part of the body. Apart from the unwanted movements the child's postures are often unusual and he is hardly ever still.

Ataxic cerebral palsy also involves purposeful movement. The child has a typical 'ataxic gait' and has difficulty sometimes carrying out intentional movements with the hands. There are not, as there are in choreo-athetoid cerebral palsy, unwanted movements. The ataxic gait is classically broad-based with high-stepping staggering movements of the legs.

While the motor disorder is the most obvious feature of cerebral palsies, it may not be the most severe aspect of the child's handicap. Epilepsy is a common feature of the condition. Approximately 50% of cerebral-palsied children are mentally retarded and a proportion of these will be profoundly retarded. Hearing disorders are common, particularly in choreo-athetosis, where there is typically a high-tone hearing loss. Visual problems, particularly squint, may involve as many as 50% of the cerebral-palsied population. Speech and language disorders are common, and dysarthric problems as well as central language problems occur. Children who are intellectually normal may have specific learning disorders.

Children with cerebral palsy have very much higher rates of behavioural problems — something like five or six times the normal. Their behaviour problems are not essentially different from those of the normal population and they may be associated with similar factors in the social environment which disturb the normal child, but the brain-damaged child is far more vulnerable than the normal child and hence behaviour problems are commoner.

DIAGNOSIS

The diagnosis of cerebral palsy involves the clinical identification of the neurological disorder and appropriate investigations to prove that the child has a static encephalopathy and not a progressive disease or some other form of mental subnormality. Clinically the early signs may well show a fluctuating neurological picture. Often both athetoid and spastic children are hypotonic in the early stages, with typically spastic features emerging slowly in the second six months of life. With the ataxic child early recognition (under the age of one) that the child has cerebral palsy may be difficult because the young child's hand movements are to some extent ataxic and only when he gets up and walks will the ataxic gait be revealed. Throughout this period, however, there will be delay in motor development and as the child gets older the more classical signs of the condition become apparent. The spastic child will have stiff hypertonic muscles which are also weak, with brisk reflexes accompanying them. Careful testing, which is not usually possible until the child is older, will demonstrate that there is usually associated sensory loss, particularly of the kinaesthesic sense together with some loss of fine sensation in a similar distribution to the motor loss.

The athetoid child develops from the floppy state into one in which the involuntary movements, sometimes spasms, of the body begin to develop during the second half of the first year of life.

As already mentioned the small baby will usually have been investigated in the perinatal period; ultrasound followed by serial CT scans may have revealed the site of an area of brain damage, and there will be developing changes over time, for example the development of a cystic lesion from a primary intraventricular haemmorhage. In other instances, where the cause of the pathology is less clear-cut, a metabolic screen, screen for congenital infections and cytogenetic studies may be undertaken.

Where the child has had a healthy intra-uterine life and neonatal period and no suspicion has arisen that there was anything wrong with the child, the parents are often the first to become anxious because of slow motor development. If the cerebral palsy becomes apparent in the second half of the first year, it is appropriate then to carry out the studies outlined above and see if any brain pathology can be demonstrated. Progressive neurological disorders may be suspected and appropriate diagnostic investigations carried out.

ASSESSMENT

Assessment of a child involves comparing his functioning and all aspects of his development with the expected norms for his age. The cerebral-palsied child will of course have delayed development as well as abnormal development. He will be late to roll, crawl, sit and walk, and the delay in the achievement of these motor milestones may well be the first thing that draws the attention of the family and the physician to the child's problems. When the child is not mentally retarded, there may be a very uneven profile of development with delayed motor development but with evidence of near-normal speech and language development. In the cerebral-palsied child with mental retardation there may of course be global delay in all aspects of development. While obviously the more profound the delay, the more ominous is the prognosis, it is not always easy to make predictions in a particular child under one year about what the likely outcome will be. As the child gets older it becomes more possible to predict what the eventual performance will be like. Table 7.1 (adapted from Bleck, 1975) gives some indication of what motor performance may be expected based on some early signs. In the child who has been born early and spent two or three months in an incubator, examination at six months of chronological age (but perhaps only three months when one allows for the prematurity) may suggest global delayed development. Within the next three months or so, as the child develops, the outlook may not

Table 7.1 Prediction of walking in cerebral palsy (after Bleck, 1975).

Test	Response
Asymmetrical tonic neck reflex Symmetrical tonic neck reflex Moro reflex Righting reflex	Persistence abnormal after 6 months
Foot placement reaction	Absence abnormal
Parachute reaction	Absence abnormal after 1 year
Extensor thrust	Presence always abnormal

An abnormal response is scored 1 point.
A score of 2 or more over the age of 2 means the prognosis for walking is very poor.

seem as gloomy as the clinician first feared.

Nevertheless the early months of management of a brain-damaged child can be extremely difficult, as the clinician is always struggling to interpret the diagnostic information in the fairest manner possible without giving rise to undue pessimism or unreal optimism about the child. As the child grows the assessment of normal development goes on alongside the observation of abnormal signs.

The child with cerebral palsy will often have poor physical growth and the affected limbs in spastic diplegia and hemiplegia are often short. Most of this failure to grow occurs during the first two years of life. In the child who has uncomplicated cerebral palsy without mental retardation, the delay in the motor aspects of development will be disproportionate to delay in other functions; thus the child may babble and vocalize at normal ages and produce language at the appropriate time. The problem is that the assessment of the child's other functions often involves a motor skill. Thus if one asks a two-year-old child who has a quadriplegia to do a puzzle (formboard) he might lack the motor skills to carry out the function. Were he able to make the appropriate movements, he might or might not have the necessary perceptual skills to do the task. Assessment therefore is a skilled process. If the child has dysarthria, that is involvement of the motor organs of speech in the cerebral palsy, he may be unable to make the responses to demonstrate that he has normal language. One can sometimes establish the extent of the child's vocabulary, by using eye-pointing at different objects suitably spaced. Often assessment of the child therefore requires lengthy observation. The clinician tries to assess function in the classical way, looking at gross and fine motor function, hearing, speech and language as outlined in Chapters 1, 3 and 4. Often others, such as physiotherapists, speech therapists, occupational therapists and psychologists, will be involved in the assessment.

In addition one has to be on the watch all the time for the development of secondary problems. In a young spastic child the tightness of the thigh adductors may have encouraged the development of subluxation or dislocation of the hips. Growth of muscle depends on them being allowed their normal stretch and a spastic muscle remains short, eventually becoming contracted so that the limb cannot be put through the normal range of movement. Thus commonly a hemiplegic child will have a tight gastrocnemius muscle and the ankles will be dorsiflexed, the knee will tend to be held in semiflexed postures, as will the hip, and at all these sites the contractures may become fixed. It is interesting to compare the standing posture of the older diplegic child, with that of a six-month baby, who tends normally to hold hip and knee slightly flexed and is often standing up on his toes. In the normal baby it is easy to overcome the preferred posture and demonstrate a full range of movement.

When the baby is born he tends to be in flexed postures, keeping knees and hips flexed with ankles extended; similarly the elbows and shoulders are kept in flexed, internally rotated postures. When the baby is placed prone in the newborn period, the knees are under the hips, whereas over the next three or four months of life, the child begins to unroll and have movements of flexion and extension. A number of the primitive responses which disappear during the first three or four months of life may persist in the spastic or athetoid child. These include the Moro response, the asymmetric tonic neck reflex and the grasp response. The persistence of flexed postures together with the primitive responses may make the child extremely difficult to handle in the early years of life.

TREATMENT

Cerebral palsy cannot be cured since the damaged central nervous system will not regenerate. This is the first fact that the clinician has to get over to the parents. In the early neonatal period specific treatments (beyond the scope of this book) may be initiated to try to prevent some of the known complications in infants of low birthweight (e.g. prevention of intraventricular haemorrhage), but, once this period is passed and a static encephalopathy has resulted, one cannot talk in terms of curative treatment of the cerebral-palsied child.

MANAGEMENT

Physical

Although it has been stressed that cerebral palsy is not simply a disorder of movement and posture, nevertheless this prime dysfunction should be very vigorously managed as soon as development is first reported as abnormal. The consequences of not providing adequate management are that the child may develop fixed contractures of the limbs and become relatively immobile. The aim of management, then, is to maintain normal posture and to maximize movement. Unfortunately the baby with cerebral palsy tends to have reduced spontaneous movements, to show persistent patterns of mass movement, such as staying in flexed postures, and to hold his limbs in postures associated with his particular form of cerebral palsy. It seems highly unlikely that sessions of treatment, however skilfully carried out, for an hour or so, even every day of the week, are going to do much to interrupt the process when, for most of the day, the baby is maintaining the postures which are innate to this pathology and is failing to make normal movements. The therapist is therefore trying to help the family handle the baby in such a way that throughout the course of his whole day of 24 hours the disability is managed so as to minimize its effects.

Growth of muscle is dependent on stretch to some extent and if, for example, the tendo Achillis is held most of the time in a degree of dorsiflexion it will not grow at the same rate as the bone and in time there will be relative shortening of the muscle and hence a fixed contracture at the ankle. In order to prevent this happening, therefore, the limbs should normally be maintained as far as possible in neutral postures. During the day this can usually be achieved by seeing that the child is sat or held standing in the appropriate position. Chairs may need special construction to see that the ankles are held at a 90° angle. At night (and during the day) lightweight orthoses may be useful in maintaining neutral positions. At the same time during the normal course of the day — during feeding, meal-times, bathing and at all playtimes — the family should encourage the young baby to move actively. Mass patterns of movements may be inhibited, for example, by seeing that the head is not allowed to flop back. In order to deal with all these intricacies of management of the motor disorder the parents clearly need and should have the support of a skilled physiotherapist.

The child may need a purpose-built chair to ensure that he is not sitting in a floppy, potentially harmful posture. If early mobilization with an electric wheelchair seems desirable a suitable moulded seat can be made. Lighweight splints can now be constructed which replace the unsightly metal calipers with which handicapped children used to be adorned. Walking frames, sticks, aids for holding spoons and other aids all need introducing to the patient and a good child development team will see this is done.

It should be mentioned here that physiotherapy in relationship to the treatment of cerebral palsy has in the past been dominated by varying schools of physiotherapy, all with a belief that the method they have devised for treatment of children with cerebral palsy is the best one and, unless the procedure is followed in the way they specify, the child will inevitably fail to improve. Undoubtedly some of the schools have, in the past, made unjustifiable claims for the treatment they have proposed. Many therapists are now trained in the UK and North America by one of the best thought out of the systems of therapy, known after its originators as the 'Bobath' method; popular in the UK too is the 'Peto' method (conductive education), which has origins in Hungary. From time to time one comes across groups of parents who have heard of the Doman−Delcato methods of treatment which were developed in Philadelphia. In this method the child and the parents are put through an intensive programme of treatment which involves groups of exercises which may take several hours a day to complete. Their efficacy is unproved.

A common reaction of parents who have a chronically handicapped child is to search for a cure or, at least as they see it, they very best form of 'treatment'. Faced with the information that their child has an incurable disease, the parents may well seek to deny the doctors' statements and look for a cure. Why shouldn't they? Doctors have often been wrong in the past and will be in the future. The problem is that parents are not likely to know all the options open to them nor can they undertake a study of human biology. Thus it is difficult for them to review objectively the options they are offered. They are likely to respond to enthusiasm rather than a more sober assessment of the likely potentials for their child. The clinician tries therefore to enthuse about what can be done while being honest about the child's problems. (This issue will be discussed under care and counselling.) People faced with bad news need to hear it from two or three different sources and the doctor should try and see that he makes it easy for the parents to consult with others, such as other parents who have had handicapped children. They are influenced by a whole range of opinions which will usually help them in making up their own minds about how they want to proceed with their own child's management.

Other aspects of management

While the child with cerebral palsy presents as a child with a motor disability he is highly likely to have other problems. Management should include the whole process of normal child-rearing, e.g. the stimulation of sound-making and listening, of speech and language, of visual activity. The family may need help over feeding difficulties early on and toileting a little later. Equally important is to stress the child's need to develop social relationships in the normal way, which has been described in Chapters 3 and 4. While the specialists are concentrating on the particular problems of a handicapped child, the primary physician may find himself as the one with responsibility for seeing the child experiences the normal processes of child-rearing within the family, at least as far as this is possible. Very often he will work in association with a health visitor: in some areas there are specialist health visitors who work largely with families who have a handicapped child.

CARE

A child with a handicap immediately becomes a member of a family with a handicapped child. The presence of the handicapped member of the family has consequences for the parents and for brothers and sisters, and indeed for the grandparents and other more distant members of the family. The clinician must be aware therefore that not only will the immediate family want to discuss what is happening to the handicapped child, but so many relatives such as an aunt who may spend quite a lot of time with the child.

Broadly, the issues of care can be divided into two. First, there are *practical issues*: these include genetic counselling, seeing that the family are aware of all the possible financial help they can obtain and providing practical help within the home, e.g. adequate nappy service. Second, there are the *emotional issues* or the need to deal with the feelings about having a handicapped child. One must not forget here the feeling of the handicapped child himself. While he is a baby, the issues cannot be discussed with the child, but as he grows it is very important to see that he has counselling about the nature of his condition, and is able to come to terms with the feelings that he has about being handicapped.

Practical issues

Genetic counselling. Although the parents are concerned with the condition of the present child, and may not be thinking about adding to the family, the early genetic counselling is very important and may prevent the birth of more handicapped children. It has been calculated that a fifth of all children with muscular dystrophy have an older brother with the condition and all these cases might have been prevented if diagnosis had been made early enough and further births avoided. Clearly the parents need to be told what the likelihood is of their having a further handicapped child and informed too of what steps could be taken to identify a potentially handicapped child in the antenatal period. The possibility of offering termination where a potentially damaged baby is identified needs discussion and the parents' views on this should be listened to with sensitivity. With the relatively rare dominantly inherited conditions the clinician is able to present the chances very clearly to the parent, but other cases may be much less clear-cut, counselling is complex and many primary clinicians will wish to invoke the experience of somebody expert in the field. The parents will often want to come back to discuss with their primary physicians the advice they have heard from the expert.

However carefully the facts are presented, the parents may find the consequences hard to appreciate for they are not as used to dealing with statistical chance in human lives as the geneticist is. Thus being told that, having had one spina bifida baby, there is an increased likelihood that they will have another, possibly in the order of one in 15, can be overwhelming to parents who have been planning a family of three or four. This, coupled with the information that amniocentesis can identify the baby and an abortion can be arranged to prevent the birth of a further spina bifida child, can raise all sorts of feelings not only about the future pregnancy but also about the circumstances which surrounded the birth of the present handicapped child. Clearly the clinician who is going to talk to the parents must have a sound knowledge of the genetic implications of the conditions himself and a general appreciation of the level of parental understanding so that he can discuss the situation with them in suitable terms.

In cerebral palsy there is a small percentage of families where a familial spastic condition is inherited; most of these conditions are rare and genetic advice will certainly be required before discussing the situation with the parents. Again a rather wider question arises as to whether the family have a greater chance of having another handicapped child, having had a first one, and what might be the reasons for this. There is certainly an increased probability in general. However, cerebral palsy has multiple causes. There may be genetic, conceptional, developmental, environmental, obstetric and neonatal factors, any or all of which have a bearing on why a baby is handicapped and whether the abnormality may or many not occur in a further pregnancy. It is not easy to guide parents through the implications of this sort of information; an obstetric consultation will often help them to reach a decision. It is not surprising to find that many parents, having had one child with cerebral palsy, are likely to decide not to have further family. It is in fact the case that the cerebral-palsied child is often the last child in the family.

Financial problems. In the early years of life the cerebral-palsied infant presents little more financial problem than an ordinary baby does. As the child grows there begin to be all sorts of expenses, from making hospital visits to buying special toys. Coupled with this, both parents are unlikely to be able to work, as one or other, usually the mother, must stay with the child because he needs so much more care than an ordinary child. The father's income is therefore not supplemented by the mother's; in addition, the father is less likely to get promoted than the father of an unhandicapped child, for he cannot easily move to new parts of the country, and it is more difficult for him to devote extra time and energy to work as he is so involved in the process of caring for the child.

There are two principal sources of state help for those caring for a dependent relative in the UK, the attendance allowance and the mobility allowance, which become available when the child reaches the age of two. The officials who assess the need may sometimes seem rather unsympathetic to the family and the parents may well look to their primary care physician for help in obtaining this support. Voluntary organizations, such as the Spastics Society, will help financially with particular problems, and the goverment-financed Family Fund will also provide help for families with severely handicapped children. This help can be very wide-ranging, from providing funds for a holiday to buying a washing-machine, or helping with the purchase of a car, and so on. The complexities of some of these methods of obtaining financial help are very puzzling to some families. Government regulations frequently change and social workers with little experience of children with handicap may not always be aware of all the facilities that are available. A good supply of recent pamphlets from both public and private sources is very useful to the doctor trying to do the best he can for families with a handicapped child.

In addition to actual practical financial help, local councils can help families with handicapped children in various other ways. They will, for example, rehouse families with handicapped children on ground-floor premises and will carry out adaptations to the house, to make the care of a handicapped person more easy. While these adaptations tend to become more important as the child gets older, they should be fully considered in the preschool years.

Therapists from the district handicap team (see next section) should visit the child in the home to identify some of the family's practical needs and give advice as to how they can be met.

Contacts with other services. It has been recommended by the government that every district should have a district handicap team, and that this team should be based on one or two child assessment centres. Not all the health districts in England and Wales yet have such a service, but two-thirds do. Many districts prefer to use the term child development team to avoid the stigma of the word handicap. A child assessment centre should be staffed by a community paediatrician, and other staff should include physiotherapist, speech therapist, occupational therapist, psychologist, nurses (often health visitors), teachers and social workers. Most moderate and severely handicapped children will attend these centres for assessment and contact there with members of the staff will then extend out into the community so that therapists will visit the home and look at the child's needs. Equally the staff should be able to help with some of the financial and social implications of handicap, discussed in other sections.

District handicap teams involve co-operation between health and social services and education, and they should provide long-term support for the child and the family. District handicap teams are backed up by regional handicap children's centres which exist in most regions now, where children with very special problems can go, particularly for diagnostic and complex assessments. In the better organized regions in the country, staff from the regional centre will visit districts on a regular basis to provide additional expertise at a local level.

In addition to these statutory provisions, many parents can be helped by parent organizations which exist now for almost every form of disability. Some parents are not keen to meet up immediately with other parents in similar circumstances, but most welcome the opportunity to talk to other families who have experienced the same problems as they have. Other parents may be able to give more practical, precise advice and counselling than the professionals can. Parents often feel that they gain more from each other than they do from even the most well-disposed professional.

Rearing a handicapped child. It is very important to share with the parents the positive attributes of the child and stress those aspects of development which are proceeding normally. Early smiling and eye interaction, suggesting good social skills developing, might be something to dwell on. Equally some of the problems such as night-waking or feeding difficulties can be lightened if one emphasizes that these problems also occur in the normal child. Enjoy with the parents the child's pleasure in some of the toys available and spend time with parents and child, commenting on his normal activities before trying to assess the child's particular problems.

The process of child-rearing with a handicapped child is usually more difficult than rearing an ordinary child. This is certainly true with a child with cerebral palsy for difficulties will start straightaway. The baby may have been in a special-care baby unit; even if he has not, he may prove to be a child who is very difficult to feed: he may be a poor sucker, and have difficulty swallowing and later difficulties in chewing. These difficulties are said to relate to later speech and language difficulties and some speech therapists will be very skilled in managing them, although again this depends on special knowledge and training.

Children with cerebral palsy are often stiff and awkward to carry, they don't mould easily to the mother's form, and they don't support themselves; they will not start sitting until much later than normal, and they will be awkward and heavy (in time) to carry. These physical characteristics alone mean that rearing a cerebral-palsied child is going to be much more difficult and if the child has additional problems, such as a vision or hearing defect, parents may well feel overwhelmed by their child's problems.

Cerebral-palsied children, like many other handicapped children, have higher rates of sleep disturbance than normal children, and the parents are liable to have broken nights (the management of sleep disturbances is discussed in Chapter 9). The children are also likely to have difficulties over simple issues like toilet training. Their lack of mobility alone may make it difficult to use a toilet, and they may be delayed in achieving dryness. It is good if these processes in child-rearing, which the handicapped child shares with the normal child, proceed normally, but they may proceed much more slowly. The mother cannot expect a cerebral-palsied (CP) child to be out of nappies by two, and consequently demands are placed on her which she does not have with an ordinary child. Clearly all these considerations have implications for management of the specific condition. Sometimes, in concentrating on the particular problems such as the motor disorder in cerebral palsy, the clinician can fail to discuss some other ordinary issue, like night-waking, which may in fact, at the time, be far more wearing for the parent than managing the night splints which have perhaps been ordered to prevent contractures. It is easy therefore, as a professional trying to be honest, to leave parents depressed about their task.

Emotional and social issues

Attention has already been drawn to Mac Keith's elegant account of the problems facing the family of a handicapped child (see Appendix A2). The following discussion is based on that account, but reviews the problem of understanding the feelings of the family, and discusses how to communicate with them. When told they have a damaged child parents often go through the classic stages of grief associated with a death.

The first crisis for the parents is the moment of realization. Where the child is born with evident abnormality or it is recognized very early on, as with Down's syndrome or cerebral palsy, the parents should be told at once what the problem is and full discussion should follow. This imparting of the diagnostic news is discussed in the following paragraphs.

Parents are often faced with a period of *prediagnostic anxiety*. They have decided the child is slow and have gone to the doctor to ask his advice. He may not be able to make an immediate decision as to whether the child has cerebral palsy and even where he is aware of some abnormal neurological signs he may want to refer the child for full diagnostic assessment and necessary investigations. During this period communicating with the parent is often extremely difficult, as it is undesirable to share with them all the alarming diagnostic possibilities. Thus a patient who has spastic hemiplegia might have a brain tumour, but it hardly seems useful to say that one reason why you are carrying out a CT scan is to exclude this relatively rare possibility. The approach that seems most positive is to share with the parents the findings on clinical examination, and then discuss with them, in rather general terms, the diagnostic possibilities and explain in some detail what further steps are necessary to clarify the situation. Where an impairment seems likely, urgent investigation should take place not only in case the child has a condition which is treatable, but also to try and allay the prediagnostic anxiety as much as possible.

Once the diagnosis is established the parents should be told what the problem is. At one time some clinicians felt that it was wise to delay the passing on of the bad news, particularly when the parent perhaps was not aware that anything was wrong. Some still wait until the parents recognize that their child is slow before agreeing with them and then admitting to the diagnosis of Down's syndrome. However, parents generally want to know and should be told as soon as the doctor knows what is wrong with the child. The amount of information the parents can take in at any one time may be limited. At the first session the parents are likely to retain not much more than the diagnostic label itself. It is obviously sensible to try and arrange this consultation when the physician can afford the parents adequate time and also at a time when both parents can be available together. With a baby it is often useful to look at the baby with the parents, demonstrating abnormal features but equally stressing the child's assets and positive normal abilities.

At later consultations it may be helpful for the child to be cared for by someone else while the parents ask all the questions they want, and share their grief with the physician. It is often helpful to provide the parents with some simple literature at the first visit and suggest that at the next consultation, which should be very soon after this initial one, the parents should come with written questions for the clinician, so that they will not forget some of the questions which are uppermost in their minds. Another useful technique is to write down for the parents in the form of a letter the essential information that you have told them, so that they can review it together more slowly at home. A home visit by the doctor may be particularly welcomed at this time. The clinician may spend two or three sessions with parents in the first week after diagnosis as they slowly begin to sort out their feelings about their handicapped child and collect the information that they want to help them understand what has happened to them and their family. Table 7.2, derived from Cunningham & Sloper (1977), outlines the main stages in this process. Particularly if there are older siblings, it is very important that they should be included in this sharing of the information at this point.

As well as wanting information at these early interviews and wishing to share their feelings of grief and anger, parents often want to try and do something for their handicapped child immediately and it is important to make a practical suggestion early on, about something useful which they can do. This can usually be based on the handicapped child's developmental level, suggesting something which may

Table 7.2 Telling the parents that they have a child with a disability (adapted from Cunningham & Sloper, 1977).

Information given by a consultant paediatrician and (if possible) a specialist community nurse (health visitor) who works with disabled children

Information given as soon as possible after the diagnosis is definitely established

Information given in a private place where there will be no disturbances

Information given to both parents together with the infant present unless the latter is seriously ill

A direct simple statement of the diagnosis with as balanced view as possible of the main consequences. Do not offer too much information at this initial interview.

Leave as much time as the parents need to ask questions but tell them that there will be a follow-up interview at once

A written statement of what has been said should be given to the parents preferably at the interview but at least within 24 hours

The parents must have a private place to be alone in after the interview

The nurse will offer to see them again as soon as they like and particularly offer them help, advice and practical things to do with the infant

The nurse will offer them a contact phone number and arrange an early home visit (if the child is in hospital, within three days of discharge)

A follow-up interview with the paediatrician will be arranged within 1−3 days

---

help him to move on to the next stage. Emphasize to the parents that, as with all children, it is their role (and not the professional's) which is the crucial one. Their love and care are essential to the child.

The primary care physician may not be first person who passes on the information about handicap, but often parents, having met a paediatrician and discussed the situation, will then want to hear the same information from another source, and will often come to the GP to discuss it.

Once the early diagnostic period has passed, the parents will often become immersed in the practical issues of caring for a handicapped child, particularly when he has cerebral palsy. Frequent hospital visits may be required together with regular physiotherapist visits: the practical details of caring seem to take up all their energy. The arrival of the firstborn normal child has a profound impact on the relationship between couples and the arrival of a child with a disability has an even greater effect. In general the data suggest that divorce and marital breakdown are not commoner among such families but, where divorce does occur, the handicapped child is often implicated as a factor and many of these divorces occur fairly soon after the child has been born. One parent may totally reject the child, while the other may be able to accept the situation. The handicapped child may serve to bind the couple together, but this may not be a very positive relationship, all the couple's energies focusing on the child while their own relationship withers.

The next 'crisis' for the parents is often when the time comes for the child to go to school. Parents who seem to have been well adjusted may suddenly reveal how they have returned to unrealistic ideas about their child. Since 1981 the process of assessment of children for all educational placement has rested firmly with education authorities. The parents are told that their child is in need of special educational provision and 'statements' are prepared about the child. One of these statements (FA2) is made by a doctor: all decisions are discussed with the parents. In discussing educational placement the physician will want to share with his educational colleagues his thoughts about the child. The clinician may be surprised by how unaware the parents still are about the nature of their child's problems which he feels he has explained so often. This reminds him how much time must be spent both explaining the problem and its implications with the parents and exploring their feelings. Some parents will fight determinedly for 'normal' school or integration for their child; others will feel their child should have special provision.

PERIODIC REASSESSMENT

Some of the foregoing discussion emphasizes the need to see that the child with cerebral palsy has periodic reassessments, and the clinician should plan the times when he will do this. At reassessment he should review the diagnosis; for example it is not unknown for a child who has initially been diagnosed as having cerebral palsy to have another disorder. Management programmes need reassessing to see how effective they have been, and whether or not a different approach should be planned or considered. The effectiveness of care and counselling needs reviewing as changes occur over time in the family and the child. This professional reassessment should be followed by a full review with the parents.

Muscular dystrophy and spina bifida

The child with cerebral palsy may have a near-normal life expectancy and the parents' energies and efforts are directed at trying to get him 'cured' or as near 'normal' as possible. For the parents of a child with a condition like muscular dystrophy the diagnosis implies inevitable early death. Coupled with this, in the preschool years there is no special treatment for the child with muscular dystrophy. Indeed, he may be functioning reasonably well in a normal nursery school, with the decline in his motor abilities becoming more prominent at school age. In consequence the parents can do nothing for the child's condition and feel helpless. Their grief is likely to be coupled with guilt as they will be told that this is a genetic disorder and therefore they may need more counselling support than the parents of a child with other types of handicap.

The medical aspects of these two common physical disabilities, muscular dystrophy and spina bifida, will not be discussed here, for they are well described in paediatric texts (see also Hall, 1984). In spina bifida, as well as the lesion on the back many children will have hydrocephalus and some may require a valve inserted. Apart from paralysis of lower limbs (and it is a lower motor neurone lesion) the child will have difficulties with bowel and bladder. In consequence of these many problems, neurosurgical, renal and orthopaedic, the spina bifida child is very likely to spend periods in hospital and have many out-patient appointments. The family often become overwhelmed by the medical attention the child seems to be needing and this exaggerates all the feelings of a family with a handicapped child (described on p. 246 under cerebral palsy). They are likely therefore to need a lot of counsel, care and support from the health services.

Developmental motor delay

A small number of children will present with motor delay or, in the older child, a degree of clumsiness where no impairment can be found and the child may simply be at the bottom range of normal. In Table 7.3 we show the numbers of children considered to have delay in gross or fine motor development at different ages. When the child presents with generalized motor delay the clinician is faced with the problem of trying to decide whether the child has a neurodevelopmental disorder or not and quite clearly any child presenting in this way deserves a most careful clinical appraisal including a family history, if possible

Table 7.3 Percentage of children regarded as having possible or definite delay at various ages. Data from our Coram Study. The number of children studied at each age was over 250.

Age (years)	Gross motor	Fine motor
1	3.0	2.0
1½	2.0	5.0
2	2.0	6.5
3	0.5	9.0
4½	3.5	6.5

obtaining information about the development of both parents when they were children, and a full physical examination. Such an examination will probably reveal in a proportion of cases some neurological signs which will suggest that further investigation is appropriate and necessary. Where there are no abnormal findings and the child seems to be normal in all respects other than motor function, the doctor has a difficult decision to make about whether to refer the child for further investigation. It seems most useful to discuss the different types of delay under different age groups.

UNDER AGE ONE

We assume here that the child presents only with delay of motor development and other dimensions of function are normal. Under the age of one, common complaints are that the child is late sitting or is not taking his weight on his legs. Failure to bear weight about six months is not an uncommon phenomenon. When lifted, the baby will often hold the lower limbs with the hips flexed at right angles and the knees extended (i.e. 'sitting on air' position). This is seen both in babies who have subsequently moved by bottom shuffling and in babies who are born by breech delivery. In both instances there seems to be some delay in the development of standing, but this is subsequently normal. In all the variants of motor development babies should certainly achieve sitting balance by nine months. In our sample mentioned in Chapter 2, over 50% were sitting by six months. If the child is not sitting without support by nine months a full neurological examination is needed in order to try and identify a cause for the delay. If the child does not seem to be sitting up at all *with* support around five to six months one would be concerned.

THE SECOND YEAR OF LIFE AND AFTER

The major milestone of the second year of life is the development of walking. Any child of eighteen months who is not walking requires full evaluation and possible investigation. We found in our sample that just over 2% of children were not walking at this age (Chapter 3). Hardie & MacFarlane (1980) studied a population of eighteen-month-old non-walking children and, while the majority of these children proved to be normal, the population did include a proportion of children with cerebral palsy and mental retardation (data from their study are presented in Table 7.4). Some children, as already mentioned, do walk late. Particularly important here are those children with a

Table 7.4 Children who were not walking by 18 months (from Chaplais and Macfarlane). Of the 127 (32%) abnormal children, 112 had been referred before 18 months. Of the normal children observed 48% bottom-shuffled.

Cerebral palsy	49
Other neurological abnormalities	9
Mentally retarded (including Downs)	25
Congenital syndromes	37
Muscular dystrophy	2
Other abnormal	5
Total abnormal	*127*
Normals	
of which bottom shufflers	116
crawlers	108
others	18
not known	17
Total normal	*259*
Not seen (presumed normal)	18

history of bottom shuffling. Of normal children who were not walking at 18 months of age, 48% were bottom shufflers. These children may walk as late as the third year and yet subsequently prove to be normal, but it is important to make absolutely sure that the child does not have some minor motor defect and Robson (1970) has pointed out the difficulty sometimes in recognizing mild spastic diplegia. Obviously the following up of the 'normal' child will continue until the clinician is satisfied that his walking is normal.

In Chapter 4 we discuss the motor assessment of three-, four- and five-year-olds and there is a progression of motor skills developing through these ages. There may be children who are rather clumsy in terms of gross motor performance at these ages but the numbers involved are very small and we think that clumsiness of movement alone is rarely of significance neurologically unless it is associated with problems of fine motor delay. Nevertheless, the child may well be at a disadvantage socially.

CLUMSINESS IN CHILDREN WITH DIFFICULTIES IN RELATION TO FINE MOTOR SKILLS

A number of children considered to be definitely abnormal at two, three and four years on fine motor skills (usually just over 1%) had in many instances general developmental problems. Clumsiness did not often present as an isolated entity. Children who are simply clumsy and who have no other defects probably represent the bottom range of the normal continuum and studies by Henderson & Hall (1982) suggest they do well.

Clumsiness needs to be recognized and accepted by the people who look after the children, who may need some help in their early school years with things like self-help skills for PE etc.; in practice these are not very serious matters if sensitively handled.

In our studies in Central London we found that 5% of three-year-old children still had a fisted grip on the pencil and 26% had not developed a full tripod grip. At four and a half only 1% still had a fisted grip and 9% still did not have a tripod grip. These children are often not clumsy but their skills are immature. Quite clearly motor function can be improved by practice and training and in assessing function the child's previous experience with, for example, crayons and paper needs to be considered. Lack of experience may have accounted for the higher rates of fisted grip found some years earlier in Deptford, in a largely immigrant population.

Jittery babies

A relatively common experience in the newborn period is to see an infant whose motor activity is high enough to be a cause for concern. The mother may observe frequent startle reactions looking like Moro responses and the baby may have a coarse tremor. On examination it may be very easy to elicit reflexes and possible to initiate ankle clonus which may be sustained for several beats. The first priority is to make sure that the baby does not have convulsive movements. These may be localized and not generalized and the beat of the tremor is uneven, that is, stronger in one direction than the other, whereas with the tremor associated with the 'jittery baby' syndrome the strength of the movement is equal in both directions. The infant may also give some feeling of increased tone. The proportion of babies who are jittery increases during the early days of life, peaking around the 9th or 10th day and then becoming less. This syndrome is sometimes referred to as the hyperexcitability syndrome and, while there have been some reports of babies with this syndrome having some minor abnormal movements later, in general the parents can be reassured that the baby will develop normally.

Mental handicap

The number of children with moderate to severe mental handicap is something over three to four per 1000, while mild mental handicap is much more prevalent, involving perhaps an additional 10% of children.

Many syndromes of mental subnormality associated with congenital malformation can be identified at birth. The best-known example of this is Down's syndrome, as the abnormal facies and the floppiness of the baby usually attract the midwife's attention. The next most common cause of mental subnormality is probably the fragile X syndrome. Many rarer syndromes are associated with obvious somatic defects in the baby. If looked for, many metabolic disorders could be identified at birth. Phenylketonuria is probably the best-known example and if identification is made treatment can be initiated. The only other 'metabolic' disorder routinely screened for in the UK is hypothyroidism. It is not, however, appropriate to screen for many of the rarer forms of metabolic disorder where no treatment is at present available. Sometimes there will be consequences of these metabolic disorders so that as the child gets older somatic signs attract the attention of the family and their doctor. This will be so with a rare condition like mucopolysaccharidosis where deposition of the abnormally accumulating substance leads to the appearance of abnormal facies. Any abnormality in a baby therefore necessitates a careful assessment of development. Many forms of mental retardation present as developmental delay. Once 'slowness' is definitely determined a full paediatric diagnostic study should be made to try and find a cause (or causes). Metabolic, cytogenetic and neurological investigations should be carried out. With the more severe degrees of mental handicap a diagnosis can be made in around 80% while in mild mental handicap a diagnosis is reached in about 50%.

Whereas in motor disorders such as cerebral palsy cognitive functions and speech and language may be normal, in the child with mental retardation it is these functions which are most severely affected and motor development may be relatively spared or normal. The difficulty for the clinician is to decide when the child's general development is so delayed that referral, diagnosis and assessment are necessary.

Assessment of the mentally handicapped child in the first year of life

In addition to children with the identifiable congenital syndromes described above, the baby who is excessively floppy in the newborn period gives cause for concern and will need careful follow-up, watching for slow development of head control, delay in the pull-to-sit manoeuvre and late sitting (after nine months is probably a reasonable cut-off point). The baby may be late rolling over, something he should normally do around three to four months. However, more important than these signs of motor delay are delays in cognitive and social function. Nine out of 10 children are smiling by six weeks and any child not smiling after eight weeks should be carefully followed. At this time the mentally handicapped baby may be reported as being 'good'. He may sleep a lot, take his feeds well, and be an easy baby to look after. As well as smiling late he is slow to enter into social interchanges with the mother. Babbling is slow to start and as the first year goes on the consonantal sounds do not appear. The 'jargon' of the normal one-year-old does not develop. Reaching and grasping are similarly delayed and the child's pincer grip may develop much later than in a normal child. Responses to both visual and auditory stimuli are slow and deliberate in the second half of the first year in contrast to the normal alert baby who turns rapidly to sound by six months, and who is busy scanning his environment much of the waking time. In the second six months, too, social slowness may be apparent: he still happily goes to complete strangers, smiles at them readily and if his parents leave him is not distressed.

Assessment of the mentally handicapped child in the second year of life

The motor delay described above becomes more evident and the child may not sit until around 13 or 14 months. More importantly now begin anxieties about speech and language. The child does not develop naming words — does not say 'mum' or 'dad' — and the flourish of vocabulary in the second half of the second year does not take place. Symbolic play does not occur. Confronted with a doll or a car the child of 18 months fails to identify their symbolic identity and treats them as objects which may be thrown on the floor or banged up and down. Mouthing objects which is so frequent at around six months may persist into the second year, as also may casting. Cognitive gains, such as posting — pushing shape forms into a 'letter-box' — banging of rods into place and so on, and early games in the second year of life are delayed. The baby may be cuddly and friendly, but not exploring his environment and staying very easy to handle well into the second and third year of life.

As the child gets older he functions at a level well below his chronological age. The mentally handicapped four-year-old may be at the level of a 'normal' 18-month-old child. In the younger age groups the clinician is often tempted to ignore or dismiss some delay. It is better to be honest and say 'he is slow' — the decision as to when to proceed to full investigation is a difficult one but is often delayed too long.

Management of the mentally handicapped child

Many of the principles discussed earlier in the chapter in relation to management are the same for the mentally handicapped child as for the physically handicapped child. The parents want diagnostic information and adequate assessment of the child. Just as with any handicap they want counselling about this slow child and about their own feelings.

The child with mental handicap must be very carefully assessed as he may have multiple problems. Thus the child with Down's syndrome is more likely than the normal child to have congenital malformation of the heart, hypothyroidism, visual and hearing defects and later orthopaedic difficulties. All these must be identified and appropriately 'treated' or managed.

The obvious and particular problem with the mentally handicapped child is the simple issue that he or she is slow to develop and all stages of childhood seem to be extended. It takes a long time to learn to handle a spoon, toilet training takes longer and so on. Some parents find it helpful to have a programme which takes them through stages and breaks up the development of one skill into small parts. Probably the best known of these programmes is the Portage system. Many district and mental handicap teams will provide a psychologist or a health visitor to help the family to use the system. The Portage worker will call on the family on a regular basis and together with the parents identify a skill which the baby might be going to acquire. For example, in the introduction of spoon-feeding, the first stage will be the child simply grasping the spoon, then he proceeds slowly through identifying that the spoon is something used at feeding time, to actually getting it into the food and picking some up. Parents and worker will identify goals which can be achieved week by week and record when these goals are reached. The system looks at the infant's behaviour under headings of general stimulation, socialization, language, self-help skills and cognitive and motor functions. The delay in the child's social development may become one of the most difficult features of the condition for the family. The child with Down's syndrome may never develop a fear of strangers and his over-friendly approach together with his immature behaviour may make him difficult to handle in social situations like shopping.

With the physically handicapped child who is also mentally handicapped the family may concentrate on the physical handicap. Some parents 'demand' more physiotherapy and try 'new cures', seeming to avoid confronting their child's mental slowness. The parents of a mentally handicapped child cannot do this and feel 'helpless' in their inability to do anything to speed their child's progress.

All handicapped children have the right to some preschool education from the age of two and parents need to begin to think about the education level appropriate for their child early on so that plans can be made. Since the 1981 Education Act, the objective is that handicapped children will be integrated into normal schools and, while this ideal aim cannot always be achieved at the moment, parents should start looking at the local situation early on and making contact with education authorities. They will often want to talk to a doctor about plans for the child's education although, as discussed earlier, the doctor does not make this decision.

Sensory handicaps

Blindness and partial sight and moderate to severe sensory-neural deafness are both rare disorders in childhood, but enormously incapacitating when they do occur (together just over 1 per 1000). Many of the conditions causing these disorders are genetic and the family history may be significant. With either of these disorders it is not uncommon for both parents to have the condition and the consequent risks for their children are therefore increased. In other examples there may be some other causative factor. For deafness the best known cause is the rubella syndrome caused by German measles infection in the early months of pregnancy. This ought to be eliminated from the United Kingdom, but has not been totally eradicated. The handicap will be identified by the routine assessment of vision and hearing in the young child and referral for diagnosis and assessment to the appropriate centre. While much sensorineural hearing loss should be identified soon after birth some congenital syndromes have onset after birth. In rubella syndrome the virus is active after birth and hearing may deteriorate. Repeated assessment of hearing must go on all through the early years of life.

Not all district handicap teams will have staff who have had experience of these relatively rare disorders and it may be necessary for the parents to visit regional centres where experience is available. Education departments have specialist teachers of both deaf and visually impaired children who will visit homes. Both the Royal National Institute for the Blind and the Royal National Institute for the Deaf have staff who will visit families in the home and give advice and help. As with all rare disorders the general practitioner may rapidly find that the parents' knowledge of the condition outstrips his own and it is important to recognize this and let the parents supply some of the information required by the doctor.

Children with visual and hearing impairment need full diagnosis and assessment, which may not be easy. Early management is important. Blind children have to be helped to use sound and touch to make meaningful communication. If appropriate, amplification should be fitted to the deaf child as early as possible and it must be carefully monitored. As with other handicapping conditions, there may be associated problems. Thus, for example, difficult behaviours may present to the primary care team and are often very difficult to manage.

Less severe visual handicap

Visual acuity errors and squint are very common disorders in early childhood. The rates that we find at three and four and a half years are given in Chapter 4. Vision testing, as described earlier (see Chapter 4), is difficult in the young child but new techniques are becoming available and both defects of visual acuity and squint, if not identified and recognized in early life, may interfere with the child's function in later life. By school age 7% of children have some disorder of vision.

Less serious hearing problems

Hearing difficulties associated with upper respiratory tract infection are extremely common in the preschool period. Their management is discussed in Chapter 8, but their identification is important. The relationship between hearing disorders and language development is a complex one and is discussed in the next section.

Speech and language disorders

Speech and language disorders are very common in preschool children. It is difficult to be certain at early ages whether the child has a speech defect or not, but the figures that we have are very similar to those of other studies. When we looked at two-year-olds, of those who responded 16% were scored as having very few words. This meant that the child possibly had only 'mum', 'dad' and other names of people in the house, but did not name common objects. In rather more than twice that number of children we did not hear a sentence, but this is perhaps not very helpful at this stage as quite a lot of the two-year-olds' utterances are not in the form of a sentence and in an inhibiting environment the child may not produce a sentence of which he may be capable. The assessment of speech and language is very much more reliable at three. Just over 10% of the three-year-olds definitely had delay in speech and language development. By four and a half, 5% were rated as definitely abnormal with a further 7% being possibly abnormal.

What is the nature of these disorders and what should one do about them? First of all, are we simply looking at a range of normal development? The answer is certainly in part 'yes'. Some of the three-year-old children when followed up to four and a half or five years seemed to have caught up and did not have any further difficulties. On the other hand numerous studies (Richman *et al.*, 1982) have now shown that if you follow three-year-old non-talkers through into school quite a proportion of them do have difficulties even though they have started to talk. They may have reading and learning difficulties. The point as to whether these represent pathology or not is in a way academic. At three if a child is not yet producing any sentences and has a limited vocabulary, perhaps under 20 words, it is time to ascertain the reason and consider some form of intervention.

Diagnosis and assessment

Speech and language disorders are sometimes associated with other problems. The most common of these are disorders of the upper respiratory tract and hearing. It may be concluded that a period of 'glue ear' has affected the child's ability to learn language and this is making him a bit late in talking, but the clinician should be a little cautious about making this rather easy assumption. It may be that there is a less direct association between frequent upper respiratory tract infections and a child's delayed speech. In our study at all ages there was some indication of a delay in speech and language development if a child had a conductive hearing loss, but this association was strongest at two years and became weaker as the child got older. The suggestion, perhaps, from these data was that, while a hearing problem during the second year of life and during the time that language is acquired may be important and certainly cause delay, it may not be enough to account for the delayed development of language in a three-year-old. A fluctuating hearing loss may mean that a child stops 'listening' to those around him and this may become more important than the actual loss. Nevertheless, anyone who sees a child with speech and language delay at three who also has a hearing problem will wish to consider the extent of the difficulty and whether amplification or other treatment might be helpful.

Speech and language disorders and mental handicap

Mentally handicapped children all have speech and language delay and when a three-year-old is seen with such delay the first thing to decide is whether this is part of a general overall developmental delay or whether other aspects of function are near normal and it is speech and language which are particularly involved.

Behaviour disorders and speech and language problems

Many studies have shown the association between speech and language problems and disordered behaviour, and this association showed up very strongly in our data at all ages. Again there is the question of what is the nature of the association. It could be that an altered relationship between the mother, father and child, or difficult behaviour on the part of the child leading to inadequate parental interaction, is a factor in the delayed development of the child's communication. Conversely, developmental delay in communication skills when other parameters of development are proceeding normally could mean that the child is frustrated and the parents' expectations similarly frustrated so that eventually this combination of circumstances has led to the development of tempers and other difficult behaviour.

Whatever the association, the nature of the disorder itself must be considered. Table 7.5, based on Bishop & Rosenbloom (1987), suggests some of the categories for a child with a speech and language problem and relates to the categories of language discussed in Chapter 2. The clinician tries to decide whether the language disorder is largely expressive in nature, only perhaps involving the transmission system while the child is developing good syntactical and semantic abilities but failing to express them, or conversely that the child's expressive side and transmission system may be functioning well but he is having difficulty with syntactical and semantic acquisition. The child needs to be observed while playing and in a relaxed manner in order to reach a decision. The speech therapist will help with the assessment and when this is complete the next issue to consider is management.

Management

Should one intervene with the child whose speech and language are delayed in the preschool period and what are the possibilities? It is first important to remember that the child learns language on a one-to-one basis. Learning in a group may help him but if he is very slow may not be very advantageous. It seems useful to us to assess what can be done at home, what can be done in the nursery school or day nursery if he is in one, and then what can be done in specific situations.

FAMILY

In relation to the family and the child it is obviously important to deal with secondary problems. If the child is having a lot of tempers and the parents are finding him difficult to manage (and it is more often a him than a her) the first thing to do is to try and help with the behaviour difficulties, in the hope that the easing of tension in the family may provide an environment in which language will naturally develop. Strategies for handling behaviour are discussed in Chapter 9. At the same time one obviously wants to discuss the way in which the family are communicating with the child. The most important element here is to ensure that once or twice a day one of his favourite adults sits down with the child and talks *with* him (not *to* him). Sometimes a parent anxious about a child's delay will desperately get him to name objects in a book or play some sort of naming game. This is a stilted style of conversation and the parents should be encouraged not to do this but rather to concentrate on developing a conversational milieu and being not too concerned about the nature of the child's reply, helping him instead to realize the importance of conversation. Many people believe reading to a child slowly or telling a simple story is a good way of attracting his attention to spoken sounds and of course this helps him to associate visual with auditory input. Play with toys between adult and child can be as good as looking at books. Most people would suggest that a parent should spend at least 20 minutes twice a day sitting with the child and talking with him. There is little direct evidence of this necessarily improving the child's performance but it can do no harm.

NURSERY

In the nursery some of the same principles apply. Is his behaviour such that the staff are finding it difficult to relate to him and only interacting with him to deal with tempers or other difficult behaviour? If so, these issues should be tackled first before the communication one. Then it is important to try and see that he is in a one-to-one situation as often as possible during the day. Investigation in nursery schools has shown that the teacher has relatively little time for direct

Table 7.5 A two-way classification of childhood language disorders with examples recently suggested by Bishop & Rosenbloom (1986).

	Structural or sensorimotor defect of speech apparatus	Hearing loss	Brain damage or dysfunction acquired in prenatal or perinatal period	Brain damage or dysfunction acquired in childhood	Emotional behavioural disorders	Environmental deprivation	Aetiology unclear
Speech limited in quality and/or quantity but other language skills normal	Dysphonia: dysarthria	Deafness acquired after language developed			Elective mutism		Developmental apraxia of speech
Generalized delay of language development		? With chronic conductive hearing loss	Common with most types of intellectual retardation			Result of neglect	? Delayed language
Specific problems with syntax and phonology		? Particularly with selective high-frequency loss		With left-hemisphere lesions in older children			Phonologic–syntactic syndrome

Specific problems with semantics and pragmatics		Cocktail-party syndrome; infantile autism (mild)		Semantic-pragmatic disorder
Poor understanding and limited verbal expression	With severe or profound prelingual deafness	Severe mental handicap	With bilateral lesions of language areas; Landau-Kleffner syndrome	Congenital auditory imperception
Severe impairment of non-verbal as well as verbal communication	Severe mental handicap; infantile mutism	Ultimate outcome of degenerative disorders		

communication with individual children, tending to communicate with them in a group. In this group situation the language-delayed child will probably not make much progress. For certain group activities such as 'story time' it is useful to see that the speech-delayed child is put near the person who is telling the story so that he or she can try and direct some of the story almost individually at him while talking to the other children. At the same time it seems reasonable to try and arrange a couple of periods during the day when he has the individual attention of the nursery teacher or nursery nurse. Will placing the child in a day nursery or nursery school help the development of speech and language? Many parents feel it will but there is little evidence to support the view that simply putting the child in a nursery school environment is an adequate treatment of speech and language delay. Where the home environment presents problems such as the mother being depressed, then clearly time in the more stimulating atmosphere of the nursery can be beneficial.

SPECIFIC TREATMENT

Specific treatment involves a skilled speech pathologist or speech thera-pist working on an individual basis with the child. There is now evidence that speech therapy can be beneficial but it is difficult to know which children to refer and when. After six months of some general advice to families and the day nursery, if a child's speech is still moderately retarded at three years, most clinicians will feel that they ought to do something to help the child and so will their speech therapy colleagues. If individual therapy is to be undertaken it is important to see that a reliable measure has been made of the child's speech and language before therapy starts (the commonest test used in this country is still the Reynell Developmental Language Scale) and that goals be set by the therapist for the achievement of certain targets, e.g. that the child is going to advance to a certain level over the next three or six months.

Therapy should be regularly monitored. Some speech therapists prefer to spend less time individually with the child and more time encouraging the adults around him, the parents and family, nursery staff and teacher, to communicate meaningfully with him. When a child seems to be making no progress with a particular form of therapy, its efficacy must be called into question. Regular reassessment of the speech- and language-delayed child is very important as the child approaches school age. If it looks as though he is going to have serious speech and language problems when he starts school, formal assessment procedures should begin before he is admitted to infant school so that appropriate extra help can be given as early as possible in his school career.

Common and uncommon forms of neurodevelopmental disorder

In this chapter we have discussed some of the commoner forms of neurodevelopmental disorder such as cerebral palsy, mental retardation (of which the classic example is Down's syndrome) and speech and language disorders. If we take any group of children with moderate to severe handicap, perhaps half of them will fall into one of these diagnostic categories. The other half will be made up of children with single diagnoses of less common conditions, of which an individual practitioner or even paediatrician may have little experience. Just as the well-known handicaps have had parent groups associated with them over the years, many of the rarer handicaps now have parent groups, some of which have made a particular point of producing literature to be given to their own doctors providing basic information about the condition. Some of the congenital disorders may not present at birth but only emerge after a year or two. The clinician should be particularly anxious when the parents report that the child's development which had been proceeding normally has regressed. Such a child might have anything from a brain tumour to a progressive metabolic or degenerative disorder. Equally disturbing is bizarre behaviour, not in the range of common behaviour problems in children. Here we include the symptoms that precede conditions like autism or some of the stereotypes or abnormal movements seen in other forms of handicap.

Services for the child with a neurodevelopmental disorder

According to how severe the disorder is, the child may be managed by the general practitioner alone or with specialist help; if the condition is moderate to severe, diagnostic assessment should be done by a paediatrician and a plan for management developed together. In addition others, such as physiotherapists, speech therapists, occupational therapists and psychologists, may need to be involved in the management of the child.

In most parts of the country, following the Court report (1976), district handicap teams have been developed and many of them are based in a child assessment or development centre. In these centres more time can be spent assessing the child than is possible in an ordinary paediatric out-patient department and most of them have the core staff described in the previous paragraph, so that a multidisciplinary approach can be made to assessment and management of the child. Possibly 1−2% of children will need to go to such a centre but many of the minor developmental disorders discussed above can be adequately managed from a family practice. It is our view that the primary care doctor should maintain close contact with the child and family even if management is largely taking place at the child development centre.

Services vary greatly in different parts of the country. Sometimes a consultant with a special interest will conduct his own clinic for children with muscular dystrophy and not refer them to the district handicap team. It may sometimes be the case that a particular paediatrician is not as aware as he should be of what is and is not available for handicapped children in his district. The general practitioner's role is particularly important with some of the rarer disorders, where the diagnosing paediatrician is at a regional children's hospital and hence can do little to support the family in their own locality. The general practitioner must then see that the family are slotted into district handicapped children's services as well as having contact with the specialist. Again, some districts lack any services for handicapped children, and where this is the case the general practitioner may want to support the family in their search for something better.

In this book we have not extended our discussion of the management of handicapped children into the school years. For the 1 or 2% of children of school age who require the services of the handicapped children's team, this should extend its service into schools and work closely with school nurses and doctors. Special schools now very commonly have a community paediatrician serving them. As and if integration develops satisfactorily there will be more moderately to severely handicapped children in ordinary schools and services must be developed to meet their needs. We are not going to discuss these issues fully here, but planning for the school years must begin in the preschool years and indeed most handicapped children benefit from going to a preschool placement. It is good for the child with a handicap to go into an ordinary nursery school or day nursery if possible, but some child development centres run nursery groups which the child can attend and fuller assessment can be made by watching him at play. It is in this situation that plans can most realistically be made for the child's education and future.

References

Bishop, D. & Rosenbloom, L. (1987) Classification of childhood language disorders. In *Language Development and Disorders* (ed. Yule, W. & Rutter, M.). Mac Keith Press.

Bleck, E.E. (1975) Locomotor prognosis in cerebral palsy. *Developmental Medicine and Child Neurology*, **17**, 18−25.

Court, S.D.M. (1976) *Fit for the future*. HMSO: London.

Cunningham, C. & Sloper, P. (1977) Parents of Down's syndrome babies: their early needs. *Child Care, Health and Development*, **8**, 1−19.

Hall, D.M.B. (1984) *The Child with a Handicap*. Blackwell Scientific Publications, Oxford.

Henderson, S.E. & Hall, D. (1982) Concomitants of clumsiness in young children. *Developmental Medicine and Child Neurology*, **24**, 448−60.

Hardie, J. De Z. & MacFarlane, A. (1980) Late walking children: a review of 106 late walkers in the Oxford area. *Health Visitor*, **53**, 466.

Mac Keith R. (1973) The feelings and behaviour of parents of handicapped children. *Developmental Medicine and Child Neurology*, **15** (4), 524−7.

Richmond, N., Stevenson, J. & Graham, P. (1982) *Preschool to School: a Behavioural Study*. Academic Press, London.

Robson, P. (1970) Shuffling, hitching, scooting or sliding. Some observations in otherwise normal children. *Developmental Medicine and Child Neurology*, **12**, 608−17.

8   Common Health Problems

THIS CHAPTER focuses on health issues which may significantly affect development and behaviour and which have important links with social and environmental factors. No attempt is made to cover the many conditions found in a paediatric textbook.

Respiratory illnesses are emphasized because we know they are linked to the child's development, behaviour and home background. Similarly, family relationships and the social environment are important in failure to thrive and sudden infant death and it may be possible to identify predisposing factors at an early and preventable stage.

Other common problems such as skin conditions, congenital anomalies and developmental orthopaedic conditions are also included because they are frequently found during routine clinical examination rather than presenting acutely and may have a bearing on other aspects of the child's progress.

Respiratory illness

Illnesses involving the upper and lower respiratory tract are responsible for 80% of consultations with the general practitioner in the under-five age-group. They are five times as frequent a reason for consultation as other common conditions like gastroenteritis, skin disease and the acute infectious diseases. On average, children experience six to eight acute respiratory illnesses each year (Dingle *et al.*, 1964) though the doctor's advice may not always be sought.

The management of acute upper and lower respiratory tract illness is well covered in standard paediatric texts. The epidemiology of these illnesses and the management of common problems are the focus of this section.

Epidemiology

INCIDENCE OF UPPER RESPIRATORY TRACT
INFECTION (URTI)

Since most uncomplicated URTIs are managed by parents at home rather than in consultation with the general practitioner, data from

Table 8.1 History of upper respiratory illnesses during three months preceding interview.

Frequency of URTI	6 month		12 month		18 month		2 year		3 year		4½ year	
	n	%	*n*	%	*n*	%	*n*	%	*n*	%	*n*	%
Less than once in 3 months	222	67	145	52	137	55	157	52	145	44	152	55
Once in 1−3 month	86	26	93	34	84	33	102	34	133	40	99	36
More than once a month	23	7	39	14	30	12	42	14	53	16	24	9
Total *n*	331		277		251		301		331		275	

studies of these illnesses in general practice underestimate the true incidence. Studies of illness in the home and information from parents themselves give a more realistic measure of these conditions. In our study parents were asked how many episodes of colds, coughs, sore throats and tonsillitis their child had had in the last three months (Table 8.1). These illnesses, which included nasopharyngitis, pharyngitis and tonsillopharyngitis, were grouped together as URTI. URTIs were least frequent from three to six months although even in this period a third of babies had at least one URTI.

The frequency of URTI increased after six months of age reaching a peak at three years, coinciding with the time most children start nursery school. Between one and three years a considerable proportion, ranging from 12 to 16% of children were reported as having colds more than once a month. This group probably represents children with 'chronic' nasopharyngitis who are having frequent infections, have some underlying nasopharyngeal condition or in some cases have allergic rhinitis. This group diminished in size by the age of four and a half. The children who had URTI more than once a month (frequent URTI) were more likely to suffer from bronchitis or ear infection as well than children with fewer URTIs, but few children suffered from both bronchitis and ear infection. URTIs were a common factor in both bronchitis and ear infection but children tended to develop either one or the other.

INCIDENCE OF LOWER RESPIRATORY TRACT INFECTIONS

There is far more information available on the incidence of lower respiratory tract infections than on that of URTIs since they are in-

Table 8.2 History of bronchitis in different age-groups of children in Camden and Westminster experimental areas.

	Age-group of child							
	0–1 year		1–2 year		2–3 year		3–4 year	
	n	%	*n*	%	*n*	%	*n*	%
Bronchitis once	24	8	11	4	14	4	9	3
Bronchitis more than once	15	5	18	6	25	7	18	6
Total *n*	274		283		328		278	

variably reasons for consulting a doctor. In all studies the peak incidence occurs during the first year of life. In Chapel Hill, North Carolina, a study of nearly 7000 children attending a paediatric group practice found the incidence of croup (laryngotracheobronchitis), bronchitis, bronchiolitis and pneumonia amounted to 250 episodes per 1000 children during the first year of life, diminishing to 180 per 1000 by the age of five years (Glezen & Denny, 1973). In a study of 2000 children in Harrow (Leeder *et al.*, 1976a) 11.5% of children had bronchitis or pneumonia during the first year, falling to 6.7% in the fifth.

In our study 13% of babies were reported to have had bronchitis during the first year, falling to 9% by the fourth year (Table 8.2).

RELATIONSHIP BETWEEN CHILDHOOD RESPIRATORY
ILLNESSES AND LATER RESPIRATORY ILLNESS

Although clinical recovery from acute respiratory illness in childhood is usual there is some evidence that there may be long-term consequences. Studies have demonstrated impaired ventilatory function in children following lower respiratory tract infection (Colley *et al.*, 1973) and in a birth cohort followed up until the age of 20 years those with a history of lower respiratory tract infection under the age of two years had a higher incidence of respiratory symptoms at the age of 20.

INCIDENCE OF WHEEZING AND ASTHMA

Asthma is a common and probably under-diagnosed condition in childhood yet its exact definition remains the subject of debate. A useful general definition is that of Scadding (1983), who states that 'Asthma is a disease characterized by wide variations over short periods of time in resistance to flow in intrapulmonary airways'. This has been expanded by Godfrey (1985) in relation to childhood asthma:

> Asthma in childhood is a disease characterized by wide variations over short periods of time in resistance to flow in intrapulmonary airways and manifest by recurrent attacks of cough or wheeze separated by symptom-free intervals. The airflow obstruction and clinical symptoms are largely or completely reversed by treatment with bronchodilator drugs or steroids.

Since wheezy bronchitis undoubtedly precedes asthma in some children studies have looked at whether these are two separate conditions or whether there is a common defect. Results have been conflicting. One study (Sibbald *et al.*, 1980) shows an increased family history of wheezing bronchitis and asthma in children with both wheezy bronchitis and asthma. Other studies show little relation between wheezy bronchitis in infants and a family history of asthma or allergic disease.

On the other hand there is a strong link between asthma and a personal and family history of atopic conditions, although the condition also occurs where there is no such history. The child with eczema has a 40 to 50% chance of developing asthma within 10 years. About 5% of children with hay fever will eventually develop asthma (Kuzenko, 1976).

Most children with asthma have their first attack under the age of five and over half before their second birthday (Blair, 1977).

Early onset does not necessarily indicate a poor long-term prognosis but severe initial attacks are associated with a higher incidence of persistent asthma 20 years later. Asthma may remit and subsequently reappear in early adult life. Studies which have followed children into adult life indicate that about half of those with childhood asthma will still be having some symptoms as adults though only about a quarter will have never stopped wheezing for longer than six months. About 5% of children with asthma will be severely handicapped by asthma as adults. Other factors which predispose to long-term asthma include the presence of associated atopic disease and a family history of atopic disease (Blair, 1977). Clearly many children will lose their asthma as they grow older, which is partly attributable to larger airways reducing the effect of obstruction. But the evidence suggests that one cannot confidently reassure parents that a particular child will grow out of it completely, especially if he has had severe wheezing at a young age. As Blair's study showed, some children enjoy a free interval during adolescence only to relapse and develop further symptoms in later years.

FACTORS INFLUENCING INCIDENCE OF RESPIRATORY
TRACT INFECTIONS

Sex

Both upper and lower respiratory tract infections and asthma are more
common in males than females during early childhood. Deaths from
pneumonia account for the male preponderance of mortality during
the first year of life. The male to female ratio was 2:1 for lower
respiratory illnesses in children under six in the Chapel Hill study
(Glezen & Denny, 1973). The ratio in asthma is approximately 2:1
(Office of Health Economics, 1976) but the sex difference disappears
towards adolescence.

Birthweight

In our study and in the British Births Study (Chamberlain & Simpson,
1970) there was a non-significant trend towards lighter babies having
more upper respiratory tract infections up to the age of three years.
Similarly lower respiratory tract infections are more common in lighter
infants (Douglas & Blomfield, 1958).

Family factors

Colds, bronchitis and pneumonia during the first year of life are more
prevalent in children with siblings (Leeder *et al.*, 1976a; Bax *et al.*, 1980).
The incidence is increased where the sibling also had bronchitis or
pneumonia, especially at school-starting age, suggesting that many
factors interact in these families such as overcrowding, poor nutrition
and poor hygiene (Brimblecombe, 1958). Other closely linked factors
act in concert to influence the effect of social class, birthweight, family
size, method of feeding, parental smoking and parental health.

   Asthma follows a somewhat different social class pattern from respiratory infections. In some studies asthma has been reported more
commonly in social classes I and II (Hamman *et al.*, 1975; Leeder *et al.*,
1976b) though severe asthma is more frequent amongst children of
manual workers (Mitchell & Dawson, 1973).

Infant feeding

There is mounting evidence that breast-fed infants have fewer illnesses
and allergic conditions during the first year of life than their bottle-
fed counterparts. In our study bottle-fed babies were four times as
likely as those who were breast-fed for more than three weeks to suffer
from bronchitis in the first six months; the difference was still significant

after controlling for social class. In Blair's study (1977) breast-feeding for up to a week improved early prognosis for asthma whereas breast-feeding for more than eight weeks significantly diminished the likelihood of long-term asthma. Another study found a marked decrease in otitis media, lower respiratory disease and vomiting and diarrhoea amongst breast-fed infants (Cunningham, 1977). There was a particularly striking reduction in pneumonia and life-threatening illness in the breast-fed group. The differences persisted within social class groups.

Parental smoking

Parental smoking has recently been recognized as a major factor in increasing the risk of lower respiratory illness in childhood. In the Harrow study (Colley *et al.*, 1974) infants whose parents smoked suffered from more frequent bronchitis and pneumonia in the first year, the pattern remaining similar within each social class. In a New Zealand study (Fergusson *et al.*, 1980) maternal but not paternal smoking increased the chances of both lower respiratory tract infection and wheezing in the first year. Presumably the duration of exposure to cigarette smoke explains the effect of the sex of the smoking parent.

The incidence of both asthma and wheezy bronchitis is increased where there is at least one asthmatic relative and there is a similar trend with a history of wheezy bronchitis. The strong similarity in family history of asthma between children suffering from both asthma and wheezy bronchitis suggests that there are some common genetic factors in both conditions (Sibbald *et al.*, 1980). However, atopy and allergy were less common in children with wheezy bronchitis than in those with asthma and it is likely that the tendency to develop asthma is influenced by the inheritance of atopy, which is not implicated in susceptibility to wheezy bronchitis.

Seasonal variation

As would be expected, there is an overall peak of upper and lower respiratory infection in midwinter though epidemics caused by particular viruses follow different patterns. In the Chapel Hill study (Glezen & Denny, 1973) respiratory syncytial virus epidemics alternated between midwinter and early spring. Para-influenza viruses were more prevalent in the autumn. *Mycoplasma* was responsible for longer epidemics continuing through the summer months. The overall winter prevalence of illness with peaks in December and March corresponds to the seasonal variation of postneonatal deaths.

Environmental condition

Exposure to air pollution, principally smoke and sulphur dioxide, has an important bearing on chest illnesses from the age of a few months onwards (Lunn *et al.*, 1967; Colley *et al.*, 1973). Colley *et al.* (1973) found that pollution was a more significant factor among children of manual workers, despite controlling for social-class-related factors. In South Wales rates for respiratory disease in children, as in adults, are well above those for English areas with comparable air pollution. It is possible that other factors such as genetic predisposition may come into play but the reason remains obscure. In areas where air pollution has been reduced a corresponding decrease in respiratory illness has been demonstrated.

Prevention of respiratory illness

Smoking is a significant factor in the incidence of respiratory disease in children and is the overriding factor in chronic respiratory illness in adults. Advice to parents should be given during pregnancy or even before conception in family planning and 'pre-conception' clinics. The dangers of smoking and taking combined 'oral contraceptives' after the age of 30 add weight to anti-smoking advice. Encouraging breast-feeding, especially where there is a family history of allergy, may prevent both asthma and lower respiratory infections. There is a strong argument for beginning health education on both breast-feeding and smoking in primary schools.

The ubiquity of respiratory viruses and the lack of any specific treatment or effective vaccine make preventive measures difficult to enforce in the community. It is not practicable to isolate children from these conditions but it is reasonable to protect the very young infant from contact with infected people. There is no doubt that the socially disadvantaged child still suffers from more illness than his affluent counterpart and in many cases improvements in the environment, especially in housing, could be justified on health grounds. Accurate diagnosis in distinguishing repeated colds from allergic rhinitis can prevent unnecessary treatment with antibiotics and allow more rational treatment with antihistamine and sodium cromoglycate.

Common respiratory problems

THE 'CATARRHAL' CHILD

The child with persistent or recurrent upper respiratory tract symptoms presents a difficult problem to general practitioners and paediatricians.

Mothers may give a history of continual nasal discharge, nasal congestion and irritating cough and say that her child is 'never without a cold'. A child under five may be expected to have three to six 'colds' a year but normally recovers between each attack. A proportion of children (about 5–10%) barely recover from one episode before developing another exacerbation. Repeated infection by one of the many different viruses accounts for many of these persistent problems, particularly when the child is in contact with a wide variety of people at home, nursery or school. In a small proportion of children chronic nasal discharge and chronic pharyngitis may reflect an underlying disorder such as nasal polyps, chronic infection of the adenoids and tonsils, foreign bodies or allergy. Allergic rhinitis frequently masquerades as chronic infection and, although more often seasonal, can also be perennial where house dust, plant allergens, foods or animals are precipitating factors. Characteristically, the child with allergic rhinitis has a watery, rather than purulent, nasal discharge, persistent sneezing, itchy eyes and nose, and lack of constitutional symptoms. The nasal mucous membranes tend to be pale and a nasal smear will often contain many eosinophils rather than the neutrophil polymorphonuclear leucocytes associated with infection. The child over three with allergic rhinitis may benefit from a corticosteroid or sodium cromoglycate nasal spray. In younger children who cannot manage a nasal spray antihistamine syrup may help symptoms. However, one has to balance the advantages of medication in alleviating symptoms with the disadvantages and possible sedating side-effects of long-term use of antihistamines.

The child with chronically enlarged and infected adenoids will present a rather different picture with signs of nasal obstruction, mouth-breathing, snoring and postnasal drip. Frequent tonsillitis and otitis media are common accompaniments. X-rays of the postnasal space may demonstrate opaque, thickened sinuses or enlarged adenoidal pad. Most surgeons are reluctant to intervene surgically in under-fives, except in the case of recurrent ear infections and 'glue ear'.

THE CHILD WITH PERSISTENT COUGH

The infant or child with a cough lasting more than a month is likely to attend the general practitioner frequently, at least once a week, especially in the winter months. Typically the parents or doctor will already have tried cough linctuses and very often one or more courses of antibiotics. Parental anxiety about serious lung disease and the child waking himself and his parents at night with coughing may be underlying reasons why the child is brought for a further consultation.

Usually, he has a loose or dry cough which is worse at night or first thing in the morning; he may be slightly anorexic but is otherwise well and active with no clinical signs of lower respiratory tract infection. Reassurance that the chest is clear and that the cough serves a useful purpose in clearing secretions from the chest may allay anxiety. Elevation of the foot of the cot to encourage drainage of secretions and increasing humidity with a vaporizer may be helpful in infants. Most persistent coughs of this kind originate from frequent upper respiratory tract infections; explanation to parents of the plethora of respiratory viruses causing such illnesses may help them accept the frequent episodes of minor illness as a normal self-limiting phenomenon. However, the child with signs of chronic infection in the tonsils or adenoids requires further evaluation.

Further investigation is indicated if the child has significant constitutional symptoms, febrile episodes or signs of lower respiratory tract involvement. Radiological examination may reveal some patchy consolidation which is most commonly caused by viral pneumonia or occasionally secondary infection with pneumococci or staphylococci. Cystic fibrosis should be considered in a child with recurrent chest infection, especially if he is also failing to thrive.

Persistent loose cough in young infants may be associated with a tendency to regurgitation, usually where there is gastro-oesophageal reflux. Aspiration of small amounts of milk may even cause repeated episodes of bronchitis and areas of aspiration pneumonia. Propping the infant in a sitting position and thickening the feeds usually reduces symptoms and the problem improves during the second half of the first year.

A persistent cough, often dry and irritating, may be due to an underlying tendency to asthma. A history of some shortness of breath on exertion may be obtained on further questioning. A history of eczema or allergic rhinitis in the child with or without a family history of allergy would add support to this diagnosis. A trial of preventive treatment with sodium cromoglycate for three months is well worth while in children from about three onwards.

WHEEZING AND ASTHMA

Parents of all asthmatic children should be advised about sensible avoidance measures to reduce exposure to precipitating factors. These will normally include regular vacuuming, especially in the bedroom, using synthetic bedding material, minimizing contact with furry animals and advising on parental smoking habits. Occasionally children wheeze in response to certain foods and additives, such as tartrazine dyes, eggs, fish, nuts and dairy produce, and these should be avoided if there is a clear history of provocation.

Wheezing in the young infant frequently occurs with an upper respiratory infection and, since this is nearly always viral in origin, antibiotics are not necessarily beneficial. There is no evidence that sympathomimetic drugs, theophyllines and corticosteroids improve respiratory function in acute attacks of wheezing in infants. The only agent which has been shown to have any beneficial effect is nebulized ipratropium bromide (Atrovent). In infants with frequent attacks a nebulized corticosteroid may help as long-term prophylaxis.

From about 18 months onward beta-sympathomimetic drugs such as salbutamol or terbutaline are the most effective bronchodilators and may be used in combination with oral theophylline in the acute attack. The syrup form of salbutamol is suited to the younger child but from three onwards the drug can be administered by a rotohaler.

The child with mild episodic asthma usually responds well to oral or inhaled salbutamol for individual attacks. If the attacks become very frequent regular administration of sodium cromoglycate is often successful in reducing frequency of attacks. In under-fives sodium cromoglycate can be administered either by spinhaler or, if this is not possible, via a mechanized nebulizer.

Over the age of four it should be possible to measure the peak expiratory flow rate (PEFR) using a Wright's peak-flow meter. Measurement before and after administration of a bronchodilator will clinch the diagnosis. Measurement after exercise may show a reduction in peak flow. The normal peak flow for a five-year-old is 150 l per min, rising to 240 l per min at 10 years.

From about the age of three onwards the use of nebulized salbutamol at home has an important place in treatment and prevention of frequent attacks and can prevent hospital admissions. However, in a severe attack close medical supervision is necessary to ensure adequate treatment and often a short course of steroids is indicated. Children who fail to respond to administration of nebulized salbutamol will require hospital admission.

If regular sodium cromoglycate or theophylline fail to control asthma there is little point in continuing them and an inhaled steroid preparation is indicated, though few children require this and only a very small number will need regular oral steroids.

The family with an asthmatic child are likely to need frequent contacts with their family doctor, both in and out of surgery hours. Easy accessibility to the doctor is essential. Most parents are able to

cope extremely well with their wheezy child provided that they have
plenty of medical support and clear advice on what to do when an
attack begins. It is likely that parental attitude can influence a child's
reaction to attacks.

Clearly, the development and behaviour of children with asthma
need careful monitoring. In severe asthma physical growth may be
retarded but there is no substantial evidence that general development
is affected. However, as we have stressed, frequent episodes of illness
and disturbed behaviour are often related.

There is no doubt that the presence of an asthmatic child can give
rise to family tensions or strains. A parent may become overprotective
towards the child and other members of the family will consequently
receive less attention. The general practitioner is ideally placed to spot
family difficulties and spend time talking about the child's relationship
within the family. There is little information on the psychological
effect of asthma on the young child but in 10–12-year-old asthmatic
children there is a slightly higher rate of emotional disorder than in
non-asthmatic children.

Otitis media

Otitis media is broadly defined as inflammation of the middle ear.
Acute otitis media implies an acute onset of inflammation and may
be associated with a collection of fluid in the middle ear (effusion).
Chronic otitis media with effusion is called by a plethora of other
terms — serous, secretory, non-suppurative, catarrhal, mucoid, allergic
or 'glue ear'. The effusion can be either serous or purulent and is un-
accompanied by signs of acute inflammation.

In our study about 15% of children from birth to five years had at
least one episode of otitis media each year (Table 8.3). Fry (1961)

Table 8.3 History of ear infections in different age-groups of children in Camden and
Westminster.

	0–1 year		1–2 year		2–3 year		3–4½ year	
	n	%	n	%	n	%	n	%
One ear infection	33	12	35	12	29	9	38	14
More than one ear infection	9	3	11	4	21	6	27	10
Total n	272		280		329		274	

Age-group of child

reported a yearly incidence of 10%. Studies from North America report a slightly higher incidence of 15–20% each year. Children who develop otitis media with effusion in the first year of life have an increased chance of having further acute or chronic episodes. The incidence of otitis media decreases after the age of six.

The incidence is higher in Wales than in England, in lower socio-economic groups, in large families and where other members of the family have a history of chronic otitis media (Teal *et al.*, 1980). The disease is particularly severe in American Indians and Alaskan and Canadian Eskimos, in children with cleft palate and other craniofacial abnormalities, in cystic fibrosis and in allergic rhinitis. In the Boston study (Teal *et al.*, 1980) breast-fed babies had a shorter duration of effusion following otitis media than those who were bottle-fed.

Acute otitis media

Characteristically acute otitis media develops after the child has been suffering from an upper respiratory infection for a few days. In 75% of cases bacteria are cultured, *Pneumococcus* in 46%, *Haemophilus influenzae* in 20% and haemolytic *Streptococcus* or *Staphylococcus aureus* in the remainder. However, some degree of inflammation of the middle ear is present in a large proportion of upper respiratory tract infections and mild otalgia and slight reddening of the ear-drum are common findings in the young child with a cold. Mild otitis media occurs in the early stages of measles whereas secondary bacterial infection occurs late in the illness.

The child presents with earache, fever, malaise, anorexia and usually runny nose. In infants vomiting and diarrhoea are frequent accompanying symptoms. Examination of the ear reveals a reddened, opaque, bulging tympanic membrane and sometimes a purulent discharge. If the child presents with a short history of earache and is only mildly febrile with a slightly reddened ear-drum, antibiotics may be withheld initially. It is reasonable to treat with paracetamol and to review the situation in 24 or 48 hours. Unless the child is prone to recurrent otitis media, it is not uncommon for earache in the early stages of a cold to settle in 24 hours. Provided follow-up is feasible, unnecessary antibiotics can often be avoided. Amoxycillin or co-trimoxazole are suitable therapy for under-fives. Some strains of *H. influenzae* are resistant to ampicillin and the antibiotic may need to be changed if there is no clinical improvement. Decongestants and anti-histamines (such as pseudoephedrine and triprolidine), either separately or as a combined preparation, are commonly prescribed for acute otitis media. However, studies have not shown any benefit from this therapy either in reducing the duration and severity of symptoms or in preventing recurrence. A substantial proportion of children suffer from side-effects, particularly from pseudoephedrine, usually irritability, poor sleeping, dizziness and general *malaise* (Bain, 1983).

Chronic otitis media with effusion (glue ear)

Middle-ear effusion is a common sequela to acute otitis media but may also develop insidiously without a clear history of acute infection. In one study of 278 two-year-olds the condition was suspected in 11% on the basis of the otoscopic findings and the flat compliance graph on tympanometry (Tos *et al.*, 1978).

After a first attack of acute otitis media 70% of Boston children (Teal *et al.*, 1980) had effusion at two weeks, 40% at one month, 20% at two months and 10% at three months. A variable degree of conductive deafness is usually associated with effusion. In another study, 55% of children with middle-ear infection had an initial hearing loss of 15 decibels or more which persisted for one to six months. Twelve per cent of children still had a hearing loss six months later.

Alteration of the mucociliary system in the middle ear associated with malfunction of the Eustachian tube is thought to be responsible for development of an effusion. Eustachian-tube blockage prevents drainage of secretions. A negative pressure develops in the middle ear causing serous or mucoid fluid to accumulate. This process may occur after frank middle-ear inflammation or with repeated upper respiratory infections. Enlarged chronically infected adenoids are thought to be one factor responsible for ascending Eustachian-tube infection and tubal blockage. It has generally been assumed that persistent effusions following antimicrobial therapy are sterile. However, some studies have found bacteria in 45% of chronic middle-ear effusions though only about 12% contained probable pathogens (Riding *et al.*, 1978).

Chronic otitis media with effusion may be diagnosed on follow-up after an attack of otitis media or may be detected at a routine examination. It should be suspected where a child has a persistently runny nose, has delayed speech development or shows any indication of deafness. Ideally all children with otitis media should have a follow-up examination and hearing test after about a month. In practice time may not allow this but any child with a severe attack, repeated attacks or suspicion of deafness should be closely watched. The appearance of the ear-drum varies enormously in chronic middle-ear disease. Typically, the membrane is opaque and retracted. A fluid level may be visible and mobility is reduced.

Impedance audiometry

Impedance audiometry is a useful technique for evaluating the function of the middle ear. The test is well suited to children as it is accurate, quick and easy to administer, creates little discomfort and is objective. A small probe is inserted into the external auditory canal of the patient and an airtight seal obtained. The probe has three small holes; one emits a 220 Hz pulse tone, the second is an air pressure outlet, and the third leads to a microphone which picks up the 220 Hz pulse tone in the canal cavity. The apparatus has three applications in children, namely tympanometry, measurement of static compliance and measurement of acoustic reflex threshold.

The compliance of the tympanic membrane of specific air pressures is plotted on a graph known as a tympanogram (Fig. 8.1). Various types of curve signify different conditions; a low peak indicates an immobile drum in otosclerosis or scarring of the drum, an incomplete peak is seen with a flaccid drum and discontinuity of the ossicles, a flat curve indicates a middle-ear effusion and a curve shifted to the left is seen where there is a negative pressure in the middle ear. Early detection of negative pressure is a valuable function of the tympanogram as early treatment can prevent the accumulation of fluid by transudation which follows reduction of middle-ear pressure. Negative pressure can also be responsible for a degree of deafness even though the cavity is 'dry'.

The second use of the apparatus is to measure 'static compliance', otherwise known as 'acoustic impedance'. Compliance refers to the mobility of the middle-ear system. A pulse tone is emitted and the sound pressure level of the tone measured via the microphone. In serous otitis media there is decreased compliance or increased impedance to sound, resulting in reduced sound intensity readings.

The third test is the determination of the sound threshold level at which the stapedius muscle contracts (acoustic reflex threshold). Normally the stapedius muscle contracts in response to loud sounds, pulling on the ossicular chain and reducing compliance of the middle ear. This reduces the sound reaching the cochlea and protects the inner ear. This reflex can be detected by the impedance audiometer as a change in compliance of the drum. The acoustic reflex can be expected to be absent if there is any conductive hearing loss as the mechanism causing the conductive loss prevents the ear-drum from showing a change in compliance.

It is likely that the application of tympanometry will become more widespread; a number of studies are currently being carried out in the community. Studies in the USA and Scandinavia indicate that up

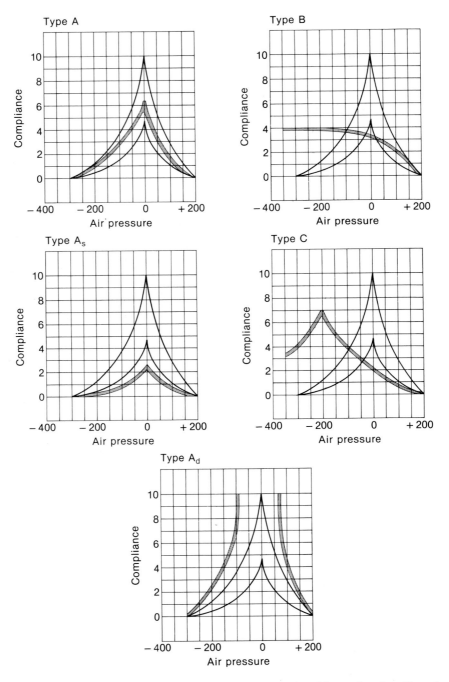

Fig. 8.1 Classification of tympanograms. Type A, normal middle-ear function. Type A$_s$ low peak — limited compliance of tympanic membrane — as in otosclerosis, scarring of tympanic membrane. Type A$_d$ flaccid eardrum with discontinuity of ossicular chain. Type B, little change in compliance of middle ear with variation in pressure in ear canal. In serous and adhesive otitis media. Type C, poor Eustachian-tube function — negative pressure in middle ear (after Jerger, 1970).

to 28% of apparently asymptomatic children may be identified by tympanometry as having middle-ear effusion during an examination period. Repeated examination indicated that the effusions resolved spontaneously in most children within a few months.

Treatment

The treatment of 'glue ear' is controversial. There are strong arguments for initiating some form of treatment early since hearing impairment may be responsible for speech and language delay, behaviour problems and educational difficulties; the disorder may also lead to more serious chronic ear disease and even sensorineural loss. Recent evidence suggests that the condition is often self-limiting (*British Medical Journal*, 1981), and it is likely that spontaneous resolution occurs in most cases eventually. Some authors therefore recommend a conservative approach initially but of course regular monitoring of hearing levels and the effect of the condition on the child are essential. A recent study found that co-trimoxazole given over three weeks was associated with more rapid resolution than antihistamine/decongestive preparations (*British Medical Journal*, 1981). Decongestants are given in the hope that they will encourage mucosal shrinking in the Eustachian canal but, as with acute otitis media, studies have found no benefit and in one study children with an allergic history fared significantly worse (Olson *et al.*, 1978). Antihistamine and nasal sodium cromoglycate are logical therapy in allergic rhinitis and are widely used though as yet there is little objective evidence in their favour.

Myringotomy with or without adenotonsillectomy is indicated if no improvement occurs with medical treatment after three months. A persistent hearing loss of 30 dB or more would be reasonable grounds for intervention. One would be more likely to intervene where the child's speech and development were affected. Myringotomy and insertion of grommets invariably improve hearing, both by withdrawal of fluid (glue) and by equalization of pressures across the tympanic membrane. Some surgeons favour myringotomy alone as an initial procedure with insertion of grommets if fluid reaccumulates. The value of myringotomy and grommets is controversial and is being currently re-evaluated by several workers. In one study of children with glue ears, one ear was treated with a grommet and one treated conservatively. After six months hearing was better in the side with the grommet but after a further six months there was little to choose between the two sides (*British Medical Journal*, 1981). Several other studies have generally concluded that hearing remains improved whilst grommets are in place although long-term results are less influenced by the procedure.

A recent evaluation of adenoidectomy demonstrated a 72% resolution of effusion 12 months after adenoidectomy, compared with 62% with adenotonsillectomy and 26% with no treatment (Maw, 1983). These findings contrast with others which have not shown any advantage of adenoidectomy in addition to myringotomy. Investigation of the immunological effects of adenoidectomy have not shown a conclusive immunological trauma but in one study otitis media continued to occur in 42.9% of children following the operation (Kjellman *et al.*, 1978). The strongest argument for the insertion of grommets is that it tides the child over a critical period of his life in terms of development and learning.

Hearing loss associated with middle-ear effusion

Generally, the degree of hearing loss associated with middle-ear effusion varies from 20 to 40 dB; it is usually conductive but sensorineural involvement can occur. In one study of children with effusion, 55% had hearing loss of 21 dB or more and 26% a loss of 31 dB or more. A typical audiometric profile accompanying otitis media with effusion is shown in Fig. 8.2. The average degree of air conduction loss through the speech frequency range is 27.6 dB.

Hearing loss is dependent on the volume of effusion rather than the viscosity. It may also accompany high negative pressure even in the absence of effusion. The hearing loss associated with effusion is

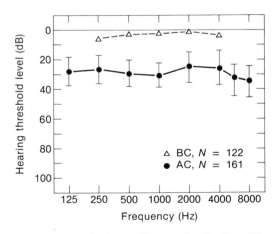

Fig. 8.2 Composite audiogram of subjects diagnosed as having otitis media with effusion. Mean air conduction (AC) values represent 161 ears, whereas mean bone conduction (BC) thresholds constitute 122 ears.

such that the child will often appear to hear normal conversational speech. He will be aware of speech but he will understand what is being said only under the most favourable conditions such as when directly facing the speaker. In the classroom he may be unable to understand much of what is said. As soon as hearing loss has been identified it is important for parents and teachers to consider the child's hearing needs.

Behavioural and developmental effects of respiratory illness and otitis media

We have focused on respiratory illnesses not only because they are commonly experienced by young children but also in view of their close relationship with the child's general development and pattern of behaviour.

It is well recognized that children with major physical and developmental handicap are more likely to have some behavioural disturbance (Bentovim, 1972; Rutter *et al.*, 1970). In our study we were able to explore the association between minor illness episodes and behavioural and developmental problems in preschool children (Hart *et al.*, 1984). Parents often report minor alterations in a child's behaviour as one of the first indications that he is becoming ill and most illnesses in young children are accompanied by some transient disturbance of behaviour such as loss of appetite, sleeplessness, irritability or difficulty in management. Our findings suggest that some illness episodes may have longer-lasting effects on behaviour and development.

When parental history of children's behaviour was compared with history of illness during the preceding six months a clear pattern of association emerged. Children who were waking at night four or more times a week were more likely to have had ear infections and frequent upper respiratory tract illnesses (URTIs). Similarly children with poor appetites, temper tantrums and difficulties in management were more likely to have had ear infections and frequent URTIs. The implication of these findings is that perhaps more consideration should be given to the broader repercussions of common illnesses. It seems reasonable that a painful illness such as otitis media may act as a trigger to night-waking. A disturbed sleep pattern may persist long after the original illness. Often this type of sleep disorder responds to a short course of hypnotics. Similarly the child who has continual colds and catarrh may have reduced appetite and this may even be reflected in a reduction of weight gain. Temper tantrums and difficulty in management are frequent in the toddler age-group and it may not always be recognized that ill health may be a relevant factor. More commonly, though, many characteristics interact to create a tense and difficult situation including not only physical health but interaction between the personalities of child and parents and the stresses of their social environment.

The view that the mother's well-being and the child's health are closely interlinked is supported by our finding that mothers who were suffering from a moderate degree of depression also reported an increased number of attacks of bronchitis in their children. Clearly a depressed mental state may alter perception of a child's state of health but it is also possible that ill health in a child, possibly associated with difficult behaviour, may contribute to a mothers low morale. Not surprisingly, depressed mothers also reported a higher incidence of behaviour problems in their children, particularly in the toddler age-group.

These findings illustrate the numerous interrelated stresses which mothers face and which need to be considered when a child is brought to the surgery with a variety of persistent health and behaviour problems. Developmental effects of illness may also be seen in the young child. Fluctuating hearing loss during the critical period of acquiring language is thought by various workers to be responsible for delay in language development. The mechanism for this effect lies in the way early language develops. Infants can make fine speech discriminations long before they produce speech; inconsistent auditory signals resulting from fluctuating hearing loss may make the input of speech sounds difficult to segment and impair the child's ability to form linguistic categories. Studies have shown that a number of children with otitis media with effusion which starts before the age of two have delayed language in the preschool period and language difficulties persisting at school age (Holm & Kunze, 1969).

In our study a history of one or more ear infections in the previous year was three times as common in children with abnormal speech at two years ($p = 0.05$) than in those with normal speech (Table 8.4). At three years ear infections were twice as common in the former group but the difference was no longer statistically significant.

There may not be a clear history of frank otitis media in some children with otitis media with effusion since the conditions can develop insidiously with frequent colds. The group of children with frequent URTIs are also at risk of hearing loss and its developmental sequelae.

The association between illness and behaviour suggests a further mechanism by which development may be affected in children with frequent illness. Problems such as difficult behaviour, tantrums and

Table 8.4 Abnormal speech and language development according to history of ear infection.

	Speech at two years*				Speech at three years			
	Normal		Abnormal		Normal		Abnormal	
	n	%	*n*	%	*n*	%	*n*	%
Ear infections at least once in previous year	49	15	6	33	43	14	7	28
Total *n*	331		18		300		25	

* $\chi^2 = 4.41$, $P = 0.05$.

night-waking may impair the quality of parent—child interaction, which is an important factor in early language acquisition. Thus the behavioural consequences of otitis media may account for some of the language problems experienced by children with this condition.

Some developmental anomalies

This section describes some conditions which may not come to light during consultation for acute illness but are more likely to be noticed in routine developmental and health checks.

Undescended testis

Descent of the testes into the scrotum normally occurs during the eighth month of fetal life. If the testes are undescended at birth natural descent should occur by the age of one year. The incidence of undescended testes is eight per 1000 male births. Unilateral maldescent is more common than bilateral; the undescended testis may be located in the abdomen, or in the inguinal canal, perineum or femoral area, or at the base of the penis (ectopic testis).

The testes are easily examined soon after birth when the cremaster muscle is relaxed. A further check should be carried out later in the first year and again at five or six years as there have been reports of ascent of previously descended testes.

Opinions on the ideal age for surgical correction have varied over the years and recent evidence points to certain advantages in early operation. Orchidopexy is technically easier under the age of 18 months and at this age there is less awareness and likelihood of psychological problems provided the parents are able to stay in hospital with the child. Deterioration in histological appearance has been noted as early as two years in undescended testes. There is a higher incidence of later malignant change in undescended testes; this risk is not altered if correction is left to 12–15 years but is probably insignificant following orchidopexy under the age of five years. It is now generally accepted that referral should take place before the age of 18 months and most surgeons would operate well before the age of five.

Hypospadias and phimosis

Hypospadias affects 103 per 1000 males and occurs in varying degrees of severity. All cases need early surgical referral as even glandular hypospadias can lead to later embarrassment as micturition in the standing position is likely to be difficult.

Phimosis is a narrowing (congenital or acquired) of the foreskin (prepuce) which prevents it being drawn back over the glans penis. At birth the foreskin is adherent to the glans, the adhesions gradually breaking down over the first three years. During this period it is not easily retracted and parents should be advised to leave it alone since retraction can be painful and can cause scarring. In some cases the foreskin remains adherent after the age of three but it will generally become retractile by the age of seven or eight. Unless there is definite narrowing of the opening, a non-retracting foreskin does not need circumcision at an early age. Phimosis may be secondary to infection; recurrent balamitis may sometimes be grounds for recommending circumcision. Phimosis or a non-retractile foreskin rarely impedes the urinary stream; drawing attention to the good urinary stream may help convince parents that circumcision is not necessary.

Umbilical hernia

Umbilical hernia is a common condition due to imperfect closure or weakness of the umbilical ring and may be associated with a degree of separation of the rectus muscles. It is more frequent in preterm and in black infants. The defect ranges in size from 1 cm to 5 cm and mostly disappears spontaneously during the first 12 months of life. Larger hernias may take longer to resolve and, unless very large, it may be worth delaying surgery until the age of four or five years or later. Centrally placed hernias are more likely to resolve naturally than supra-umbilical hernias where the defect lies above the umbilicus.

Strapping is ineffective and possibly deleterious. It is helpful to reassure parents that the hernia is painless, despite bulging associated with crying, and that strangulation is virtually unknown.

Developmental orthopaedic conditions

Wide variations in the normal range of limb posture and walking pattern exist in young children. Parents can be reassured that most of these do not affect the age of walking, are self-correcting and do not usually necessitate special footwear or exercises. Full examination of the limbs and observation of walking are essential to convince parents that all will be well and to pick out the few children who require further evaluation. Overall only 5 to 15% of untreated lower-limb abnormalities persist beyond skeletal maturation. (Congenital dislocation of the hip is discussed on p. 34.)

ROTATIONAL VARIATION OF THE LOWER LIMBS

As the limbs grow there is a wide range of normal physiological rotational variation. Mild degrees may give rise to parental concern but it is only the extreme cases of limb rotation which need intervention. All children with a rotational variation should be examined to exclude cerebral palsy or other neurological disorders. Assessment of the lower limb includes examination of the foot, the tibia and the femur for rotation or bowing, measurement of the range of movement at the ankle, knee and hip, and observation of walking in the older child.

IN-TOEING OR PIGEON TOES

In the newborn in-toeing is most commonly due to in-turning of the front part of the foot (metatarsus varus or metatarsus adductus) or in-turning of the entire foot due to medial tibial torsion. In toddlers two further conditions are also responsible for in-toeing, namely, persistent femoral anteversion and talar torsion; many children have more than one of these disorders.

Metatarsus varus

Many infants are born with the front part of the foot turning inwards (metatarsus varus) and the condition may be related to intra-uterine positioning (Fig. 8.3). If the forefoot can be moved into 45° of abduction and dorsiflexed so that the top of the foot touches the tibia anteriorly there is no need for concern and parents can be reassured that the

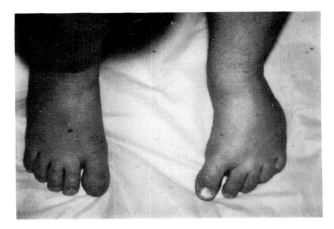

Fig. 8.3 Metatarsus varus.

posture will resolve spontaneously.

In metatarsus varus the metatarsals are adducted at the metatarsal—tarsal joint and inspection of the sole of the foot reveals that the lateral border is convex. Of children with this condition, 5—10% have been noted to have congenital dislocation of the hip.

The majority of cases of metatarsus varus resolve spontaneously by the age of three. However, it can be difficult to determine in which children this will occur. Initially, if the forefoot can be abducted to 30°, passive abduction by the parents can be effective treatment. If a moderate or severe degree is still present at three to four months, plaster-cast treatment is recommended. After this correction becomes more difficult.

Mild cases do not need treatment as most will correct spontaneously and any remaining deformity is of no consequence. There is no evidence that special corrective shoes are of any value.

Medial tibial torsion and lateral tibial bowing

In medial tibial torsion the whole foot points inwards as a result of medial rotation of the tibia (Fig. 8.4). The appearances can be accentuated if lateral bowing of the tibia is present. Both tibial torsion and lateral bowing have a natural tendency to correct spontaneously. Medial tibial torsion even up to 20° does not usually impair function. Toddlers may have a tendency to trip over their feet but this usually disappears at the age of four or five. Surgery is only rarely indicated in this condition.

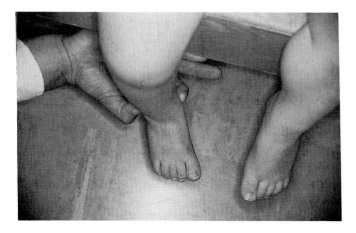

Fig. 8.4 Medial tibial torsion.

Persistent femoral anteversion

Persistent femoral anteversion is a cause of in-toeing which usually becomes apparent after the child reaches two years. Parents report that their child has a marked in-toe gait and walks clumsily, often throwing his heels out to the sides. A characteristic sign is that children sit in the so-called 'w' or television position with the hips internally rotated and the legs out sideways (Fig. 8.5). The condition improves naturally in 80% of the children by the age of eight. Surgical treatment is rarely required and best left as late as 10; special footwear is unnecessary.

EXTERNAL ROTATION

Some infants may show a marked degree of external rotation of the hip and legs. There may be as much as 180° of external rotation which may be associated with some contracture of soft tissue round the hip. Parents can be reassured that correction will occur when the child begins to walk and can be advised to carry out stretching exercises by internally rotating the legs when nappy-changing. Radiographic examination of the hips is indicated to exclude congenital dislocation of the hip.

GENU VARUM (BOW-LEG)

A mild degree of bow-leg is common in infants and usually corrects itself by about 18 months, sometimes even progressing to knock-knees

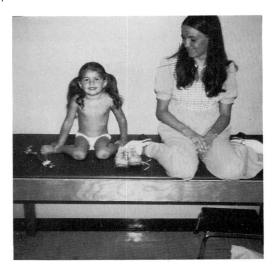

Fig. 8.5 Mother and daughter with persistent femoral anteversion sitting in 'W' position.

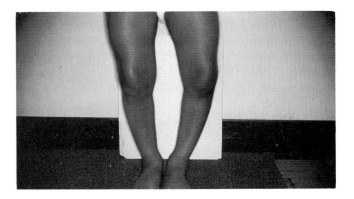

Fig. 8.6 Genu varum (bow-legs).

for a time (Fig. 8.6). The legs gradually develop toward their final shape at around nine years. The appearance of bowing may be exaggerated when the child is just beginning to walk as he adopts a broad-based gait. If bowing is marked and progresses after 18 months further evaluation is necessary. Rickets, either dietary or renal, should be considered in a child who appears to have swollen joints and who has short stature or failure to thrive. The severity of bow-legs can be assessed with the child standing with the medial malleoli together. If the distance between the medial femoral condyles is 4 cm or more then treatment would normally be recommended. Initially night-splinting is used and only very few children eventually need osteotomy. Early treatment of severe cases of both bow-legs and knock-knees is worth while to prevent the development of osteo-arthritis of the knee joint in adulthood due to the abnormal stresses and strains imposed by the deformities. Some children with untreated bow-legs can develop Blount's disease (tibia vara), in which there is a disorder of growth of the medial part of the proximal tibial epiphysis, resulting in extreme tibial bowing.

GENU VALGUM (KNOCK-KNEE)

In young children there is a natural progression from bow-legs to knock-knees (Fig. 8.7). Correction of knock-knees usually occurs by the age of nine and at skeletal maturity the normal degree of genu valgum, expressed as the angle between the femoral and tibial shafts, is 5° to 7°.

The progress of knock-knees can be followed by measuring the distance between the medial mallioli. There is no need for special treatment, arch supports or shoes. Pes valgus (flat foot) may be secondary to genu valgum and parents may complain that the child 'goes over' the medial aspect of his shoes. Even then there is no convincing evidence that shoe supports protect the feet from pronation.

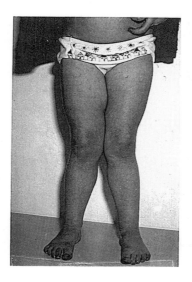

Fig. 8.7 Genu valgum (knock-knees).

Increasing knock-knees after the age of six or seven need further evaluation but only 1% of children with this condition eventually need surgery in the form of stapling of the medial femoral condyle.

Some toddlers have a dramatic degree of genu valgum and parental reassurance can be difficult. It may help to point out that one rarely sees adults with this deformity.

PES VALGUS (FLAT FOOT)

Parents frequently consult their doctor with anxiety about flat feet during various stages of childhood (Fig. 8.8). When the child first stands and walks flat feet are normal as the medial arch does not develop until the second or third year. Typically he stands with his feet wide apart and everted and the appearance of flat feet is also accentuated if the legs are externally rotated. Assessment of the shape of the foot is more meaningful after a stable walking pattern has developed. Several conditions are easily confused with true pes valgus. The normal toddler's foot is chubby and the medial fat pad frequently obscures the longitudinal arch — a 'fat' rather than 'flat' foot. Similarly, enlarged and prominent malleoli can give the appearance of flat feet.

After the age of two children who present with loss of the longitudinal arch but a normal heel and forefoot are unlikely to have long-term problems with their feet and this form of flat foot is painless. A simple test is to ask the child to stand on tiptoes. In most cases the longitudinal arch will appear due to the action of the long flexor muscles of the foot. This is a useful procedure to convince parents that

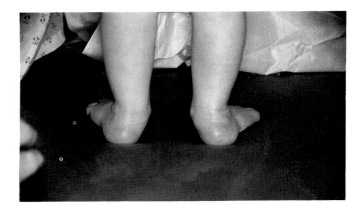

Fig. 8.8 Pes valgus (flat foot).

the feet will develop normally. Simple exercises to strengthen the muscles of the feet may be recommended although co-operation may be poor in the young child. Special footwear does not alter the shape of the foot and is not indicated.

CONGENITAL TALIPES EQUINOVARUS (CLUB-FOOT)

Club-foot is an abnormality that occurs in about one per 1000 live births, with a sex ratio of about two males to one female (Fig. 8.9). There may be a family history of the condition, which seems to have a multifactorial mode of inheritance. It may be associated with intra-uterine positioning problems and oligohydramnios. The entire foot is inverted and the heel is in the equinus and varus position. The deformity is ideally corrected as soon as possible after delivery when the infant's tissues are most elastic. Serial manipulation and taping or casting successfully corrects about two-thirds of cases. Surgery may be indicated at two to three months of age if stretching and casting are no longer improving the foot.

TOE-WALKING

Many toddlers begin to walk on their toes and some may continue doing this as a habit. If the child is observed for a while he will usually be seen to toe-walk intermittently with periods of normal gait indicating that there is no underlying abnormality.

Spastic cerebral palsy and tight Achilles tendons are the two pre-

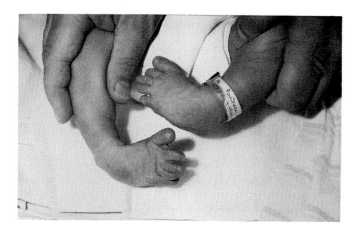

Fig. 8.9 Bilateral talipes equino varus (club foot).

dominant conditions giving rise to toe-walking. The former condition may be mild and clues to the diagnosis include limited abduction of the hips due to adductor spasm, brisk reflexes, ankle clonus and limited dorsiflexion of the foot. Tight Achilles tendons may be congenital in origin or secondary to cerebral palsy. Normally the child's foot should be capable of dorsiflexion to 20° above the right angle. If this cannot be achieved stretching exercises should be attempted. Some children may need immobilization in plaster or if this is not successful surgical lengthening of the tendon. Generally speaking a child is unlikely to require surgery if he can stand with both feet flat on the ground.

Skin disorders

Skin disorders commonly present in chronic forms in the surgery or child health clinic. Quite clearly they may involve long-term management but of further importance is their association with behaviour problems and the child's environment.

Atopic eczema

The incidence of atopic eczema in the general population has been reported to be as high as 20% (Matthew *et al.*, 1977). A family history of atopy is found in about 70% of patients with atopic dermatitis. If one parent is affected the chances of an offspring being affected is 50%, rising to 66% if both parents are affected. About 30% of children with atopic eczema are likely to develop asthma by the age of seven. Likewise there is a higher incidence of allergic rhinitis in atopic children.

The role of allergens in the development of atopic eczema is a subject of controversy. Allergy tests on eczematous children show that many have elevated IgE antibodies to various foods and react positively to patch tests with a wide variety of allergens, such as house-dust mites, grass pollens and animal dander. About 80% of atopic patients have serum IgE levels increased to 5−10 times over normal but the level is not consistently related to the severity of the disease. Undoubtedly some children with eczema experience exacerbations after contact with dairy produce and eggs and avoidance of these foods improves the condition. As yet there is no conclusive evidence that strict food-avoidance regimes are beneficial in childhood eczema and there is a danger that over-enthusiastic diets can result in malnutrition. Evidence is also mounting for the value of avoidance of cow's milk, dairy produce and eggs in the first six months of life in preventing atopic eczema and other allergic conditions (Burr, 1983). As early as 1936 a study of 20 000 infants found that in comparison with breast-fed infants eczema was twice as common in partially breast-fed infants and seven times as common in bottle-fed infants (Grulee & Sandford, 1936). In another study (Matthew *et al.*, 1977) infants of allergic parents developed less eczema when following an allergic avoidance regime than infants who were conventionally managed. These authors concluded that it is worth while advising allergic parents to breast-feed or only use soya milk and to delay weaning until three months, avoiding cow's milk, dairy produce, eggs and fish during the first six months. Goat's milk is unsuitable as it is similar to cow's milk, is unpasteurized and is not modified to meet the dietary needs of infants under six months. Recent evidence offers some explanation of the finding that breast-feeding does not provide infallible protection against eczema and other allergies (Cant *et al.*, 1985). Breast-fed babies can become sensitized to both milk protein and egg albumen by foods eaten by their mothers which pass into breast milk. Neither does soy feeding offer complete protection since soya protein can cause sensitization.

CLINICAL PICTURE

Atopic eczema is an inflammatory skin disorder characterized by itching, redness, excoriation, exudation and crusting. It commonly begins between the ages of two and four months with lesions on the face and scalp often spreading over large areas of the body, typically affecting the popliteal fossa, wrists and elbows. In contrast to seborrhoeic dermatitis in infancy it spares the axillary and inguinal flexures and the nappy area. Remission occurs in a large proportion of children by the age of three to five but the condition may persist in a childhood form, typically involving the antecubital and popliteal fossae with lichenification. The two most persistent aspects requiring particular attention are dryness of the skin and irritation. When irritation is not controlled, secondary infection commonly occurs which prevents remission until treated.

TREATMENT

Some children with eczema may need long-term treatment, and success will depend on a satisfactory relationship between parent and doctor. Parents need encouragement to help them through the many relapses. Stress can play a large part in triggering relapses and the general practitioner needs to be aware of family circumstances. Advice should be given on avoidance of irritating agents such as woollen clothing, fabric softeners and bubble baths. Occasionally contact with animal dander can produce exacerbations but advice against keeping furry pets should perhaps be restricted to those children where there is a convincing link. The theoretical advantages of avoidance of cow's milk, dairy produce, egg and fish in the first six months have been discussed. After the age of six months avoidance of dairy produce and eggs may need to be continued for a long period if there is continuing evidence that ingestion of these foods exacerbates eczema. In severe cases of eczema strict avoidance diets are probably worth trying for a trial period of three weeks. Continuation of an avoidance diet is worth while if a definite improvement occurs and supervision by a dietitian is then advisable. Foods which are least likely to cause sensitization are lamb, peeled potatoes, carrots, lettuce and pears. Once improvement of eczema has occurred foods can be gradually reintroduced.

Most atopic patients suffer from dry skin, and improved hydration produces symptomatic improvement by relief of itching. Emollient creams may need to be applied as frequently as two-hourly during the day to prevent dryness and irritation. A 50/50 mixture of liquid paraffin and white soft paraffin is excellent but a wide variety of other preparations are available such as aqueous cream — E45 cream and a soap substitute such as unguentum emulsificans is ideal for bathing the child and bathing is recommended at least once a day. Hydrocortisone cream (1% and 0.5% for the body and face respectively) is effective in most cases and the stronger fluorinated steroid preparations are best avoided. Secondary infection frequently accompanies acute exacerbation and requires treatment with systemic antibiotics such as erythromycin or flucloxacillin. Itching, especially at night, is likely disturb sleep and exacerbate the condition. An antihistamine such as trimeprazine syrup has an effective antipruritic action with some sedative effect.

Infantile seborrhoeic dermatitis

This condition may begin as early as the first month of life and characteristically involves the scalp, retro-auricular areas, face, neck axillary flexures and napkin area. It consists of scaly areas on an erythematous background which may occur in patches or spread over a large area of the body. Unlike atopic eczema the dermatitis is non-pruritic and the presence of irritation and weeping may suggest a coexistent atopic tendency.

Seborrhoeic dermatitis of the scalp (cradle cap) can be treated with antiseborrhoeic shampoo or the crusts may be loosened before shampooing by the application of cetrimide solution, salicylic acid cream or olive oil. Elsewhere the condition usually clears promptly with a weak topical steroid combined with an antifungal and antiseptic agent to prevent *Candida* and bacterial infections which are liable to occur.

Nappy rash

The principal factors responsible for this common condition are prolonged contact with a wet or soiled nappy, retention of moisture inside plastic pants, or a seborrhoeic or atopic skin and secondary infection. Prolonged or recurrent nappy rash may be associated with infrequent nappy changing and cleansing and the possibility of parental neglect should be borne in mind.

Nappy rash usually begins as erythematous areas of the skin creases. It may become papular and excoriated, causing discomfort to the infant. A seborrhoeic type of rash is typically red, shiny and involving the skin folds and often associated with patches elsewhere on the baby. Atopic dermatitis is irritating and may weep. Secondary infection, mainly by *Candida albicans* (thrush) but also by *Staphylococcus aureus*, is frequent. Thrush nappy rash may be associated with oral and gastrointestinal candidiasis. Isolated 'spots' are likely to be due to thrush infection, but frankly pustular lesions are a result of bacterial infection.

Frequent nappy changing, cleansing of the skin, exposure to the air and application of a simple emollient preparation such as zinc and castor oil ointment BP help prevent and treat nappy rash. A variety of other preparations are popular such as Drapolene and Sudocreme. In addition to these measures most persistent rashes, being due to thrush, are cleared up with nystatin cream. Coexistent oral thrush needs treatment with nystatin drops. A combined weak topical steroid, antifungal and antiseptic cream is helpful in a seborrhoeic or eczematous rash. Bacterial infection may require topical antibiotics.

Socially related health problems

Failure to thrive

The infant or child who fails to achieve a reasonable rate of growth is a frequent cause of concern to the general practitioner, paediatrician and health visitor. The term 'failure to thrive' is usually reserved for infants, whereas 'growth retardation' is applied to older children. However, the approach to the problem is similar in all age-groups. Between 1 and 5% of children admitted to paediatric wards are suffering from failure to thrive. Of those who are investigated in paediatric departments less than a quarter are found to have important organic disease. In a further quarter the children have obvious feeding difficulties or an inappropriate diet. Over half the children are classified as non-organic failure to thrive because no sufficient pathophysiological cause for the condition can be found. In the past it has been assumed that these children are suffering from maternal rejection and neglect but recently a more balanced view of the mother–child relationship has been put forward. The factors which result in inadequacy of nutrition and failure to thrive involve a complex interaction between the child and the caregiver. Characteristics of both the mother and the child interact and may generate a cycle of incompatibility resulting in failure of adequate nutrition.

INITIAL ASSESSMENT

Measurement

Parents frequently express anxiety about their child's weight gain or stature. Plotting the child's weight and height on a percentile chart will establish whether there is a genuine problem and help to reassure parents where the measurements show that growth is within normal limits. More often, perhaps, it is the doctor or health visitor who is concerned by the observation that a child is failing to gain weight adequately or that there has been a falling off of weight gain. Some of the more deprived children may not be brought for regular weighing and the doctor and health visitor may suspect under-nutrition at a surgery or home visit.

Generally, a child is considered to be failing to thrive if the weight and/or height falls below the 3rd centile or if there has been a significant deviation from a previously accepted pattern of growth. Accurate serial measurements of growth are much more valuable than measurements taken at a single point in time, as they demonstrate changes over time and enable velocity of growth to be determined. In practice growth velocity involves complicated calculation and is usually reserved for growth clinics. More simply, the standard percentile charts indicate roughly when a child crosses percentile lines and it may be possible to relate these changes to precipitating factors such as illness or the introduction of gluten. Change in rate of weight gain is a sensitive index of health and nutritional intake. Recent studies have shown that a deceleration of weight gain precedes sudden infant death in some cases. This has led to an increased awareness by health visitors and doctors of the importance of monitoring weight.

Under-nourished children have a low weight in relation to their height or length. In severe malnutrition both height and weight are reduced but weight is more affected than height. Children with growth-hormone deficiency usually have heights below the 3rd centile but are relatively heavy for their height. In the constitutionally small child, who typically has smaller-than-average parents, weight and height are correspondingly low. Head growth may be relatively spared in failure to thrive so that the infant may appear to have a large head. However, prolonged under-nutrition in infancy impedes brain growth and may prejudice later intellectual performance. Small head size may occur when failure to thrive is associated with a primary CNS deficit such as birth injury, chromosomal abnormality or intra-uterine infection.

Weight gain in the first two years of life is related to birthweight and antenatal and perinatal factors. Birthweight is largely determined by maternal influences which regulate intra-uterine growth. Looking at infants' weight charts it may be noted that some infants cross percentile lines during the first year to level out along their genetically determined growth pathways by 12–24 months. This weight adjustment is distinct from failure to thrive when the weight falls off progressively and the infant usually appears far from well. The preterm baby undergoes a period of catch-up growth in the first year but some of the smallest infants may not achieve their ultimate growth pathway until two years. Their weights can be plotted on a chart which takes gestational age into consideration. Light-for-dates babies are more likely to show growth retardation. Most manage to grow to between the 10th and 25th centile by the age of two but the majority will never attain heights within the taller half of the population.

History

A detailed dietary history is necessary to determine calorie intake and feeding behaviour. Mothers are often sensitive about feeding and weight gain as these are seen as indications of success as a mother. If the doctor is able to avoid seeming critical of the mother's care of the baby he will probably obtain a more realistic account of what is happening at home. The breast-fed baby who is failing to thrive may be receiving inadequate amounts. Practical advice on increasing the frequency of feeds along with support from the health visitor may be all that is needed to remedy this problem. Intake is easier to measure in the bottle-fed baby. The requirements should be calculated relative to the baby's expected weight rather than his actual weight. Other relevant points in the history are interval between feeds, length of time the baby takes to feed, sucking difficulties, regurgitation and whether the baby tires easily. From six months onwards it is important to establish whether the child is able to chew. The mother may describe her child as having a poor appetite or even as being a voracious eater. Anorexia may stem from emotional deprivation whilst a baby who is being underfed will be ravenously hungry at meal-times, giving the impression that he is a good feeder. Appetite can also vary in some physical conditions leading to failure to thrive. The child with cystic fibrosis is typically an enthusiastic feeder whilst the child with coeliac disease tends to dislike meal-times. A home visit by the health visitor may provide further valuable information especially if she is able to be present during feeding time. The management of common feeding problems which may contribute to failure to thrive are further described in Chapter 6.

In the older child the emphasis should be on the kind and amount of food offered to the child, the amount actually eaten and meal-time behaviour. A useful approach is to enquire exactly what the child consumed the previous day and perhaps to ask the parents to complete a dietary record card for a short period. Some emotionally deprived children may show bizarre feeding habits, known as pica. Pencils, soil, wood, paper and many other inappropriate substances may be ingested.

The medical history should include enquiring about episodes of illness, breathlessness whilst feeding, cyanotic attacks, vomiting, and the character of the stools. Persistently loose stools suggest an intestinal infection or intestinal allergy. Bulky, pale offensive stools are characteristic of malabsorption. Loose stools may also be seen in environmental failure to thrive particularly when feeding is erratic. A large intake by a hungry infant may cause reactive diarrhoea due to impaired absorption. The doctor will begin to form an impression about the relationship between mother and child. The mother may admit to finding the baby very difficult to manage. She may appear uninterested in the baby and fail to respond to his signals of distress. The doctor should enquire about temperament, crying, colic and night-waking as well as about feeding behaviour. In the older child temper tantrums, aggressive behaviour or enuresis may accompany emotional deprivation. The mother may be suffering from depression or premenstrual tension which prevents her from responding to the needs of her child.

Observation of the mother's behaviour in the clinic or surgery may give clues to the quality of interaction. Eye contact between mother and baby, holding the baby so that he moulds to the mother's body and sensitive responses to signals such as crying are examples of interaction which are easily observed. However, the mother may not behave in her normal manner in the clinic and observations made in the home surroundings are likely to be more revealing. Where non-organic failure to thrive is suspected a much fuller evaluation will be needed, as discussed in the following section.

Examination

A developmental examination forms part of the initial assessment of failure to thrive. The child with non-organic failure to thrive may show delay areas which depend on social interaction and stimulation, such as speech and language and social/adaptive behaviour. The child with a primary CNS deficit is likely to be delayed in all areas of development.

Physical examination should be carried out with the child undressed. The state of clothing, cleanliness and presence of nappy rash would indicate the standard of maternal care. The child should be checked for bruising since non-accidental injury may accompany failure to thrive. Examination of the heart, abdomen and chest and observation of the child's head shape and facial appearance should be included. The child with malabsorption characteristically though not invariably has a protruding abdomen with wasting of the buttocks.

Initially urinalysis and culture of urine and stool are worth while, the latter particularly if there is a history of abnormal stools. Stool culture may reveal infection with *Campylobacter* or giardiasis. A full blood count could be carried out before hospital referral and may reveal nutritional anaemia or rarely more serious disease.

EVALUATION OF NON-ORGANIC FAILURE TO THRIVE

The traditional viewpoint that under-nutrition leading to failure to thrive stems from maternal neglect and rejection over-simplifies a more complex problem. Clearly there are some families where severe deprivation, disorganization and social disadvantage seem to be obvious causes for a child's malnourishment. Failure to thrive is associated with non-accidental injury in a proportion of cases and it would appear that these two share similar psychosocial patterns. But even in severely deprived families one child may stand out as being more affected than his siblings and equally many children emerge from apparently disadvantaged backgrounds emotionally and physically unharmed. There is no universal picture of the kinds of mother who fail to nurture their children adequately. A combination of subtle characteristics of both mother and child is involved in the generation of a behavioural cycle which results in under-nutrition and emotional deprivation. Many cases of non-organic failure to thrive are puzzling to the doctor. In order to intervene effectively the nature of these characteristics and the way they generate certain responses in mother and child need to be identified.

It is widely accepted that under-nutrition is a unifying theme in non-organic failure to thrive rather than a psychologically induced defect in absorption of metabolism. For example, the infant may be offered insufficient milk at infrequent intervals due to the caretaker's lack of awareness of the infant's appetite and requirements. Food may not be available due to disorganization or preoccupation with aspects other than child care and the mother may not notice how much the child actually consumes. The under-nourished child may appear to be a good feeder but chronic underfeeding may result in irritability and apathy towards meal-times.

In the early months the most intimate moments between mother and child occur at feed times and it is not surprising that mismatch between personalities of mother and child results in unsuccessful feeding. In the older child meal-times can become a battlefield sustained by emotional tension and conflict.

It may take a while for a mother to 'tune in' to her infant's style of behaviour. A mother may feel surprised by a highly active, non-cuddly baby and may regard this behaviour as rejection of her mothering skills. However, a sensitive mother will soon realize that the baby can be consoled by diverting his attention for example with a toy or biscuit or by carrying him round. In fact these infants are constantly seeking stimulation and thrive providing that they receive a high level of attention. On the other hand an apathetic, inactive baby may frustrate an impatient mother. He may like to take his time over feeding but she may be anxious to complete it as soon as possible. The inactive baby may become increasingly ignored and spend long periods in his cot. He may demand little and receive little attention. Some infants appear to be content spending long periods between feeds without crying but they are actually underfed and starving. As a general rule mothers should be advised to wake a baby for a feed during the day if he's still asleep five hours after the last feed. Sleeping for long periods during the day and reducing feeds to four a day before three months many indicate that the mother is not responding to the baby's needs.

Maternal depression is a well-recognized factor which may have behavioural consequences in the child. The mother's symptoms may be aggravated by the child's difficult behaviour and sleepless nights. Single parenthood and marital, housing or financial problems are among environmental factors which make mothers more vulnerable to depression. Hormonal influences may also play a part as in postnatal depression and the premenstrual syndrome. Over-anxiety is a common accompaniment of depression and may be reflected in tension in the infant or toddler, resulting in poor feeding. The mother's emotional state may make her intolerant of difficult behaviour and she may not spend sufficient time coaxing the baby to feed; he will remain hungry, crying and irritable, thus generating a cycle of anger, frustration and feelings of failure.

Failure to thrive may be difficult to diagnose and require patience and persistence to remedy. Practical help on feeding technique accompanied by close support by a health visitor may help to restore confidence and generate more positive mother—child feelings. Some mothers may reject help and it may require considerable tact and sensitivity for a health visitor or social worker to be accepted. Sometimes systematic advice on family budgeting and organization of the day and close supervision by a family aide are needed though some parents may resent such intervention as an intrusion of privacy. In severe neglect where social services are involved, the provision of such supervision may be a condition on which the parents' continued care depends.

Long-term follow-up of children with non-organic failure to thrive has shown that a substantial proportion manifest developmental and educational difficulties. They are also at considerable risk of continued growth retardation and later physical abuse. This suggests that more long-term help for such children is needed.

Unless the initial clinical assessment points to an obvious cause such as coeliac disease, most paediatricians would admit the child to hospital for a trial of feeding before embarking on more invasive tests.

The response to a trial of feeding illustrates a useful classification of failure to thrive. One group of children will feed well with a good intake and show a large weight gain, indicating that they were receiving insufficient calories due to feeding difficulties or maternal deprivation. A second group may achieve a good intake of food but a poor weight response will suggest malabsorption in the presence of abnormal stools (cystic fibrosis, coeliac disease or intestinal infection) or abnormal utilization of nutrients when stools are likely to be normal (inborn errors of metabolism) (Table 8.5).

A third group of children fail to achieve a good intake in hospital

Table 8.5 Some causes of organic failure to thrive.

Condition	Initial investigation
Gastrointestinal	
Hiatus hernia	Barium meal
Pyloric stenosis	Examination of abdomen during a feed
Cystic fibrosis	Sweat test
Coeliac disease	Stool fat, intestinal biopsy
Intestinal infection	Stool culture
Cow's milk allergy	Milk challenge/exclusion
Central nervous system abnormalities	
Birth injury	Neurodevelopmental examination
	brain scan, skull X-ray
Chromosomal abnormality	Chromosomal analysis
Cardiovascular	
Congenital malformation of the heart	ECG, chest X-ray, cardiac catheterization
Endocrine	
Hypothyroidism	Thyroid function tests
Growth-hormone deficiency	Bone age, growth hormone estimation
Metabolic	
Inborn errors of metabolism	Urine chromatography
Idiopathic hypercalcaemia	Serum calcium
Renal tubular acidosis	Urinalysis, blood electrolytes
Chronic infection	
Urinary tract infection	Urine culture, renal ultrasound, IVP
Tuberculosis	Mantoux, Heaf test, chest X-ray
Renal	
Renal insufficiency	Blood urea, creatinine and electrolytes,
	IVP

and consequently fail to gain weight. Some children appear to feed well but regurgitate, vomit or ruminate excessively. This picture occurs commonly in emotional deprivation but may also be a sign of hiatus hernia, pyloric stenosis, metabolic disease or raised intracranial pressure (see Table 8.5).

Poor intake may be due to poor sucking and swallowing secondary to CNS disorders and neuromuscular immaturity. The baby who feeds excessively slowly may have an underlying infection or hypothyroidism. Tiring during feeding is seen in congenital malformation of the heart and respiratory disease.

Unexpected childhood deaths

The sudden unexpected death of a child is a devastating event for the family and may have a profound effect on those who cared for the child medically. Sadly the number of children dying in this way has remained relatively constant in recent years, averaging 1 in 415 live births. A substantial proportion of these deaths remain unexplained even after the most detailed postmortem examination. Since 1970 these deaths have been termed sudden infant death syndrome (SIDS) rather than the older term cot deaths.

Young children who die unexpectedly form a heterogeneous group. They share the common feature of being unforeseen, usually with little in the way of untoward symptoms, but when the cases are investigated further a wide spectrum of clinical conditions emerges.

Two recent studies, the DHSS Multicentre Study of Post Neonatal Mortality in England and the Cot Death Study in Scotland (Arneil *et al.*, 1985), looked in detail at the clinical histories, medical care and necropsy findings in postperinatal deaths. The deaths of 17% of children in the Multicentre Study compared with 41% in Scotland were totally unexplained by clinical and pathological examination; these were true SIDS. In a further 57% in the Multicentre Study and 38% in Scotland they found mild disease, metabolic upset or a minor abnormality of a degree not normally associated with a fatal outcome and these were termed partially explained deaths.

In 26% of deaths in the Multicentre Study and 16% in the Scottish Study postmortem revealed previously unsuspected serious conditions such as congenital abnormalities, serious acquired disease (mainly pneumonia, bronchiolitis and meningitis) and gastrointestinal pathology.

The Multicentre Study looked in detail into the parents' account of the child's symptoms before death. A striking finding was that some babies who subsequently died of unrecognized serious illness and some with SIDS had shown some signs of illness such as coughs, colds, wheeziness and non-specific behavioural symptoms such as drowsiness, irritability, excessive crying or an altered character to the cry, vomiting feeds or sweating.

In about a quarter of cases it was felt that earlier action by parents might have influenced the outcome and in a similar proportion the treatment given by the GP was considered inadequate.

In the Sheffield Study (Taylor & Emery, 1982) a third of all children who died had evidence of possibly treatable disease. These children were suffering from illnesses which are occasionally fatal, but normally respond well to early treatment. This group includes conditions such as bronchitis, pneumonia, meningitis, gastroenteritis and otitis media. Notably, many of the possibly preventable deaths took place in socially disadvantaged families. A further small group of babies were thought to have been 'gently battered'. This diagnosis was only made after extensive discussion with parents when it became apparent during the interview that the parents' account of events was inconsistent and implausible. Generally speaking these families suffered an excess of adverse social factors such as psychiatric and physical illness and marital problems.

These findings suggest that there may have been preventable factors in a substantial proportion of deaths. Different actions by parents and professionals might have altered the outcome.

Background characteristics of children who die unexpectedly

Epidemiological data about the children and their families offer some clues to the circumstances contributing to childhood mortality and highlight areas where preventive measures might be effective.

Unexpected deaths have a peak incidence between four and 11 weeks, only 10% occurring after 28 weeks. Along with respiratory illnesses they occur more often in the winter months, particularly in the January–March quarter. Not surprisingly they occur largely at home between the hours of midnight and noon and are normally discovered after 6 a.m. Some children have been left for long periods unobserved before being found dead. In 12% the interval was 10 hours or more.

The Multicentre Study compared background factors of children who died with a group of healthy control children. Mothers of children who died were younger, had a higher parity and were more likely to smoke than controls. The infants who died were lighter at birth or of shorter gestation and more likely to be a twin and to have been admitted to a special-care baby unit. They were also less likely to have been breast-fed and received solid foods earlier than controls.

Factors representing social disadvantage were more prevalent amongst families of dead infants. Larger, poorer families living in overcrowded, poorly repaired accommodation were more likely to experience infant death.

The two groups differed in their use of medical services. The dead infants had more out-patient attendances and hospital admissions. The general practitioner had more often visited at home but had not seen the infant more often in the surgery.

Interestingly the characteristics of the 20% of children in whom no pathological evidence of disease was found (SIDS) were somewhat different from those of children whose deaths were associated with disease. They shared the risk factors of low birthweight and short gestation but were not strongly associated with bottle-feeding and maternal smoking and in other social aspects were not easily distinguishable from surviving controls. This perhaps explains why the use of risk-score systems to select children for intervention has been more successful in preventing deaths associated with disease than the smaller proportion of wholly unexplained deaths.

Prevention of infant deaths

Studies in Sheffield and subsequently the DHSS postneonatal study have demonstrated several areas where some preventive measures might reduce the incidence of infant mortality. However, the absence of a national decline in postneonatal and unexpected deaths in recent years suggests that the problem needs to be tackled more vigorously in the future.

PARENTAL ADVICE

Both the Sheffield and DHSS studies indicate that parents may fail to recognize important signs of illness in their child. Parents need information about the changes in behaviour and clinical symptoms to look out for. Drowsiness, irritability, altered cry, failure to take feeds, vomiting, diarrhoea, fever, dehydration, breathing difficulties and weight loss were common symptoms and signs seen in babies who died.

Education may be achieved through specially designed books and leaflets but some mothers are unlikely to read such literature. The health visitor is the ideal source of information for parents and needs to be accessible to discuss symptoms and anxieties when they arise.

MEDICAL CARE

Quite clearly, parents of young children need easy access to their general practitioner and this is recognized by most practitioners, who will readily see any sick child within a short time. However, some parents have experienced difficulty in obtaining prompt help and in certain communities this is a great cause for concern.

THE HEALTH VISITOR

The health visitor has a vital role to play in parental education on infant feeding. She is in the best position to assess how the mother and baby are faring. Apart from encouraging breast-feeding she can keep an eye on how the mother is making up milk formulas. She can enquire about the frequency and amounts of feeds and the time taken to feed. Most health visitors have portable baby scales to monitor weight gain. Studies have shown that a falling off in the rate of weight gain sometimes precedes SIDS.

The health visitor provides an important link between the mother and the general practitioner and hospital. Some mothers may need advice on how to obtain medical help. A practice-attached health visitor can easily discuss any concerns about a child with the doctor, who can then take prompt action.

Frequency of visits depends on the health visitor's judgement of how much support a mother needs. Risk-scoring systems have been advocated to help decide which babies need extra visits. The evidence suggests that increased contact with the health visitor can prevent some infant deaths, particularly those associated with unrecognized serious illness. Totally unexplained deaths (SIDS) have not been appreciably reduced. Both kinds of unexpected deaths share low birthweight and short gestation as risk factors but SIDS is more difficult to predict from background factors.

Many health visitors would argue that they are already identifying mothers in need of extra support without a scoring system. One drawback of concentrating services on a supposedly high-risk group is the danger of services being too thinly spread over the rest of the population. In the Sheffield Study visits were made fortnightly until 14 weeks of age and then three-weekly up to 20 weeks. Some mothers need more frequent visits at certain periods while some probably manage with fewer visits. There are strong arguments for increasing the number of health visitors so that all babies can receive more visits.

APNOEA ALARMS AND REGULAR WEIGHING

Doctors may receive enquiries from parents about the use of apnoea alarms especially if the family has had a previous cot death or the baby has had breathing difficulties after birth. Their use in the home is controversial and their value in preventing unexpected infant deaths is not yet established.

Some alarms use a sensor placed beneath the baby's mattress and others a capsule attached to the baby's abdomen. The sensor is designed to detect breathing movements. One drawback is that they do not immediately detect a blocked airway as breathing movements can continue for some time even if no air is reaching the lungs. Parents need to be instructed on techniques of resuscitation if using an alarm.

False alarms occur frequently and are a distressing experience for parents. This has to be balanced against the reassurance provided by the alarm.

There is insufficient evidence that cot death is preceded by apnoeic attacks in the majority of cases. Therefore there is no indication for their use in normal babies. There may be a certain group of babies for whom, for various reasons, a paediatrician may recommend an alarm. The group would include infants of low birthweight, babies with a history of apnoeic attacks and siblings of cot-death babies.

A study has been carried out (Emery *et al.*, 1985) to compare the relative values of apnoea alarms and regular weighing as preventive measures in siblings of cot-death babies. Findings suggest that regular weekly weighing, together with recording the child's symptoms and weekly visiting by the health visitor, are as acceptable as apnoea alarms to parents, as a method of monitoring babies at high risk of cot death. Looking back at the weights of children who died unexpectedly, a clear pattern of diminishing weight gain before death is apparent. Special weight charts are available which indicate when weight gain falls to below an acceptable level. If this occurs prompt medical attention is recommended to determine the cause. This may be readily apparent, as in gastroenteritis or otitis media, but hospital admission is required if no obvious diagnosis can be made. Clearly regular weighing is not feasible or desirable for all babies, but the evidence suggests that weighing, together with health visitor support, is a useful tool in monitoring babies whose health gives cause for concern.

Support for families who have an unexpected infant death

Parents whose child dies suddenly not only experience shock and distress at the loss of their child but may also suffer further trauma by the events which follow the discovery of the death. The way the situation is handled by doctors, police, ambulancemen and hospital staff can deeply affect the parents' reactions. Subsequent support from family, friends, the health visitor and the general practitioner can assist the parents in coming to terms with their bereavement.

The Foundation for Study of Infant Deaths is involved in the support of families of cot-death infants and has a network of support groups in various areas of the country. Many parents find it helpful to meet with others who have undergone a similar experience. The Foundation also runs study days and supplies information leaflets for parents and doctors. It funds research into reasons for and prevention of cot deaths and has also carried out a survey of parents' reactions and views on the way the death was handled. These findings are of interest when planning ways of helping such families.

The vast majority of SIDS occur in the home and may be confirmed either by the general practitioner or at hospital. Most parents feel that the doctor offered sympathy and practical help. They may fear that they were in some way responsible and need explanation that some babies do die completely unexpectedly. When the ambulance is involved, the ambulancemen should handle the dead baby considerately and allow the parents to accompany the baby to hospital. In the accident and emergency department, parents need privacy and should be given the opportunity to hold the baby if they wish. It may be suggested that brothers and sisters are taken to see the baby in a chapel of rest as children often find it reassuring to see the baby looking peaceful and happy.

The general practitioner or paediatrician has to inform the parent that the death must be investigated by the coroner and that a post-mortem will be needed. Most parents are anxious to know why their baby died and appreciate the need for a postmortem. The investigation will involve a statement to the police and often a visit to the home by the coroner's officer. In the survey most parents were satisfied by the way the police handled the case but 10% were angered and distressed by their experience and felt that they were being treated with insensitivity and suspicion. The general practitioner should visit as soon as he or she learns about the death. Parents may need to explore their feelings of guilt and grief over several visits. The doctor can advise them about the kind of feelings they may experience, such as hearing the baby cry, distressing dreams, loss of appetite and sleeplessness. Listening to parents express their feelings of anger, grief and guilt and allowing them to relate in detail the events of the last few hours or days are perhaps the most valuable ways in which the doctor can help initially. At a later date when the postmortem findings are available parents will wish to discuss the cause of death. In some areas the paediatrician arranges to counsel the parents. If a mother is breast-feeding she will need medication and advice on suppressing lactation. The reaction and health of siblings need careful assessment. Twins carry an extra risk of cot death and the surviving twin may be observed in hospital for a time. The health visitor will be closely involved with the mother and all the health care team will need to give extra attention and support with subsequent children. (The Foundation for the Study of Infant Deaths is located at 15, Belgrave Square, London.)

References

Arneil, G. *et al.* (1985) National Post-Perinatal Infant Mortality and Cot-death Study, Scotland 1981–82. *Lancet*, 30 March, 740–3.

Bain, D.J.G. (1983) Can the clinical course of acute otitis media be modified by systemic decongestant or anti-histamine treatment? *British Medical Journal*, **287**, 654–6.

Bax, M., Hart, H. & Jenkins, S. (1980) *The Health Needs of Pre-school Children*. Thomas Coram Research Unit, London.

Bentovim, A. (1972) Handicapped pre-school children and their families — effects on the child's early emotional development. *British Medical Journal*, **3**, 634–7.

Blair, H. (1977) Natural history of childhood asthma: 20 year follow-up. *Archives of Disease in Childhood*, **52**, 613–19.

British Medical Journal (1981) Secretory otitis media and grommets (editorial) *British Medical Journal*, **282** (6263), 501.

Burr, H.L. (1983) Does infant feeding affect the risk of allergy. *Archives of Disease in Childhood*, **58**, 561–5.

Cant, A., Marsden, K.A. & Kilshaw, P.J. (1985) Egg and cow's milk hypersensitivity in exclusively breast fed infants with eczema, and detection of egg protein in breast milk. *British Medical Journal*, **291**, 932–7.

Chamberlain, R. & Simpson, R.N. (1979) *The Prevalence of Illness in Childhood. Report of the British Birth Child Study into Illnesses and Hospital Experiences of Children During the First 3½ Years of Life*. Pitman Medical, Tunbridge Wells.

Colley, J., Douglas, J. & Reid, D. (1973) Respiratory disease in young adults: influence of early childhood respiratory tract illness, social class, air pollution and smoking. *British Medical Journal*, **3**, 195.

Colley, J., Holland, W.W. & Corkhill, R.T. (1974) Influence of passive smoking and parental phlegm on pneumonia and bronchitis in early childhood. *Lancet*, **ii**, 1031.

Cunningham, A.S. (1977) Morbidity in breast fed and artificially fed infants. *Journal of Pediatrics*, **90** (5), 726–9.

Dingle, J.H., Badger, G.F. & Jordon, W.S. Jr (1964) *Illness in the Home: a Study of 25 000 Illnesses in a Group of Cleveland Families*. Press of Case Western Reserve University, Cleveland.

Douglas, J. & Blomfield, J.M. (1958) *Children Under Five*. George Allen & Unwin, London.

Emery, J., Wait, A.J., Carpenter, R.G., Limerick, S.R. & Blake, D. (1985) Apnoea monitors compared with weighing scales for siblings after cot death. *Archives of Disease in Childhood*, **60**, 1055–60.

Fergusson, D.M., Horwod, L.J. & Shannon, F.T. (1980) Parental smoking and respiratory illness in infancy. *Archives of Disease in Childhood*, **55**, 358–61.

Fry, J. (1961) *The Catarrhal Child*. Butterworth, London.

Glezen, W.P. & Denny, F.W. (1973) Epidemiology of acute lower respiratory disease in children. *New England Journal of Medicine*, **288** (10), 498.

Godfrey, S. (1985) What is asthma? *Archives of Disease in Childhood*, **60**, 997–1000.

Grulee, C.G. & Sandford, H.N. (1936) The influence of breast and artificial feeding on infantile eczema. *Journal of Pediatrics*, **9**, 223–5.

Hamman, R.J., Hakil, T. & Holland, W.W. (1975) Asthma in schoolchildren. Demographic associations and peak expiratory flow rates compared in children with bronchitis. *British Journal of Preventative and Social Medicine*, **29**, 228–38.

Hart, H., Bax, M. & Jenkins, S. (1984) Health and behaviour in pre-school children. *Child: Care, Health and Development*, **10**.

Holm, V.A. & Kunze, L.H. (1969) Effect of chronic otitis media on language and speech development. *Pediatrics*, **43**, 833.

Jerger, B. (1970) Clinical experience with impedance audiometry. *Archives of Otolarygology*, **92**, 311–24.

Kjellman, N. (1978) Allergy, otitis media and serum immunoglobulins after adenoidectomy. *Acta Paediatr Scandanavica*, **67**, 717–23.

Kuzenko, J. (ed.) (1976) *Asthma in Children*. Pitman Medical Publishing Co., London.

Leeder, S.R., Corkhill, R., Irwig, L., Holland, W.W. & Colley, J. (1976a) Influence of family factors on the incidence of lower respiratory illness during the first year of life. *British Journal of Preventative and Social Medicine*, **30**, 203–12.

Leeder, S.R., Corkhill, R., Irwig, L.M. & Holland, W.W. (1976b) Influence of family factors on asthma and wheezing during the first five years of life. *British Journal of Preventative and Social Medicine*, **30**, 213–18.

Lunn, J.E., Knowelden, J. & Handysich, A.J. (1967) Patterns of respiratory illness in Sheffield infant schoolchildren. *British Journal of Preventative and Social Medicine*, **21**, 7.

Matthew, D.J., Taylor, B., Norman, B.P. & Turner, M.W. (1977) Prevention of eczema. *Lancet*, 12 February, 321–4.

Maw, R. (1983) Chronic otitis media with effusion (glue ear) and adenotonsilectomy: prospective randomized controlled study. *British Medical Journal*, **287**, 1586–8.

Mitchell, R.A. & Dawson, B. (1973) Educational and social characteristics in children with asthma. *Archives of Disease in Childhood*, **48**, 467.

Office of Health Economics (1976) *Asthma*. Office of Health Economics, London.

Olson, A. *et al.* (1978) Prevention and therapy of serous otitis media by oral decongestant: a double-blind study in paediatric practice. *Pediatrics*, **61** (5), 679–84.

Riding, K., Bluestone, C., Michaels, R., Cantekin, E., Doyle, W. & Poziviak, C. (1978) Microbiology of recurrent and chronic otitis media with effusion. *Journal of Paediatrics*, **93** (5), 739–43.

Rutter, M., Tizard, J. & Whitmore, K. (1970) *Education, Health and Behaviour*. Longman, London.

Scadding, J.G. (1983) Definitions and clinical categories of asthma. In *Asthma* (eds Clark, T.J.H. & Godfrey, S.), 2nd edn, pp. 1–11. Chapman & Hall, London.

Sibbald, B., Horn, M. & Gregg, I. (1980) A family study of the genetic basis of asthma and wheezy bronchitis. *Archives of Disease in Childhood*, **55**, 354–7.

Taylor, E. & Emery, J. (1982) Two-year study of the causes of post-perinatal deaths classified in terms of preventability. *Archives of Disease in Childhood*, **57**, 668–73.

Teal, D.W., Klein, J.O. & Posner, B.A. (1980) Epidemiology of otitis media in children. *Annals of Otology and Laryngology*, **89** (suppl. 68), 5–6.

Tos, M., Poulser, G. & Borch, J. (1978) Tympanometry in 2 year old children. *ORL*, **40**, 77–85.

9 Behaviour Problems in the Younger Child

UNTIL RELATIVELY RECENTLY behaviour problems in pre-school children have received little attention, although all those working with young children would agree that they are common. Certainly by primary school age they cause more concern in the classroom than other health problems, and there is some evidence that rates of behaviour problems are increasing, particularly in inner city schools.

In the preschool child behavioural difficulties are often closely related to health and developmental disorders, and also to family stress, particularly maternal depression. Stevenson & Richman (1978) described close correlations between speech and language difficulties and child behaviour in a large study of three-year-olds in Waltham Forest, and this has been confirmed in other studies such as those from Newcastle and Dunedin (Fundundis et al., 1979; McGee et al., 1984). A close association between recurrent minor health disorders and children's behaviour has also been described (Bax et al., 1983). For many children the problems are not transient; follow-up of the Waltham Forest children showed that a considerable proportion of them had behaviour disorders and school difficulties at the age of eight. Hence these are not problems to be lightly dismissed with the platitude 'she will grow out of it'. Rather a thorough assessment of the child is called for, with an indication to the parents that you do take their concern seriously. Time spent on handling what may appear to be a minor problem with tact and sensitivity will pay dividends, as parents are then more likely to come back with other concerns about their child at an early stage rather than waiting until they become more serious. Although behaviour problems in the preschool child are a common source of anxiety to parents, they may well not be taken to the general practitioner, or may present masquerading as medical problems. Because behaviour is usually situationally determined, the child described by parents as impossible to cope with at home may well behave angelically in the surgery. Other children may exhibit difficult behaviour in the clinic or surgery, in which case the parents' concern is more likely to be taken seriously. Relatively small numbers of preschool children are referred to the child psychiatric services for help whereas

315

health visitors, general practitioners and paediatricians are commonly involved in discussing behavioural aspects of child-rearing.

Prevalence of behavioural and emotional disorders

Epidemiological studies in childhood have demonstrated considerable numbers of children with behaviour problems. The Waltham Forest study of a large number of three-year-olds found 22% to have significant behaviour problems (Richman *et al.*, 1975) and studies of older children, notably the Isle of Wight survey of 10- and 11-year-olds (Rutter *et al.*, 1970) again found about 20% showing significant psychological problems.

Particular groups of children have been shown to be especially at risk, for example those with chronic physical disorders or learning difficulties, as well as children in particular settings such as day nurseries (see Chapter 10). Research into the work of district handicap (or child development) teams found that around 50% of children with handicapping conditions of all types had additional behaviour problems or psychiatric disturbance requiring some form of intervention (Bax & Whitmore, 1985). Paediatricians too estimate that around one-third of their out-patient referrals are for predominantly emotional or behavioural problems, and these are also a major consideration among children admitted to paediatric wards.

Within general practice the rate of consultation specifically for psychological reasons is low (3.5% of all attendances in one study) but in around a quarter of attendances there is considered to be a psychological component to the presenting problem (Bailey *et al.*, 1978).

Hence many health professionals in addition to child psychiatrists will have contact with young children manifesting behaviour problems and it is important that they are adequately trained in this field.

Good basic techniques for assessment and management are essential for child health doctors (Graham & Jenkins, 1985) and for health visitors, who are increasingly gaining expertise in behavioural management (Perkins & Linke, 1984). Health visitors are often the first health professionals to be consulted when there is anxiety regarding a child's behaviour and are in an ideal position both to observe the child when visiting the home and to discuss methods of management with parents.

In this chapter we consider some of the common problems of behaviour presenting in young children, how they relate to other aspects of the child's health and development, and an approach to management. Data from the Thomas Coram study form the basis of this chapter.

Interestingly it was found that behaviour problems were about as common as health problems although parents were far less likely to have sought help from their general practitioner in managing them. In the initial sample, less than 2% of practice consultations had been for behaviour or management problems, although of course these may have masqueraded as physical disorders.

Data on behaviour were collected throughout the study, by using a behaviour questionnaire (see Table 3.1) which was presented to the parents at the time we saw the children for their development examinations, the questions following on from those relating to the child's health and development. Separate questionnaires were used for children under two years and over two years, relating to individual items of behaviour and finishing with a question to the parent as to whether any aspect of their child's behaviour was a worry to her or him; if so this was described in more detail.

As with any information obtained by interview rather than observation, the question is raised of how far the information obtained is accurate, and whether parents perceive problems which would not be borne out by observing the children at home. Some reassurance on this point comes from a study by Dunn & Kendrick (1980) in which they found close correlations between the child's behaviour as reported by the mother and observed behaviour in the home. As with a medical history, there is no reason to believe that the majority of parents deliberately misrepresent their children's behaviour, and where we had the opportunity to observe the child either at home or in the nursery the parents' description of their child's behaviour was nearly always borne out by observation. These considerations aside, where parents are expressing anxiety about their child's behaviour this is reason enough to take them seriously.

The numbers of parents in our study who were worried about their child's behaviour are shown in Table 9.1. It can be seen that problems reach a peak around three years when 15% of parents were worried,

Table 9.1 Prevalence of parental concern.

	6 month		1 year		18 month		2 year		3 year		4½ year	
	n	%	*n*	%	*n*	%	*n*	%	*n*	%	*n*	%
Parents worried about behaviour	11	3	23	8	15	6	34	11	45	15	35	13
Parents not worried	321	97	254	92	236	94	268	89	283	85	243	87
Total *n*	332		277		251		302		328		278	

with a slight fall at four and a half years when 12% were worried. We ourselves made an assessment of whether we considered the child had a behaviour problem (based both on history and observation at the time) and graded problems as mild, moderate or severe. There was high agreement between doctors' and parents' rating of problems; the majority of behaviour problems fell into the mild category but 6% of children at three years and 5% at four and a half years were rated as having moderate or severe problems. This is very similar to the prevalence rates of behaviour problems described in the Waltham Forest study, where 7% were rated moderate to severe and 15% mild (Richman *et al.*, 1975).

Problems at six weeks

At six weeks the problems reported reflected early management difficulties experienced by some mothers in adjusting to the demands of a small baby, and their often unrealistic expectations of establishing a 'routine' in the early weeks. Twelve per cent of mothers described their babies as being 'colicky' after nearly every feed, and a further 17% reported 'colic' most days ('colic' was a descriptive term used where mothers reported the baby as being in discomfort and unsettled after a feed associated with screaming and drawing up the legs). Six per cent of babies were reported as crying a lot most days; the majority of these were also described as 'colicky'. Other worries at this age related to the common lack of day and night routine, the demanding of frequent feeds by the baby and, less commonly, difficulties with the baby actually taking feeds. Management of these and other problems at later ages is discussed further on in this chapter.

Problems at six months

At six months few parents (3%) were worried about their baby's behaviour. Concern mainly centred around difficulty in settling the baby to sleep (8% difficult most nights) and night-waking (13%), with feeding difficulties being less common. Only 1% of babies were reported as crying or being miserable most days, but these babies would obviously be a cause for professional concern.

Problems in the under-twos

In the children under two years the most commonly reported problems were those of feeding and sleeping, with feeding problems becoming more common after the age of 18 months.

SLEEPING

Sleeping problems, particularly night-waking, are extremely common between six months and two years and are a considerable source of anxiety and exhaustion to parents. They are strikingly more common than feeding problems, and the highest rate of night-waking (on four or more nights a week) was at one year when it was 21%. It was only slightly less common at 18 months (17%) and additionally at each age there were a further 6 to 9% of children who were waking on two or three nights a week (see Table 9.2). Very often it was the same children who were also difficult to settle to sleep, so the night-time disruption to parents was often considerable. No sex differences were found at any age in rates of night-waking, nor did we find social class differences.

Similar rates of night-waking have been reported in other samples of children, namely 17% of 14-month-olds in Cambridge (Bernal, 1973), 23% of 15-month-olds in London (Blurton Jones *et al.*, 1978), and 24% of 18-month-olds in Oxford (Ounsted & Simons, 1978).

Continuities of night-waking

There is a tendency when confronted with a child who wakes at night to reassure the parent with the advice that 'he will grow out of it'. This is undoubtedly true, but the clinician should be aware of how long this may take, and how much support may be required in the mean-

Table 9.2 Sleeping problems.

	6 month		1 year		18 month		2 year		3 year		4½ year	
	n	%	*n*	%	*n*	%	*n*	%	*n*	%	*n*	%
Settling to sleep												
Easy	289	87	228	83	211	85	247	82	270	82	230	84
Difficult 2 or 3 nights a week	16	5	15	5	13	5	20	6	25	7	22	8
Difficult most nights	28	8	34	12	26	10	36	12	36	11	22	8
Total *n*	333		277		250		303		331		274	
Night-waking												
Hardly ever	268	81	201	73	183	74	244	79	261	79	229	84
2 or 3 nights a week	19	6	17	6	23	9	18	6	30	9	16	6
Most nights (4 or more)	44	13	58	21	43	17	44	15	40	12	27	10
Total *n*	331		276		249		306		331		272	

time. We examined the continuities of night-waking from six months onward and found that, of babies who were waking four or more nights a week at age six months, 44% were still waking this frequently at one year. Of the night-waking babies at one year, 41% were still waking on four or more nights at 18 months, and from 18 months to two years 54% of wakers continued waking. A far smaller proportion of children at each age (10–15%) developed a night-waking problem which was not present at the previous age. Five per cent of children whom we were able to follow from six months to two years had persistent night-waking throughout this period.

Night-waking in infancy is probably far less common in cultures where children traditionally sleep very close to their parents, although most reporting is anecdotal; the majority of studies have attempted to relate sleep disturbance to perinatal events rather than environmental factors such as where the child sleeps. Maturational factors in the child are certainly important, and it is known that sleep patterns change considerably over the first few months, with longer periods of sleep and wakefulness being established, and a diurnal pattern emerging. There are wide individual differences in the amount of sleep needed by different infants, and this shows some consistency over the next two years (Bernal, 1973).

Electrophysiological studies of infants again show maturational changes; at term infants spend about half their sleep time in active 'rapid eye movement' sleep (REM sleep) and around 40% of their sleep time in quiet sleep (non-REM sleep). These proportions change with age so that by eight months there is twice as much quiet sleep as REM sleep, and this proportion gradually increases until by 10 years the normal adult proportions of 20% REM sleep to 80% quiet sleep are reached. The REM sleep state represents physiological arousal and its control mechanisms lie in the pontine nuclei. Non-REM sleep appears to serve the function of restoration and anabolism, and is regulated by the forebrain.

These changes in proportion of sleep states are thought to be due to CNS maturation and are probably not influenced by environmental factors. Adverse perinatal factors can, however, affect the organization of sleep patterns, although polygraphic sleep studies of brain-damaged and high-risk infants have produced disparate results (see Anders & Weinstein, 1982). Two clinical studies have, however, shown an association between obstetric factors, early infant behaviour, and night-waking during the second year (Bernal, 1973; Blurton Jones *et al.*, 1978) (Table 9.3). Other studies have failed to show such an association (Ounsted & Simons, 1978).

Table 9.3 Night-waking: prevalence and associated factors.

Study	Prevalence	Age	Associated factors
Bernal (1973)	17%	14 months	Perinatal factors
Carey (1974)	25%	6–12 months	Temperament Prolonged breast- feeding
Blurton Jones *et al.* (1978)	23%	25 months	Perinatal factors
Ounsted & Simons (1978)	24%	18 months	None
Jenkins *et al.* (1980)	21%	12 months	Ear infections Upper respiratory tract infections Maternal stress

The child's individual temperament is also important. Carey demonstrated an association between certain temperamental characteristics (a low sensory threshold) and night-waking; he also found a significantly higher proportion of night-wakers among infants who had prolonged breast-feeding, compared with bottle-fed infants (Carey, 1974). In our study night-waking was found more commonly in breast-fed than bottle-fed infants but the difference was not statistically significant. There is some evidence that an over-responsive parent may reinforce a baby's demands for attention during the night and so encourage the persistence of the problem in a baby who is already predisposed to wake at night.

Many other factors can contribute to the development of waking, including birth of a sibling (Dunn *et al.*, 1981), illness (Bax *et al.*, 1983) and stress. In our preschool study we found recurrent upper respiratory tract infections and a history of ear infections to be significantly related to night-waking, while hospitalization for any reason was not. It is well known that environmental stresses, including maternal depression and psychiatric illness, influence children's behaviour, and vice versa. One might expect sleep problems to be particularly associated with stress, and there was evidence from our study of a strong association between night-waking and maternal stress. The association is almost certainly in two directions, since night-waking undoubtedly induces exhaustion in the parents, and this underlines the need for support and help for families with such problems. Difficulties in settling to sleep may reflect problems of separation or of over-arousal. These are further discussed under management later in this chapter.

FEEDING PROBLEMS

The two aspects of feeding which we asked about in our study were appetite and food fads. The prevalence rates of problems reported in each of these areas are shown in Table 9.4. Both persistently poor appetite and marked food fads were most prevalent at the age of three years, when 16% of children were reported as always having a poor appetite and 12% reported as very faddy. As might be expected there was considerable overlap between these, with approximately half the children with poor appetites also being reported as very faddy. In the London study by Richman and her colleagues (1975) food fads were reported in 13% of three-year-olds.

Although feeding problems are less common in very young babies (2% at six months) they are a cause of considerable concern to mothers. A baby who is difficult to feed may be perceived as rejecting and, as in other aspects of early child-rearing which do not go smoothly, this is very undermining to a mother's self-confidence. It can also result in a chronic situation where intake is inadequate and the child fails to thrive. Successful feeding is felt to be an integral part of 'good' mothering, so early feeding difficulties can result both in maternal tension and a loss of self-esteem. Much of the early communication between mother and baby centres around feeding, so it is in the interests of both mother and child that this should be a positive and enjoyable experience. In relation to breast-feeding, there is evidence that early experience is important, in that babies put to the breast soon after delivery are more likely to be successfully breast-fed than those who waited eight hours or more (Martin, 1978).

Table 9.4 Feeding problems.

	6 month		1 year		18 month		2 year		3 year		4½ year	
	n	%	*n*	%	*n*	%	*n*	%	*n*	%	*n*	%
Appetite												
Usually good	316	96	251	91	204	81	213	71	223	67	181	66
Sometimes poor	8	2	16	6	32	13	56	18	56	17	68	25
Always poor	8	2	10	3	15	6	34	11	52	16	26	9
Food fads												
Not faddy	292	88	242	87	212	84	231	77	231	70	185	67
Few fads	25	8	24	8	30	12	43	13	60	18	65	24
Very faddy	10	3	11	4	9	4	29	10	40	12	25	9
Not on solids	4	1	1	0.4	—	—	—	—	—	—	—	—
Total *n*	332		278		251		303		331		275	

Continuities of feeding problems

We did not find such strong continuities with feeding problems as with sleep problems. Of the children at 18 months with very poor appetite, 23% had persistently poor appetite at two years. Between two and three years continuities were stronger; 65% of two-year-olds with poor appetite were reported unchanged in this respect at three years. 25% of the children who were reported very faddy at 18 months were still faddy at two years, and between two and three years faddiness persisted in 31%. At all ages more children were likely to present afresh with feeding problems than those in whom the problems persisted. There was some evidence that babies who were small at birth (either preterm or small for gestational age), weighing less than 2500 grams, had more feeding problems at the age of two than babies of a normal birthweight and there is no doubt that some preschool feeding problems begin in early infancy.

Problems in the over-twos

In children over two years a rather different clinical picture emerges, with sleeping problems becoming relatively less common and management difficulties emerging. Children at this age are becoming increasingly exploratory, mobile and independent, and parents of these older children commonly find their children difficult to manage, and report them as having frequent temper tantrums or being too dependent. Problems in this age group may also arise due to the birth of a sibling, and aggression towards peers or adults may also develop around this age. Between two and four and a half years, 5–9% of children were said to be frequently difficult to manage or too demanding, while around a quarter of children, as might be expected, were sometimes demanding a lot of attention (see Table 9.5).

CONTINUITIES OF MANAGEMENT PROBLEMS, DEPENDENCY AND TEMPER TANTRUMS

Few of the children reported as being frequently difficult to manage at two years were still considered difficult at three years and similarly three-quarters of the very attention-demanding two-year-olds were considered not demanding by three years.

Temper tantrums were commonly reported from the age of two years (we did not ask about them at 18 months), with 19% of two-year-olds, 18% of three-year-olds and 11% of four-and-a-half-year-

Table 9.5 Problems over two years — management.

	2 years		3 years		4½ years	
	n	%	*n*	%	*n*	%
Management difficulties						
Easy to manage	203	68	209	64	188	68
Sometimes difficult	81	27	92	28	69	25
Frequently difficult	14	5	26	8	18	7
Dependency						
Independent	189	64	216	66	183	66
Sometimes demands a lot of attention	79	27	83	25	75	28
Demands too much attention	28	9	28	9	16	6
Temper tantrums						
Hardly ever	148	50	176	54	184	67
1–4 a week	93	31	92	28	60	22
Nearly every day	38	13	44	13	24	9
3 or more a day	18	6	15	5	6	2
Total *n*	298		327		275	

olds having tantrums at least once daily. There were no sex differences in the rates of temper tantrums at any age; but at two years significantly more boys than girls were reported as frequently difficult to manage. These rates again are very similar to findings in other studies (e.g. Ounsted & Simons, 1978). Temper tantrums were quite likely still to occur at the later ages. In this study 20% of all two-year-old children were having frequent tantrums (at least daily) and at three years 45% of them were still having frequent tantrums. Of those children having frequent tantrums at three, one-third were reported as still having frequent tantrums at four and a half, so, although the likelihood of tantrums persisting from three to four and a half is not as high as from two to three years, it is still significant.

Associated factors

Most people consider temper tantrums to be a normal expression of behaviour in the age group 18 months to three or four years. The majority of parents cope well with tantrums and are not too concerned. Frequent tantrums can be quite difficult to manage, however, and can undermine the confidence of even the calmest of parents. Tantrums are most likely to occur when children are tired or hungry, and also when they are unwell (Goodenough, 1931). The majority of tantrums at younger ages are provoked by conflict with a parent, but as children get older disagreements with playmates become more common. In this study we found significant associations between episodes of illness and tantrums; thus children who had recurrent upper respiratory tract infections or earache were more likely to have frequent temper tantrums at all ages. It was also found that the children who had more minor illnesses were reported as more difficult to manage.

The question of causality is a complex one, but the relationship of common behaviour problems and childhood illnesses is important to underline. It emphasizes that different aspects of the child cannot be separated when considering management of a presenting symptom. Family and environmental factors, particularly maternal stress and depression, must also be taken into account. A highly significant association was found between measures of maternal stress and children's temper tantrums, difficulty in management and behaviour problems reported by parents, illustrating again the complexity of the subject.

TOILETING PROBLEMS

Toilet training is a gradually achieved process, with the child attaining control through a series of stages which will vary from one individual to another. Most children are clean and dry during the day sometime during their second year, with night-time bladder control usually achieved sometime between two and four years. A classic American book on child care states that 80% of children are clean and dry during the day by two and a half years. In our study 44% of two-year-olds, and 86% of three-year-olds were always dry by day, and complete bowel control had been achieved by 54% of two-year-olds, 93% of three-year-olds, and 98% of four-and-a-half-year-olds.

The epidemiology of nocturnal enuresis shows considerable variation from one population to another. In surveys of three-year-olds, 87% were dry at night in Sweden, 77% in Newcastle and 64% in Baltimore. By the age of five years the overall percentages who were dry at night were Sweden 94%, Newcastle 91% and Baltimore 72% (from Kolvin *et al.*, 1973). In this preschool study 23% of two-year-olds, 62% of three-year-olds, and 79% of four-and-a-half-year-olds were almost always dry at night, and on the whole there was very little anxiety expressed by the parents of the four-and-a-half-year-olds who were wetting the bed (Table 9.6).

Soiling was a less common problem at four and a half, occurring in

Table 9.6 Achievement of bladder control.

	Percentage of children		
	2 years ($n = 302$)	3 years ($n = 331$)	4½ years ($n = 278$)
Reliably dry by day	44	86	94
Almost always dry at night	23	62	79

only 3% of our sample. However, it was a cause of much concern, and the majority of children who were soiling at this age had other associated behaviour or management problems. Intervention is always indicated in this situation.

The effect of gender

Studies of behaviour problems in children of primary school age report higher rates among boys, and this is certainly true in older age groups (Rutter *et al.*, 1970; Chazan & Jackson, 1971; McGee *et al.*, 1984). In a study of three-year-olds in London (Richman *et al.*, 1975) there was some evidence of higher rates of moderate and severe problems in boys, but the difference was not significant. In our study we looked both at individual items of behaviour and parents' ratings of problems, to see if there were any sex differences. At no age were behaviour problems more common in boys. For most items of behaviour the rates were the same for boys and girls, the only exception being that rates of feeding problems were slightly higher in girls, and at two years more boys were reported difficult to manage. There were no differences between sexes in rates of night-waking. So it seems that, whatever factors are operating to influence the higher rates of problems amongst boys in older age groups, they are not influential in the preschool period.

Relationship of behaviour with development

Both physical handicap and chronic illness in childhood are known to be associated with higher than average rates of behaviour disturbance, and where there is central nervous system dysfunction (as with epilepsy or cerebral palsy) the rates are particularly high. In the classic Isle of Wight study, Rutter and colleagues (1970) found that children with a physical disorder such as asthma had twice the rate of psychiatric disorder compared with the general population of 11-year-olds, while the rates among children of this age with epilepsy or neurological disorder were four times those of the general population. This has again been confirmed recently in a study of children with epilepsy and with diabetes, where the children with chronic epilepsy were found to be significantly more disturbed than those with chronic diabetes (Hoare, 1984). The rates of disturbance among children with newly diagnosed epilepsy were also significantly higher than among children with newly diagnosed epilepsy were also significantly higher than among children with newly diagnosed diabetes and in the general population.

Young children with developmental disorders are also at increased risk of developing behaviour problems, and several studies have now reported an association between speech and language disorders and behaviour problems (Stevenson & Richman, 1978; Fundundis *et al.*, 1979; Bax *et al.*, 1983). At two years, 45% of the children in our study with behaviour problems also had speech and language delay or abnormality, compared with 18% of the children without problems (Table 9.7). Conversely Stevenson & Richman (1978) found that 58% of three-year-olds with language delay also had behaviour problems compared with 14% in the general population. In their follow-up of these children it was found that behaviour problems were more likely to persist until age eight in the children who had earlier speech problems. This association may reflect some underlying neurophysiological mechanism which is responsible for both the language delay and the behaviour disorder, or may in part be explained by the frustrations in communication experienced by a small child with language delay. It is

Table 9.7 Relationship between speech and language and behaviour problems.

| | Speech and language at 2 years | | |
	Normal	Possibly abnormal	Definitely abnormal
No problem ($n = 263$)	215 (82%)	43 (16%)	5 (2%)
Behaviour problem to parents ($n = 33$)	18 (55%)	7 (21%) $p < 0.001$	8 (24%)
No problem ($n = 264$)	219 (83%)	41 (16%)	4 (1%)
Behaviour problem to doctor — mild ($n = 21$)	12 (57%)	5 (24%)	4 (19%)
Behaviour problem to doctor — moderate ($n = 9$)	1 (11%)	2 (22%) $p < 0.001$	6 (67%)

probable that both mechanisms play a part, in many cases compounded by social disadvantages and stress.

One study in a general practice setting found that the two-year-old with speech delay was much more likely to come from a family where there was social or emotional deprivation (Starte, 1975). Of course, recurrent ear infections may result in hearing loss and contribute to both speech delay and behaviour problems. Whatever the mechanism, all aspects of the child's functioning must be assessed, including an assessment of the family environment, before planning any intervention. Only then can the role of speech therapy, play group, nursery or other help be decided on.

Later outcome of behaviour problems

It is now clear from follow-up studies that some behaviour problems do persist from preschool to school age, although many disappear with maturity. In our study less than a third of the three-year-olds with behaviour problems (on parent and doctor assessment) had problems at four and a half years, and it would obviously have been interesting to follow those who had stable problems at these ages to see whether they were in trouble in the primary school setting.

Coleman et al. (1977) have demonstrated poor correlations between early childhood symptomatology as perceived by parents when their children were aged three and four, and behaviour problems perceived by teachers at age five. However, Richman and colleagues (1982), who followed up three-year-olds with behaviour problems, found that between 40 and 55% of them had problems in school at the age of eight (on both parent and teacher ratings) compared with 20% in the control group. Factors associated with a higher likelihood of persistence of problems were male sex of the child, the presence of speech problems at age three, and maternal psychiatric disorder, particularly depression. The relationship of preschool speech and language disorder and later behaviour problems has also been reported in the Newcastle study by Fundundis et al. (1979). Both early speech and language problems and behaviour disorders are strongly associated with later learning difficulties in school, particularly related to reading. A further large follow-up study from New Zealand (McGee et al., 1984) found some stability between behaviour problems at age five and age seven, the most prevalent problem being antisocial behaviour, which was more common among boys. Twelve per cent of the sample of seven-year-olds were thought to have a significant behaviour problem, and stable behaviour problems were associated with specific reading retardation at age seven and with the use of professional services for help. As yet there is little evidence on the value of early intervention in preventing some of these later problems, and such evidence is urgently needed.

Effects of maternal depression and stress

More attention has been focused on maternal depression and stress than on the paternal psychiatric state, although clearly fathers are also important to the family. The fact that it is commonly the women who spend most of their time at home as the main caretakers of young children has justified this attention, although studies are now increasingly looking at the father's influence on the social and emotional development of their children (see Chapter 5).

Women with young children are particularly vulnerable to depression, and Brown and Harris (1978) have reported rates of depression of between 30 and 40%. This is not only the classically accepted 'postnatal' depression, but commonly depression occurring in the second or third years after the birth of a child, which may be prolonged or recurring. The nature of depressive symptoms makes it highly likely that child-rearing abilities will be affected, as has been shown in studies that have attempted to look at this. Maternal psychiatric state has been shown to relate both to concurrent child behaviour problems and to the likelihood of behaviour problems persisting (Richman *et al.*, 1982). Another recent longitudinal study in London has also found relationships between child behaviour and maternal and family stresses, and has particularly related maternal depression to later occurring child problems (Ghodsian *et al.*, 1984). As mentioned in Chapter 5 poor quality housing and financial anxieties arising from poverty contribute to both depression and difficulties with child-rearing.

Depression among mothers of preschool children was found to be common in our study (Moss & Plewis, 1977), with close correlations being found in this as in other studies between maternal stress and concurrent child behaviour problems, although our data did not allow us to examine this relationship longitudinally. Factors which seem to be 'protective' against depression are having a supportive partner at home, and the mother going out to work at least some of the time. Middle-class women are less at risk of depression than working-class women, probably because they are likely to have both more support systems and fewer adverse factors such as poor housing conditions and inadequate income to cope with. It follows that health care professionals should be alert to the presenting symptoms of depression in mothers of young children. Very often there is a strong element of anxiety in the presentation, as well as classic symptoms of poor appetite, sleep disturbance, early morning waking and lack of self-esteem.

Assessment and management

When a child presents with what predominantly appears to be a behaviour problem, a systematic approach is required just as for a child with a physical symptom such as cough. A careful history should be taken and the child examined fully, including a check on developmental status.

History-taking

Eliciting a full history may take some time, but is essential in understanding the problem, and involves listening carefully to what the parent says and enquiring specifically about family and environmental factors which influence the child. With babies and young children the health visitor may often offer helpful insights, and in most cases will have visited the family several times at home. Some parents may seek reassurance or help early on, while others appear to tolerate difficult behaviour for some time before consulting anyone, and then it is useful to ask what prompted them to come to see you at this particular juncture. The health and development of the child should be asked about, as there is often an association between recurrent mild illness and behaviour problems, and also with developmental deviation, particularly speech and language delay.

A detailed history of the presenting behaviour problem should include how long the parent has been concerned, how often the behaviour occurs (every day or night, several times a day, only at weekends, etc.), where the behaviour occurs, what else is going on at the time (mother trying to cook lunch, feeding another baby, visitors to the home, etc.) and so on. It is helpful to go through a diary of the child's typical day, as this will help to clarify periods when the child is happy and not presenting problems. Sometimes parents have become so focused on the child's unacceptable or difficult behaviour that they forget about the good times of day and this may need to be pointed out to them. It is important to know who else is in the family and whether there are worries about other children, or perhaps about a husband recently made redundant, or an ill grandparent.

Some sort of assessment of the mother must be made, particularly whether or not she is depressed. Hence a full personal and psychosocial history is needed if the problem is to be adequately understood and helped. Sometimes it is not appropriate to gather all the information at once and the story may unravel over several visits, but this is usually less satisfactory and takes a longer time.

On the basis of the history the seriousness of the problem is assessed, including how far the child's social and emotional life is affected and to what extent family life is disrupted by focusing on this child's behaviour. Many problems can be successfully helped or alleviated in a primary care setting, but for some specialist help is needed, and indications for this will be discussed later in this chapter. In any event the child should be examined, including looking in the ears with an auriscope — in a surprising number of children 'glue ear' contributes to the symptoms. The child's development should also be assessed. With most behaviour disturbances, and particularly where the presenting problem appears to be essentially one of management, it is helpful to see both parents together, and this may require a specific appointment. Sometimes the difficulty stems from the fact that the parents cannot agree on how to respond to the child; perhaps one likes to be lenient and the other is more disciplinarian, resulting in inconsistent handling and a somewhat confused child as well as tension between the parents. Many times it is the mother who is the main caretaker, and she may lack the support of her partner on certain issues. Joint interviews can help air these issues, and clearly there is more likelihood of successful management when both parents agree on an approach.

The early weeks

Difficulties in the first few weeks of a baby's life are common and perhaps should not be viewed as behaviour problems. Some of the difficulties have already been discussed, but feeding problems, colic, excess crying and difficulty in establishing a routine can be worrying to a parent, particularly when this is the first baby. Even more worrying are disturbances of mother—infant attachment, with rejecting be-haviour, and crisis management is then needed, with intensive skilled support involving social or psychiatric services as well as health visitor and doctor. Experienced health visitors are extremely skilled at assessing the mother—infant dyad, and where they express concern about the couple this must be taken seriously.

Management difficulties in the early weeks are more likely where there has been a difficult pregnancy, a premature delivery or other adverse perinatal factors. A baby may recover from a neonatal illness remarkably quickly, but anxiety generated by the illness may persist for many weeks. Where the father of the baby is not supportive, unsurprisingly there are likely to be more difficulties early on, with sleeping and feeding patterns being more erratic and the mother less confident in her handling of the baby.

Colic

Colic is a self-limiting condition occurring in a large proportion of normal healthy babies, usually improving or disappearing between three and four months of age. It manifests as paroxysmal screaming attacks in which a baby draws up her legs, clenches her fists and cannot be soothed by cuddling or feeding. Symptoms may occur after any or all feeds but are more common in the evenings, and many parents describe their babies as crying and being inconsolable for several hours each evening. Some studies have shown that colic is somewhat more common in breast-fed babies and a French study implicated parental smoking as a contributory factor. It has been suggested that eliminating cow's milk and milk products from the mother's diet helps some severely affected breast-fed babies, although another study showed that excluding cow's milk from maternal diets had no effect on the incidence of colic.

Management of the condition includes sympathetic support for the parents, with reassurance that the baby is healthy, and information on the self-limiting nature of colic. Parents should be advised about handling the baby, who will often be most comfortable being rocked on either a knee or a shoulder. Maintaining body contact by carrying the baby in a sling is often helpful and many mothers find this both comfortable and convenient since they can perform other tasks while carrying the baby. Increasing the amount of time a baby is carried has been demonstrated to reduce the amount of crying in a nice study from Boston (Hunziker & Barr, 1986). It is not usually helpful to tell a mother that her tenseness is contributing to her baby's symptoms. Of course babies react to their caregiver's tensions, but helping the baby's symptoms will do a lot to reduce anxiety and restore parental confidence. Dicyclomine (Merbentyl) should not be given to babies under six months old, in view of recent reports of apnoea, cyanosis and even death attributed to its use in young babies (see also Chapter 6).

Crying for other causes

Babies may cry for a large number of reasons, the commonest being hunger, discomfort, boredom, lack of contact, drop in temperature (as with a cold wet nappy), pain and tiredness. Older babies may also cry from anxiety, insecurity or frustration. It takes a little time for parents to discern the differences in cry of their baby which will often give them a clue as to the cause.

Some babies cry a lot more than others for no apparent cause and this is clearly distressing for both baby and parent. Medical advice is often sought to rule out physical illness and of course otitis media or more severe illness in a small baby may present this way. Parents may need a lot of reassurance, and to be told positively that the baby should be picked up and comforted when she cries — the myth of 'spoiling' a baby still hangs on. A home visit from a health visitor is indicated when a baby seems to be crying excessively and it is important to assess the parents' capacity to cope in this situation. Single parents are particularly vulnerable as there is no one to hand the baby to and share the caring, and this can generate extreme tension. It may be necessary to monitor the situation closely over days or weeks, offering a lot of support, and always remembering that a crying baby can be a powerful trigger for child abuse in an already fraught household. Some districts run a 24-hour 'crying baby' on-call service, with health visitors prepared to visit as an emergency: even the knowledge that there is someone on the end of a phone prepared to help and take the situation seriously can often diffuse the tensions.

Feeding difficulties

Feeding difficulties in the first few weeks are usually due to inexperience and lack of confidence or poor feeding techniques, and will be helped by a skilled and supportive health visitor. Management of early feeding and organic causes of poor feeding are discussed in Chapter 6.

When a mother or father brings an older baby with a feeding problem, as well as taking a history and examining the baby it is helpful to see the baby feed, and if bottle-fed to check the flow of milk from the teat. It is surprising how often a baby's difficulty or discontent is due to too small or too large a hole in the teat. A common anxiety with breast-feeding mothers is that the baby is not getting enough milk, and regular checks on the baby's weight combined with reassurance and encouragement to feed on demand will help. The physiology of lactation should be explained and it should not be assumed that the midwife will have already done this. Many mothers having difficulty with breast-feeding will be putting the baby to the breast at infrequent intervals, and may then become discouraged and offer a bottle between breast feeds, which of course makes the situation worse. Other aspects to consider are rest and diet — it may need a professional to 'prescribe' rest to a mother who is attempting to keep up her standards of tidiness and cooking as well as feed her baby, a situation common in our society where some fathers still opt out of sharing the responsibilities.

Babies are quick to pick up on their parents' feelings, and it is not unusual for a baby of a depressed mother to become withdrawn and refuse feeds or take only small amounts. While health care workers may recognize this in a toddler of 18 months or so, they may be more sceptical when the baby is only three or four months old. Measures which support the mother and help to alleviate her depression should also help the feeding problem although it may be a slow process. Obviously the weight of the baby will need careful monitoring. Anxiety is a potent cause of feeding problems and the baby may also be somewhat irritable and cry a lot, which in turn will discourage contented feeding. Since the cause of the anxiety may well be related to feelings of insecurity in the role of mother, the baby's feeding behaviour can set up a vicious circle of events which can be difficult to break. Counselling and support groups of other mothers with children who have perhaps experienced similar difficulties can be helpful in both these situations. Early intervention of this sort may prevent feeding difficulties persisting as the child gets older.

Solids are usually introduced from around the age of four or five months, and if introduced very gradually do not usually give rise to difficulties. Some babies, however, seem determined to feed themselves even as early as seven months and frequently by nine months. This can mean refusal to feed from a spoon, and after hours of loving preparation the parent concerned may justifiably feel resentful, or sometimes angry. Tensions can build up which exacerbate the problem, and one should afford parents the opportunity to discuss their feelings in this situation. Sometimes it is helpful for the father to feed the baby for some meals if he is not already doing so, and allowing the baby to finger-feed rather than be spoon-fed for a period may get over the difficulty. Some parents with high standards of cleanliness and tidiness find the stage of messy finger-feeding very hard to cope with. They may want to persist with feeding a child who is trying to be independent, because they cannot tolerate the mess. A discussion of the child's developing skills and need to explore is helpful, as well as practical tips like putting a plastic table cloth or newspapers on the floor under the high chair. It is important to avoid conflict at meal-times, which should be happy sociable occasions, and babies should never be force-fed.

Difficulties of this sort are more common when solids are introduced late — after around nine months — and where late weaning is the cultural norm as in many Asian families, and can be a real worry when the child's weight begins to drop on the percentile chart due to insufficient breast milk and the refusal of solids.

Food fads are increasingly common from around the age of two, but are often short-lived. Most children go through a stage of being faddy and parents may find this worrying and perplexing, particularly where the child will only eat one or two favourite foods. As with other feeding problems, it is helpful to reduce the anxieties and tensions that may build up around meal-times by discussion of the problem, and reassurance that the child's diet is adequate. A look at the percentile chart should indicate that weight gain is satisfactory and this in itself is usually reassuring. The child should not be made to eat food that is currently disliked — and, within reason, the child's likes and dislikes should be respected. They will often change dramatically from one month to the next, and even from one situation to another. A food refused at home may be eaten in a friend's house, and some parents take this very personally and feel 'got at'.

It is sensible to put only small amounts of food on the child's plate at meal-times, including one item which is liked, and remove whatever is left at the end of the meal. The presentation of food can be quite important, and a plate piled high can be very discouraging to a child with a small appetite. Avoidance of snacks and sweet drinks or milk between meals should help to increase appetite at meal-times. Interestingly, it has been shown that, if children are given a free choice and allowed to select their own diet, they will choose a balanced diet, and dietary deficiencies due to faddiness do not occur, except in extremely disturbed situations.

Temper tantrums

These are extremely common from about 18 months on, although some babies do start them as early as one year. Most parents cope well with tantrums, accept them as part of normal child development, and handle them appropriately. When tantrums are distressing or occurring very frequently, then professional advice may be useful, firstly in trying to understand the cause and secondly for help in management. The child may be unwell, or have a developmental problem such as speech delay and this will become apparent from history and examination.

The history should focus in some detail on the tantrums — when they occur, what happens, who responds and how, and what happens when the tantrum is over. This approach — looking at the antecedents and consequences of a behaviour — will usually give a clue as to management. Many tantrums occur only in certain circumstances, and can perhaps be avoided by diversion tactics. Others are responded to inappropriately — by anger or by offering rewards such as sweets or bribes. Often the subject that provoked the tantrum — a packet of Smarties in the supermarket — will be used as 'reward' to stop the tantrum, thus reinforcing the undesired behaviour. Once this is pointed out, parents can be helped to think of a more appropriate way of responding. Parents may want reassurance that ignoring a tantrum is the correct thing to do, and are often anxious that children may hurt themselves with kicking and head-banging, or be 'psychologically damaged' by being ignored. Being locked in a room is obviously punitive and inappropriate — but being calmly taken to a quiet place to cool off, with reassurance that the parent will come back as soon as the child is quiet, is a sensible approach. It is helpful later in the day, once the child is calm and happy, to discuss what provoked the tantrum — this both reassures the child that she or he is still loved and accepted despite their previous behaviour, and this may help to verbalize some of his or her frustrations.

Sleep problems

As we have said earlier in this chapter, sleep problems are one of the commonest causes of parental anxiety in the first two years of life, and disturbed nights may impose a continuing strain on many parents. This may result in irritability and exhaustion as well as feelings of helplessness and an inability to cope with relatively minor daytime crises.

In some families difficulty in sleeping can be a response to more generalized stress, and management may need to be directed towards alleviating the wider problems. In cases where there are no other significant factors, management can be directed solely towards the disorder. Regardless of aetiology, parents very often want help in alleviating the immediate burden of broken nights and disturbed evenings. They may also be feeling guilty or anxious about their current management, either believing it is 'wrong' to have the child in bed with them, or perhaps feeling guilty that they would rather have evenings to themselves. They may think that being firm about bedtime will make the child feel rejected, and then will need reassurance that setting limits is in the child's interest and does not imply lack of love and affection. Some parents may, for a variety of reasons, be especially

attentive to the child at night and unwittingly reinforce waking behaviour. Two situations in which this commonly occurs are when the
child is the long-awaited precious baby of older parents, and when the
mother is working during the day and perhaps feeling somewhat
guilty about this, over-compensating with attention in the evenings
and at night. Hence, a sympathetic discussion of how parents feel
about their own behaviour is as crucial to management as taking a
history of the problem itself.

THE HISTORY

A full developmental and medical history should be taken, as well as
family and social history to assess whether there may be any factors
here contributing to the problem. It is important too to know about
the physical environment of the child, including sleeping arrangements,
play space, worries about neighbours hearing any noise and other
such environmental factors. A detailed 'diary' of the child's day should
help demonstrate which are the most difficult times of day and also
highlight the periods when the parents are enjoying the child. If there
are two parents, ascertain who deals with any difficult behaviour —
for example, getting out of bed and coming into the living-room after
being put to bed — and whether both parents have the same approach
to dealing with it. Often one parent will want to put the child back to
bed, while the other is saying 'let her fall asleep on the sofa', in which
case the child will be getting confused messages as to what is expected
of her.

Following a detailed history and discussion, the problem and how
the parents feel about it should be fairly clear. It is then usually helpful
to talk about the variations in children's sleep patterns and some of
the possible reasons contributing to the current problems, before
discussing possibilities of changing the behaviour, if that is what the
parents want. It is important neither to give dogmatic views as to how
children should behave at night nor to tell parents how they should
handle any particular problem. The approach should rather be to share
current knowledge with the parents and to agree an approach with
them which they are comfortable with, and which acknowledges their
needs as well as those of the child. Wherever possible, and certainly
over the age of two, the child should be involved in discussions about
management. Before planning with the parents any change in management, one should be quite clear that they do want help with the
problem. Some parents cope well with what may seem like intolerable

sleeping patterns from their child, and clearly intervention should not be suggested in this situation; indeed, it would be quite undermining to do so.

DIFFERENT MANAGEMENT APPROACHES

Apart from minor adjustments to the child's routine, such as cutting down daytime sleep, giving more food in the evening, having a bedtime routine and so on, the three main approaches to sleep problems have been prescribing drugs, taking the child into the parents' bed, and behavioural management techniques.

Drugs, such as antihistamines (promethazine, trimeprazine) and hypnotics (Trichloral, chloral hydrate) should, in our view, only be used rarely and with discretion. They are not usually helpful where there is a persistent night-waking problem, habituation rapidly occurs, they do not provide a long-term solution, and they are potentially open to abuse. Although these medications may provide temporary improvement, there is usually no lasting benefit (Richman, 1985). Not uncommonly idiosyncratic responses can occur, particularly to promethazine, with the child becoming over-excited instead of sleepy. They are occasionally useful when night-waking has been recently triggered by an illness, such as otitis media or a hospital admission. If used, an appropriate weight-related dose should be used for a few successive nights, and then the drug should be tailed off fairly quickly.

Taking the child into the parents' bed often provides immediate relief from a wakeful night. Many parents try this, and where parents and child sleep contentedly together it is a good solution. It is undoubtedly very reassuring for the child, and is the norm in very many cultures. Frequently, however, there are parents who do not sleep well with their child in their bed, and who resent the child's presence there. What may be tolerated for a few nights or weeks is no longer tolerated after a couple of months, and it may then be difficult to settle the child back to sleeping in her own bed. Hence, what is a good solution for one family may not be appropriate for another family.

Behavioural management techniques are usually the treatment of choice for sleep problems, and have been demonstrated to be effective (Richman *et al.*, 1985). Some training in the use of these techniques is required and clinical psychologists are increasingly involved in training health visitors and primary care doctors in using them. Initially (after a full history as described earlier) parents are asked to keep a diary or chart of the child's sleep pattern and their own response to it over a one- to two-week period. This can then be used as a basis for discussion, and will usually suggest the changes to be made. Often it will be found that the parents are responding inappropriately to the child, perhaps by giving quantities of drinks or by playing and talking to the child for long periods in the night and thus reinforcing the waking pattern. The diary will also reveal if the response to the child is inconsistent from one occasion to the next, so that the child never learns what is expected of her.

Alterations in management can be discussed with the parents and decisions jointly made as to how to proceed. Sometimes small changes are suggested at first, such as the parent sitting with the child instead of lying on the bed, and then gradually withdrawing from the room. The frequent drinks of orange may be replaced by water; the child may be taken back to her own bed each time she wakes instead of being allowed to fall asleep in the parents' bed, and so on. What is important is the consistency of response and a firm approach to the problem.

With an older child a system of rewards such as a chart with stars or stickers for staying in their own bed can be helpful. Initially parents may need a lot of help and support to maintain their approach, and weekly (or even more frequent) visits may be needed. Sometimes telephone contact is adequate to support the programme, with less frequent appointments. A time limit is normally set, with perhaps four or six sessions offered, and this is normally enough to produce definite improvements.

This behavioural management approach is very effective in the majority of cases but some selection is needed. A child with widespread emotional or behavioural difficulties would not be appropriately helped by such an approach in isolation. Where there are additional problems such as parental depression or marked anxiety, or adverse social circumstances, these may prevent parents from carrying out a consistent programme. To embark on such a treatment in these circumstances may be inviting failure, which can further undermine a family's self-esteem.

There are several publications, useful to both parents and professionals, on the topic of sleep disturbance, and it is sometimes helpful to direct a parent to one of these (e.g. Douglas & Richman, 1984).

Referral to a child psychiatrist

The decision to refer to a child psychiatrist, and when to refer, will obviously reflect both the seriousness of the presenting problem and the experience and resources of the referring doctor (Graham, 1984). Many of the less serious behaviour problems can be successfully managed in a primary care setting, where the doctors concerned have been appropriately trained and are prepared to afford the necessary time. Management usually requires a lot more time than managing a physical disorder such as otitis media, both for the initial assessment and for follow-up. When time and skills are not available, referral elsewhere for help will be indicated, as it will also be when the child's symptoms are serious and long-standing, or when gross family pathology is evident. When there are serious anxieties about the parent–child relationship and a possible risk of rejection or child abuse, skilled social work help will be needed, and early referral to a child psychiatry unit may be indicated.

Choice of referral will obviously depend on the available local resources but ideally referral should be to a psychiatrist who offers a variety of approaches (rather than, say, a purely analytic approach) and who can offer an early appointment once the decision to refer has been made. In some cases it may be more appropriate to refer direct to a psychologist or social worker, and the former may be the most appropriate for a child with perhaps a marked sleep disturbance where a behavioural approach is thought to be indicated.

The decision as to whether referral is indicated may not always be made until a child and family have been seen several times; where it is clear that no improvement is occurring and the problem is evidently more complex than at first thought, it may then be appropriate to discuss with the family referral for more specialized help.

A crucial consideration is whether the parents are prepared to receive psychiatric help, as there is a high rate of failed appointments with psychiatric referrals. To some extent this reflects the skill of the referrer in explaining the service on offer, as there are many parents to whom referral to a psychiatrist carries an implication of madness, or failure in their role as parents. If pressurized to accept a referral, there is a strong likelihood of failed appointments. Where the child concerned is attending a nursery it is sometimes helpful for the initial interview to take place at the nursery, which is familiar territory to both parent and child, and many child psychiatry units now offer this flexible approach.

Child abuse

Incidence

The spectrum of child abuse ranges from minor bruising and neglect, including emotional neglect, to repeated severe injury, sometimes resulting in death. The incidence of all forms of abuse is difficult to assess since some episodes go undetected and others may only be regarded as suspicious. Recent studies (Addy, 1985) suggest that the incidence of severe abuse is 1 in 1000 children under five with a death rate of 1 in 10 000. Figures from the NSPCC's child abuse register have shown steady increases in the past five years, with between 150 and 200 children dying following abuse and neglect each year in England and Wales.

Diagnosis

Children who die as a result of non-accidental injury nearly always have a history of earlier injuries. Awareness of the pattern of injuries which suggest child abuse may bring about earlier detection and prevention of serious consequences. Very minor injuries may precede severe abuse and may be noticed by an observant doctor or health visitor. Ounsted (1975) has described 'open warnings' when mothers demonstrate a minor injury to the doctor, the significance of which may only be realized retrospectively if further injuries occur. Kempe (1971) suggested that mothers tend to bring their children to the doctor with a variety of minor complaints before an episode of injury.

The behaviour of the parents and child at home and in the surgery may raise concern about possible abuse. The health visitor may be the first person to sense that the relationship between parents and child is not progressing happily. This concern should always be taken seriously and the situation closely monitored. Lack of eye contact, failure to respond affectionately to the child's demands and negative or critical feelings towards the child are cause for concern. The child may appear frightened, withdrawn and passive, exhibiting 'frozen watchfulness'. In this characteristic behaviour the child keeps still and gazes intently at adults but maintains a fixed expression as if wary of provoking any response. On the other hand, a proportion of children may demonstrate highly active, aggressive behaviour which provokes hostile reactions in the parents.

Physical neglect, failure to thrive and developmental delay are frequently associated with child abuse and reflect a basic disturbance in the parent—child relationship, resulting in inadequate nurturing (see section on failure to thrive, pp. 299—306). Emotional neglect is less easily substantiated than physical abuse but may have equally damaging long-term effects. Non-accidental injury should be suspected if parents give an unrealistic or inconsistent account of how an injury has arisen. Delay in seeking medical attention is a suspicious factor as is repeated injury or an unusual reaction to the child's injury.

If non-accidental injury is a possibility, opportunity should be sought to examine the child unclothed. The practice of undressing all babies for weighing at clinics allows examination without conveying suspicion to the mother. Any bruising in an infant is unusual. Bruising of the head and neck and lumbar region is common in abused children and bruising on the face and ears is particularly suspicious. Fingertip marks may be visible on the trunk where a child has been held tightly and shaken. A ring of bruises indicating a bite mark is not uncommon.

Fractures may present as recent injuries or multiple fractures of different ages, or be detected on skeletal survey. Skull fractures are the most common bony injury and are typically wide and depressed. Other fracture sites include the ribs, humerus, radius, ulna, femur, tibia and fibula where the characteristic metaphyseal chip injury occurs. It is estimated that around a quarter of all fractures in children under two years are non-accidental and the proportion in children under one year is higher.

Intracranial haemorrhage, usually in the subdural region, may accompany skull fracture or arise without bony injury as a result of a blow or vigorous shaking. Retinal haemorrhages are characteristic (from shaking) and may result in visual impairment and squint. Burns from cigarettes cause small circular marks and may occasionally be confused with impetigo. Other characteristic burns or scalds are to the buttocks, legs or feet, from immersing them in hot water or holding the child against a hot object. Asphyxia, poisoning and drowning are encountered occasionally.

Careful history-taking and accurate charting of any injuries are essential in cases of possible abuse. Meadow (1982) has described a form of abuse, 'Munchausen syndrome by proxy', in which the mother fabricates illness in her child. For example a child may be reported fictitiously as having fits or abnormal bleeding. A mother may believe that her child is suffering from severe allergy and drastically restrict his diet. The syndrome may be suspected if a mother seems unconcerned about her child's illness, if she is the only witness to the symptoms or if there is evidence that she is interfering with the child, for example, causing persistent wound infection or bleeding.

Certain conditions may occasionally be mistaken for non-accidental injury, causing considerable distress to parents. For example Mongolian blue spot, bullous impetigo and erythema multiforme can be diagnostic pitfalls. Bruising below the knees is commonly seen in normal active children. Testing for bleeding disorder should usually be carried out when bruising presents but very seldom proves positive.

In all cases of child abuse the main concern must be the future safety of the child. Often this has to be ensured by taking legal action and reception into care. If non-accidental injury is suspected the doctor has to decide the most appropriate action to take to protect the child and should contact the local social services team. A case conference may follow to collect further information and plan future management. The conference will decide whether or not to place the child on the at-risk register and who to appoint as key worker. Although the family health visitor may be closely involved in monitoring a younger child, it is generally a social worker who is the key worker. Where definite or probable non-accidental injury is diagnosed removal into care or hospital is usually necessary to safeguard the child and allow further investigation of past and present injury. Admission to a paediatric ward is very often the most useful course of action, particularly for younger children. It is essential that the general practitioner, health visitor and any other professionals who know the child are consulted where there is any doubt. If it seems likely that the parents may remove the child prematurely back to a dangerous environment, a Place of Safety Order can be arranged.

Under Section 28(1) of the Children and Young Persons Act 1969 any person (usually a hospital or social services social worker) may apply for a Place of Safety Order to a magistrate at any time and any place. If the problem arises out of normal working hours the emergency duty social worker is available and a magistrate can be contacted at his or her home if necessary. Physically injured children may be placed in safety on one of three grounds:

1 'his or her proper development is being avoidably prevented or neglected',
2 'his or her health is being avoidably impaired or neglected', or
3 'he or she is being ill-treated'.

Siblings can also be covered by this order, which allows detention for up to 28 days. Unless an interim care order (for a further 28 days) is taken before the end of the period, the abused child and siblings cannot be detained after 28 days but must be returned to their parents.

Anxieties have been expressed that Place of Safety Orders are too easily obtainable, resulting in a tendency to play safe, causing undue separation of parents and children. Other fears are that taking legal action destroys parental trust, prejudicing future co-operation and effectiveness of therapy. Lynch's study (1975) found that, on the contrary, many parents, though initially exhibiting anger, subsequently felt relief that the situation had been recognized and decisive action taken. Initial hostility about an order was seen as a healthier sign than complete indifference to the whereabouts and welfare of the child.

Generally about a third of abused children are the subject of Place of Safety Orders and over half of these are involved in further care proceedings.

Care proceedings in cases of child abuse are brought before the juvenile court under Section 1 of the Children and Young Persons Act 1969. The choice usually lies between a Care Order and a Supervision Order. A Care Order places the child in the care of the local authority until the age of 18 unless the court decides to discharge the order earlier. Regular reviews are required. The authority decides whether the child remains in a children's home or a foster home or is allowed to return to the parental home 'on trial'. Sometimes the child will be placed with another close relative such as a grandparent. When a Supervision Order is granted the child normally stays at home under the supervision of the local authority for up to three years. However, the parents are not legally obliged to allow the supervisor into the house to see the child and in practice regular surveillance is better achieved with a Care Order. However, it is the court which makes this decision.

Children can also be received into voluntary care at the request of their parents under Section 1 of the Children's Act 1948. Parents can remove their children at any time and if this action causes concern about their safety a Place of Safety Order followed by a Care Order is necessary.

The background of abused children

Groups of parents with an increased potential for abuse can be broadly defined but the problems arising between individual parents and children are generated by interaction of personal characteristics. It is well recognized that frequently only one child in a family may suffer from non-accidental injury or emotional deprivation. Parents may admit that this particular child seems different, difficult and unrewarding. Frequently the abusing parent is not the child's natural parent. The parents are more likely to be young, to have had an unhappy childhood, and to have less social support than non-abusing parents (Baldwin & Oliver, 1975). Biological factors such as illness and certain patterns of behaviour may provoke unreasonable parental responses. Social and economic factors may influence parents' capacity to be adaptable so that they cannot respond to their child's varying needs in an appropriate way. Poor mental and physical health have been shown to be important factors in parents of abused children. In the Park Hospital study (Lynch, 1975) of severely abused children, over half the mothers had suffered from psychiatric or emotional ill health since the birth of the abused child, often with a history of suicidal gestures. Fewer of the fathers had a history of psychiatric illness but a sizeable group had disturbed personalities.

Nearly a third of mothers suffered from physical health problems, for example, gynaecological complaints. Psychosomatic symptoms such as migraine, backache and fainting attacks were frequent. It is likely that mothers who are depressed or unwell are less likely to cope with difficult behaviour in a child.

Abnormal pregnancy, delivery and neonatal period have all been associated with later child abuse. In one study as many as 40% of abused children were separated from their mother after birth in the special-care baby unit (SCBU) for two days or more. It has been suggested that, if the mother and child are prevented from developing a close bond in the early days, there is a greater risk of the relationship failing to flourish later on. However, it must be pointed out that babies who are in an SCBU are more liable to suffer from health and developmental difficulties which may affect their parents' ability to cope with them. With greater awareness by staff of SCBUs of the need for parents to be closely involved in the care of their sick or low-birthweight infants, problems originating from this period are diminishing.

Both serious and recurrent minor illnesses and congenital abnormalities are reported more commonly in abused children. Preterm birth, neonatal illness, pneumonia, bronchitis, pyloric stenosis, cleft palate and harelip, cerebellar ataxia, and convulsions are amongst conditions reported. Persistent irritating complaints, such as eczema, colic and vomiting, are more frequent in abused children than in their siblings. Frequent night-waking is another factor which can be a trigger to child abuse. It is not surprising that certain parents whose backgrounds, personalities and social circumstances increase their potential for child abuse find it extremely difficult to cope with an infant who is small or unwell or has a congenital abnormality. Furthermore, a handicapping condition such as cerebral palsy not only may be a precursor of child abuse but may arise as a consequence of injury. Parents of handicapped or chronically sick children need extra support and some relief from the relentless demands which fall upon them.

Child sexual abuse

Prevalence

Child sexual abuse is becoming increasingly recognized as a widespread and disturbing problem. Since a large proportion of cases occur within families and are veiled in secrecy, accurate estimates of prevalence are difficult to obtain; many cases do not come to light until several years after the offence has occurred. Research on community samples in the USA have indicated that 19% of women and 9% of men experienced sexual abuse as children, which appeared to have harmful long-term effects on their sexual relationships. Another study from the USA suggests an even higher incidence, 38%, of women who suffered sexual abuse before the age of 18 years (Russell, 1983).

The number of cases coming to professional notice in the UK is considerably less, but is increasing yearly as health professionals and others have become more aware of the issue and more prepared to intervene. Undoubtedly, though, many cases remain unreported and true incidence figures are not available.

In one district in the UK, in a two-year period 337 cases were diagnosed as having been sexually abused (out of 608 referrals where this was thought to be a possibility). Just over two-thirds of cases were girls; 38% were under the age of five at diagnosis, with the mean age being eight years (Hobbs & Wynne, 1987). This is a considerably younger age of presentation than in previous studies but is confirmed by other people's recent experience. As awareness increases and child care staff in places like day nurseries receive training in this field, it is likely that cases will be diagnosed at younger ages than previously. Alongside this, many children will be referred with the suspicion of sexual abuse where it turns out to be a false alarm. A careful balance is needed, as investigation can in itself be harmful to children and families, and many legal and ethical issues have yet to be resolved. Where the allegation comes from the child or parent, 70 to 80% of cases will be found to be true abuse, whereas in most recent experience only 50% of all investigated cases were positive. It is postulated that with a higher index of suspicion there will be a rise not only in wrongly investigated cases, but also in missed cases (Zeitlin, 1987).

Perpetrators

Most studies reveal that 50–60% of perpetrators are related to the child, half of them being natural fathers. Stepfathers and mothers' boyfriends are also commonly found to be the perpetrators. Other family members implicated have been older siblings, grandparents, uncles and mothers. Very often the perpetrator is known to the child, and teenage baby-sitters are increasingly implicated. Strangers are responsible in less than a quarter of cases.

Definitions

Sexual abuse is not a consistent diagnostic entity, and most definitions have their limitations. A commonly used definition is as follows:

> Sexual abuse is defined as the involvement of dependent, developmentally immature children and adolescents in sexual activities that they do not fully comprehend, to which they are unable to give informed consent, or that violate the social taboos of family roles. (Kempe & Kempe, 1978.)

This is a broad and useful definition, covering aspects of sexual abuse from incest to fondling, and activities such as photography for pornographic purposes. There is wide variation in the nature, frequency and intrusiveness of the acts involved in sexual abuse, and variation too in both the psychological and physical trauma involved.

It is not always possible to predict the effect on the child of any particular act, but reports from the literature reveal an increasing number of both short-term and long-term harmful effects. These include the capacity to form later satisfactory sexual and marital relationships, effects on mental health and self-esteem, and effects on parenting ability. However, it is also clear that not all individuals suffer harmful sequelae from sexual abuse. Long-term adverse effects are particularly likely where there has been forceful, repeated or prolonged abuse or severe physical violation. It is also common after abuse by fathers or stepfathers.

As Zeitlin says:

> This is not to condone any form of sexual abuse or to suggest that the less harmful variants do not progress to more harmful if ignored. We must, however, give thought to the impact when proposing any intervention that might itself have long-term harmful effects. (Zeitlin, 1987.)

Presentation

Sexual abuse may present to the clinician acutely as trauma, or as obvious genital interference or infection but often the situation is chronic and frequently the problem masquerades as a variety of behavioural disturbances. The child may also be brought to a clinician following disclosure of abuse.

Clearly the presentation will vary according to circumstances and whether the situation is acute or chronic. Very often there is only a suspicion of abuse, and these children present the greatest difficulty in management.

Sexual abuse is presumed where the child is found to have a sexually transmitted disease, to be pregnant, to have anal or genital trauma, or to disclose the abuse. Children do not fantasize about specific sexual activities, and fictitious reporting by children is rare, although it has been reported in disturbed teenagers. The rule therefore should be always to believe the child's story.

The diagnosis should be suspected if a child presents with recurrent vaginal discharge or irritation, genital or anal inflammation, painful micturition or urinary tract infection, or pain on sitting or walking. However, vaginal soreness and discharge occur quite commonly in girls of all ages and only a small proportion of these children will have experienced sexual abuse. Whilst it is important to be alert to the possibility of abuse, over-zealous questioning and investigation can cause extreme distress with deleterious effects on the child and family as well as undermining the doctor's relationship with the family.

Enuresis, encopresis, abdominal pains and headaches can be psychosomatic symptoms of sexual abuse. They may be an expression of the stress, guilt and conflict experienced by the child or may result from pain inflicted during sexual experience.

Certain behavioural patterns may suggest that a child is the victim of abuse. In the preschool period the child may present because of inappropriate sexual behaviour such as excessive masturbation or genital play, perhaps with another child. Other suggestive behaviour changes may be excessive clinging or withdrawn behaviour, sleep or appetite disturbance, sudden mood changes or fearfulness.

However, there are often other underlying causes of such behavioural changes and caution is clearly needed to avoid over-interpretation of symptoms. Masturbation and genital play are common in preschool children, and it may be hard to decide where to draw the line between normal and disturbed behaviours.

In the school-age child similar behavioural changes may be suggestive; in addition school performance may fall off, or seductive behaviour may be noted. Truancy and withdrawal from friends may occur, and psychosomatic complaints may be present. Sexual abuse may drive a child to drastic actions such as running away from home and suicide attempts. This is more common in adolescence, where drug abuse, promiscuity or anorexia may also occur.

The history of abuse may be extremely difficult to obtain as the child is likely to feel guilty and afraid of divulging a secret about something he or she knows is wrong. Skilled interviewing is needed and should be carried out by someone who can relate well to children and who is trained and comfortable in this role. Flexibility of approach is needed and ways of communicating will vary with the child's age and developmental level. Play with anatomically correct dolls or drawings may reveal knowledge of sexual activity inappropriate for the age of the child and is one of the most successful ways of encouraging a younger child to talk about her experiences. Disclosure may only occur months or even years after the event.

A variety of abnormal patterns of family functioning are seen in cases of sexual abuse within the family. Often there are marital problems with a lack of a satisfying sexual relationship between the parents. One or other parent may be over-identified with the child. The mother may have ceased to show affection to her family and be unable to cope with running a household, often as a result of her own overwhelming problems such as depression or social isolation. In this situation the husband may turn to his children for affection. In other families the father may be authoritarian or conversely excessively weak. Alcoholism or drug addiction and unemployment resulting in the father spending a lot of time around the home may be factors leading to sexual abuse in the family.

The relationship between mother and daughter may be distant and the mother may suppress her suspicion or knowledge of an incestuous relationship between father and daughter. The father becomes dependent on the mother in case the abuse is reported resulting in punishment and family breakdown. Fear of family breakdown is a likely reason why so many cases of incest remain undisclosed.

Management

Suspicion of sexual abuse demands sensitive handling by trained, experienced professionals. The general practitioner, paediatrician or clinical medical officer may well be the first person to suspect possible abuse. In some cases it may be obvious that abuse has taken place and prompt action needs to be taken. More often, though, the problem requires cautious and thorough investigation before suspicion can be confirmed and formal action taken. Consultation between all professionals concerned with the family, including the health visitor, nursery or school teacher, social worker and paediatrician, is essential to substantiate the diagnosis.

Difficult ethical questions may be raised if the suspect is also the doctor's patient. However, protection of the child is the overriding concern and must be the major factor influencing the doctor's actions. Admission of the child to hospital may be appropriate to ensure the safety of the child and to allow investigations to begin. The social services department should be informed so that a case conference can be arranged and if necessary a Place of Safety Order obtained. Social services are obliged to inform the police of suspected or alleged abuse and specially trained police investigations should coexist with therapy which aims to alter family relationships and to help the victim come to terms with his or her experiences.

MEDICAL EXAMINATION

This should only be done if there are clear indications that it is likely to be helpful. Examination should include a complete assessment of the child's growth, health and development. This includes behavioural and emotional aspects, and care should be taken to note how the child reacts during examination. Medical evidence of abuse is not always present, particularly in chronic or past abuse, and specific forensic evidence is normally only useful if collected within 48 hours of the last contact.

Examination should be conducted with extreme care, and only by a trained examiner, and should be seen as part of the treatment process. It should never be necessary to examine a child on more than one occasion, and examination should never be experienced by the child as an assault. Thought must be given to where the child is seen. The practice of examining children at police stations is to be deplored, and many police surgeons now work closely with paediatricians and social workers and use designated treatment rooms in hospitals or clinics.

Details of the examination have been well described (Hobbs & Wynne, 1987) and the hazards of making assumptions based on physical signs alone have been highlighted by the Cleveland enquiry.

Outcome of child abuse

Sexual abuse

The extent of the long-term effects of child sexual abuse depends on its early recognition and treatment. Studies of adults who were abused as children identify a high risk of abnormal sexual behaviour, with promiscuity, drug and alcohol abuse being common. Another manifestation is coldness in sexual relationships, with a failure to form long-lasting sexual and emotional relationships. Low self-esteem and depression are frequent findings among adult women who suffered childhood abuse. It is, however, difficult to find control populations who were abused in childhood but have no later adverse effects, since much of the research has been amongst populations of women attending for psychiatric treatment.

There is some evidence from surveys of college students that a good outcome in adulthood is more likely where there has been good support during childhood and the child has not been blamed for the abuse. Whether or not a sympathetic and understanding partner is found in adulthood also clearly affects outcome.

Physical abuse

Follow-up studies of the abused child demonstrate a high level of neuro-developmental and psychological impairment. About half of seriously abused children are likely to be left with some degree of neurological disability, ranging from cerebral palsy, epilepsy, mental retardation and visual impairment to mild clumsiness and incoordination.

In Lynch and Roberts' study (1982) over half the abused children under five showed developmental delay, particularly in the area of language development. Oates *et al.* (1984) found that school-age children who had suffered abuse had lower IQs and had difficulties with language and reading.

The outlook for abused children's emotional development appears to be equally gloomy for they rapidly become disturbed and difficult individuals. They may show aggressive destructive behaviour or in contrast be withdrawn, depressed or uncommunicative. These deviant behaviour patterns result in inability to make relationships with their peers and to respond to help from adults and contribute to failure at school. The findings highlight the need for long-term child-centred intervention even after the 'abusing' situation has been corrected.

Intervention in terms of placement can markedly affect the child's prospects. A study in a deprived area of Liverpool (Hensey *et al.*, 1983) found that the children fared best when an early decision was made to sever contact with the parents and to place the child permanently with a substitute family. Factors associated with an unsatisfactory outcome included increasing age when taken into care, increasing time spent in care before returning to natural parents and several placements while in care. Children returned to their parents run an appreciable risk of further abuse and rehabilitation must involve intensive, long-term support and therapeutic intervention.

References

Addy, P. (1985) Talking points in child abuse. *British Medical Journal*, **290** (6464), 259–60.
Anders, T.F. & Weinstein, P. (1972) Sleep and its disorders in infants and children. *Pediatrics*, **50**, 312–24.
Bailey, V., Graham, P. & Boniface, D. (1978) How much child psychiatry does a general practitioner do? *Journal of the Royal College of General Practitioners*, **28**, 621–6.

Baldwin, J.A. & Oliver, J. (1975) Epidemiology and family characteristics of severely abused children. *British Journal of Preventative and Social Medicine*, **29**, 205–21.

Bax, M. & Whitmore, K. (1985) *District Handicap Team Report to the DHSS*. Community Paediatric Research Unit, St Mary's Hospital, 5a Netherhall Gardens, London NW3 (work supported by DHSS).

Bax, M., Hart, H. & Jenkins, S. (1983) The behaviour, development and health of the young child: implications for care. *British Medical Journal*, **286**, 1793–6.

Bernal, J. (1973) Night waking in infants in the first 14 months. *Developmental Medicine and Child Neurology*, **15**, 760–9.

Blurton Jones, J., Rossetti Ferreira, M.C., Farquar-Brown, M. & Macdonald, L. (1978) The association between perinatal factors and later night waking. *Developmental Medicine and Child Neurology*, **20**, 710–19.

Brown, G. & Harris, T. (1978) *Social Origins of Depression*. Tavistock Publications, London.

Carey, W.B. (1974) Night waking and temperament in infancy. *Journal of Pediatrics*, **84**, 756–8.

Chazan, M. & Jackson, S. (1971) Behaviour problems in the infant school. *Journal of Child Psychology and Psychiatry*, **12**, 191–210.

Coleman, J., Wolkind, S. & Ashley, L. (1977) Symptoms of behaviour disturbance and adjustment to school. *Journal of Child Psychology and Psychiatry*, **18**, 202–9.

Douglas, J. & Richman, N. (1984) *My Child Won't Sleep*. Penguin, London.

Dunn, J. & Kendrick, C. (1980) Studying temperament and parent–child interaction: comparison of interview and direct observation. *Developmental Medicine and Child Neurology*, **22**, 484–97.

Dunn, J., Kendrick, C. & MacNamee, R. (1981) The reaction of first born children to the birth of a sibling. *Journal of Child Psychology and Psychiatry*, **22**, 1–18.

Fundundis, T., Kolvin, I. & Garside, R. (eds) (1979) *Speech Retarded and Deaf Children: Their Psychological Development*. Academic Press, London.

Ghodsian, M., Zajisek, E. & Wolkind, S. (1984) A longitudinal study of maternal depression and child behaviour problems. *Journal of Child Psychology and Psychiatry*, **25** (1), 91–109.

Goodenough, F.C. (1931) *Anger in Young Children*. University of Minnesota Press, Minneapolis.

Graham, P. (1984) Paediatric referral to a child psychiatrist. *Archives of Disease in Childhood*, **59**, 1103–5.

Graham, P. & Jenkins, S. (1985) Training of paediatricians for psychosocial aspects of their work. *Archives of Disease in Childhood*, **60** (8), 777–80.

Hensey, O.J., Williams, J.K. & Rosenbloom, L. (1983) Intervention in child abuse: experience in Liverpool. *Developmental Medicine and Child Neurology*, **25** (5), 606–11.

Hoare, P. (1984) Does illness foster dependency? A study of epileptic and diabetic children. *Developmental Medicine and Child Neurology*, **26** (1), 20–4.

Hobbs, C.J. & Wynne, J.M. (1987) Child sexual abuse — an increasing rate of diagnosis. *Lancet*, 837–41.

Hunziker, U.A. & Barr, R.G. (1986) Increased carrying reduces infant crying: a randomized control trial. *Pediatrics*, **77** (5), 641–8.

Jenkins, S., Bax, M. & Hart, H. (1980) Behaviour problems in preschool children. *Journal of Child Psychology and Psychiatry*, **21**, 5–17.

Jenkins, S., Owen, C., Bax, M. & Hart, H. (1984) Continuities of common behaviour problems in pre-school children. *Journal of Child Psychology and Psychiatry*, **25**, 75–89.

Kempe, C.H. (1971) Paediatric implications of the battered child syndrome, *Archives of Disease in Childhood*, **46**, 28–37.

Kolvin, I., MacKeith, R.C.O. & Meadow, S.R. (1973) *Bladder Control and Enuresis*. Clinics in Developmental Medicine, Nos. 48/49, Spastics International Medical Publications and Heinemann, London.

Lynch, M. (1975) Ill health and child abuse. *Lancet*, 16 August, 317–19.

Lynch, M. & Roberts, J. (1982). *Consequences of Child Abuse*. Academic Press, London.

McGee, R., Silva, P.A. & Williams, S. (1984) Behaviour problems in a population of seven year old children: prevalence, stability and types of disorder. *Journal of Child Psychology and Psychiatry*, **25** (2), 251–9.

Martin, J. (1978) *Infant Feeding 1975: Practice and Attitudes in England and Wales*. HMSO, London.

Meadow, R. (1982) Munchausen syndrome by proxy. *Archives of Disease in Childhood*, **57**, 92–8.

Moss, P. & Plewis, I. (1977) Mental distress in mothers of pre-school children in Inner London. *Psychological Medicine*, **7**, 641–52.

Oates, K., Peacock, A. & Forrest, D. (1984) The development of abused children. *Developmental Medicine and Child Neurology*, **26**, 649–59.

Ounsted, C. (1975) Gaze aversion and child abuse. *World Medicine*, **10**, 17–27.

Ounsted, M.D. & Simons, C.D. (1978) The first born child: toddler problems. *Developmental Medicine and Child Neurology*, **20**, 710–19.

Perkins, T.S. & Linke, S.B. (1984) Management of behavioural disorders: a joint approach by parents, health visitors and a psychologist. *Health Visitor*, **57**, 108–9.

Richman, N. (1985) A double-blind drug trial of treatment in young children with waking problems. *Journal of Child Psychology and Psychiatry*, **26**, 591–8.

Richman, N., Stevenson, J. & Graham, P. (1975) Prevalence of behaviour problems in three year old children: an epidemiological study in a London borough. *Journal of Child Psychology and Psychiatry*, **16**, 277–87.

Richman, N., Stevenson, J. & Graham, P. (1982) *Pre-school to School: a Behavioural Study*. Academic Press, London.

Richman, N., Douglas, J., Hunt, H., Lansdown, R. & Levere, R. (1985) Behavioural methods in the treatment of sleep disorders — a pilot study. *Journal of Child Psychology and Psychiatry*, **26**, 581–90.

Russell, D.E.H. (1983) The incidence and prevalence of intrafamilial and extrafamilial sexual abuse of female children. *Child Abuse and Neglect*, **7**, 147–54.

Rutter, M., Tizard, J. & Whitmore, K. (1970) *Education, Health and Behaviour*. Longman, London.

Starte, G.D. (1975) The poor-communicating two year old and his family. *Journal of the Royal College of General Practitioners*, **25**, 880–7.

Stevenson, J. & Richman, N. (1978) Behaviour, language and development in three year old children. *Journal of Autism and Childhood Schizophrenia*, **8**, 299–313.

Zeitlin, H. (1987) Investigation of the sexually abused child. *Lancet*, 842–5.

10 Use of Services

I N THIS CHAPTER we review health service needs in preschool children, describe preschool social and education provision with which all health professionals need to be familiar and discuss how health care should interrelate with this provision.

Parents of young children need easy access to sources of advice, expertise and reassurance on a variety of topics related to child care, as well as sympathetic medical care. The provision of preventive care, including immunization and child health surveillance, is only one part of this service and we need to recognize that reassurance and support in the difficult business of child-rearing are as valuable to a parent as, for instance, routine developmental checks — indeed more so, since they are asked for and sought in time of need. In planning services for preschool children, there is a constant need to balance what health professionals may perceive as being important for children with what parents require from the service. Increasingly, at a local level, parents are coming into partnership with professionals in planning and developing the services for children and this is a welcome development, although in most areas health boards are slower to recognize this potential than some other aspects of children's services. The move towards parent-held child health records, as pioneered in Oxfordshire and recommended in the 1987 National Children's Bureau report *Investing in the Future*, acknowledges that parents (rather than professionals) should hold the relevant information about their child's health, and hence accepts their key role in child health.

Parents are the main providers of primary health care for their children, although this role of the parent is often forgotten and the focus in the UK has generally been on the parent as a user or consumer of services with the professional as provider. As Graham & Stacey (1984) put it:

> Services are designed to maximise the flow of information and expertise from doctor to patient. Other inputs, typically, flow the other way: it is parents who travel, it is parents who sit and wait, and it is parents who return home confused.

In fact, most illness experienced by children is dealt with outside the medical services, with studies from the USA and UK showing that medical advice is only sought for between 10% and 17% of reported symptoms (Alpert *et al.*, 1967; Spencer, 1984). Coping with illness in a young child involves a complex process of observation, recognition of symptoms, assessment of severity, and decisions about the appropriate action to take. Frequent reassessment is needed and outside advice may be sought from friends and relatives before any decision is taken to consult a health professional. Clearly, circumstances such as coping with more than one young child, isolation, depression or family stress can affect the decisions made. Similarly, although there are high rates of accidents in young children, the majority of these are dealt with by parents and only a small minority ever reach the doctor's surgery or hospital accident and emergency department (Mayall, 1986).

Parents, then, need to exercise a fair degree of skill in both diagnosis and treatment, and in recognizing when it is appropriate to consult a health professional. It is important that health professionals recognize and reinforce parental skills rather than (as often happens) undermining the parents' confidence in their role as health providers.

Maintaining the family's health, as any parent knows, is one of the most fundamental roles of parenting. It is time-consuming and demands skills which should be recognized. When Graham studied the daily life patterns of women within families, she concluded that 80% of a mother's main activities were concerned with promoting and protecting her children's health (Graham, 1984).

Much information on health care is now available from books, magazines and the media. It is not surprising, then, that mothers have considerable knowledge of what constitutes appropriate health care, and their views about appropriate nutrition, tooth care, accident prevention and so on are closely similar to those of professionals. This has been clearly shown by detailed studies such as that of Mayall & Grossmith (1985).

However, poor material circumstances as well as cultural and environmental factors can hamper the ability of parents to put their knowledge into practice. Hardly surprisingly, there is a relationship between income and diet, and between income and ownership of safety gadgets such as stove-guards and stair-gates.

Lack of social support, low self-esteem and depression can clearly also hamper parenting abilities in relation to health care. The interactions of depressed mothers and their children have been described in several studies and well reviewed recently by Cox (1988).

Against this background, this chapter looks at the provision of community child health services and day-care provision for the pre-school child.

Use of child health clinics

The role of the child health clinic should be evolving to meet the changing needs of users, while continuing to be a source of reassurance and advice, providing preventive care in the form of immunizations and screening, and providing ongoing health surveillance for young children. Increasingly, health visitors, CMOs and general practitioners are working closer together, with more general practitioners now running child health clinics within their own practices or intending to do so. In 1985 a survey of general practitioners found that 24% of them were actively providing such a service, while 65% thought that they should be doing so (Burke & Bain, 1986). General practice is gradually changing, with those now entering practice having a more comprehensive training in paediatrics in both hospital and community settings. Many are keen to take on preventive aspects of care, and it would seem likely that uptake of preventive surveillance programmes will increase when these are part of the overall health care of the child. With the appointment of more consultant paediatricians with an interest in community child health it is likely that increased training and support of general practitioners in this aspect of their work will be offered, with a consequent raising of enthusiasm and of standards.

In the past, attendance rates at child health clinics have been disappointing, with fairly high take-up at the early check-ups (six weeks and then six to eight months) but often only 50% or less after the age of two, by which time primary immunizations are complete. Attendance rates at child health clinics run by general practitioners vary widely, from very high rates in one home counties practice (Curtis Jenkins *et al.*, 1978) and at a Glasgow health centre (Barber, 1982) to lower rates elsewhere. Clearly, this reflects the energy and enthusiasm of the health workers concerned, as well as organizational issues such as up-to-date age−sex registers, follow-up of non-attenders and so on. Some consultant community paediatricians are now running joint clinics with general practitioners, a service which appears popular with patients and which may help to encourage a higher uptake of appointments for developmental surveillance (Crouchman *et al.*, 1986). Attendance rates also reflect the perceived value of the service on offer to parents and children. Where parents find a service which comes close to matching their needs and expectations, attendance rates are high, as shown in our own Thomas Coram study.

The Thomas Coram study

Before the start of the Thomas Coram study, at the child health clinic in Camden there was a 70% attendance rate at six weeks, with drop-

Table 10.1 Attendance for routine examination.

	Age at examination						
	6 weeks	6 months	12 months	18 months	2 years	3 years	4½ years
Camden							
No. of children due to be seen	203	192	163	161	174	195	169
No. of children seen	203	190	162	156	170	191	167
% Attendance	100%	99%	99%	97%	98%	98%	99%
Westminster							
No. of children due to be seen	103	89	74	70	78	86	60
No. of children seen	103	89	72	67	76	85	58
% Attendance	100%	100%	97%	96%	97%	99%	97%

off to 58% at one year, 49% at two years and 47% at three years. During the research study, attendance rates at the selected ages were over 96% at all ages; there were no significant social class differences between parents who were high attenders and those who were low attenders, nor was there any social class variation in the number of clinic visits in the first year (Table 10.1).

Attendance at the clinic was high too between routine visits for developmental checks, and on these occasions the mothers saw the health visitor and, where appropriate, the doctor. The average number of visits to the clinic (excluding developmental checks) was 13 in the first year of life (Table 10.2). One reason for the high attendance was the enthusiasm of the research health visitors, who had relatively small case loads (200–240 families), knew the families well and maintained high rates of home visiting.

Table 10.2 Clinic attendance between routine developmental examinations during the first three years.

	Camden mean number of visits	Westminster mean number of visits
First year	12.5	14.8
Second year	2.7	6.7
Third year	1.9	2.4

Note: At these visits the mother always saw the health visitor and often also the doctor.

This contrasts with an earlier study of child health clinic attendance in York (Graham, 1979), which found that, although initially attendance rates were high for all mothers, by five months only 40% of working-class mothers continued to attend, compared with 87% of social class I and II mothers. Interviews with mothers suggested some reasons for the drop-off, with some mothers perceiving the approach of the clinic staff to be critical or judgemental, as well as finding the advice given less than helpful. Hence, it was not surprising that these parents failed to return to the clinic.

The danger, however, is that these parents will be judged by health professionals to be uninterested in their children's health and labelled 'non-attenders', with no attempt to address the question of why people may choose not to come.

Why do parents attend child health clinics?

Apart from attending to ensure that their child is immunized and for developmental checks, parents commonly attend for advice and re-assurance on a wide variety of topics. When considering the use made of the child health clinic, this must be viewed in the context of other sources of advice and availability of other medical services for parents of young children. Many parents attend because they enjoy the social contact at the clinic and the opportunity to meet and talk with other parents. Anxieties over behaviour are common reasons for consulting the health visitor or doctor, and in the Coram study we found that around 10% of doctor consultations were for behaviour reasons (see Chapter 9).

Concerns about children's development are a further reason for attending, particularly regarding speech and language development and hearing problems, and it is worth noting that speech delay is the commonest developmental problem in the two to four age group (see Chapter 4). As parents become more knowledgeable about the norms of child development they are increasingly seeking advice on developmental aspects of child-rearing.

Depression and anxiety in the mother is often the real reason for bringing a child to the clinic or surgery, with a variety of minor complaints. It is crucial to be on the look-out for this, for it is well recognized that frequent attendances, ostensibly for advice about a child, may be the presenting symptoms of a depressed mother. Frequent attendances may also reflect uncertainties of child-rearing by an in-experienced parent, or the clinic may be providing a social milieu for isolated parents to meet in an informal and friendly setting.

Standards of general practice in inner urban areas are still very variable, as reflected by the fact that many parents prefer to bring a sick child to the clinic rather than to their GP despite being discouraged from doing this. Some of the difficulties experienced by patients in access and use of general practitioner services in London were highlighted in the Acheson report (1981).

This is not of course universally true, and as standards of general practice in inner city areas are improving the situation is changing. Reports have also drawn attention to the considerable number of people in inner city areas who are not registered with general practitioners and the considerable difficulty some of them have in being accepted on to a general practitioner's list. This is particularly true of mobile families and homeless families, whose numbers are increasing drastically and for whom registering with a general practitioner is often impossible. Hence, clinics and accident and emergency departments will, for these families, be the most readily accessible source of primary health care.

We found in our study (Hart *et al.*, 1981) that many attendances at the clinic were for illness (see Table 10.3) and clearly, here again, combining the 'preventive' and 'curative' aspects of the service is beneficial to parents and children. Advice from the clinic is sought too on a variety of family and social problems, particularly housing problems in urban areas, and also on preschool provision for children.

As can be seen from Table 10.3 developmental and behavioural aspects of child care were commonly discussed as well as illness, and aspects of housing and preschool provision were discussed by 11% and 16% of mothers respectively (Hart *et al.*, 1981). The level of satisfaction with the two clinics in the Coram study in terms of advice and help given was high, with 75% of parents satisfied, 7% dissatisfied and the rest equivocal.

Parents particularly like a welcoming and friendly atmosphere, staff who are clearly interested and have time to listen and to give thorough explanations, the lack of need for appointments, and careful examinations of their children. Clinics are often able to provide reassurance about a wide variety of aspects of child-rearing, and this role of child health staff should not be underestimated. Social aspects of child health clinics are also important to many parents. Criticisms are usually about length of waiting time and inability of clinic doctors to prescribe, but these are normally considered to be outweighed by the advantages and social aspects of the clinic. At one clinic held in a children's centre, parents were able to talk, relax and drink tea while the children played under adult supervision in a room at the other end

Table 10.3 Reasons for consulting the clinic doctor during a four-month period by mothers of 909 children (from Hart *et al.*, 1981). Some children were brought for more than one reason.

	Children (*n* = 909)	
	No.	%
Routine examination	301	34
New baby check	31	3
Respiratory tract infection	117	13
Skin problem	95	11
Vomiting or diarrhoea	40	4
Feeding	35	4
Teething/colic	17	2
Thrush	8	1
Constipation	14	2
Sight	12	1
Orthopaedic problem	7	1
Surgical problem	13	1
Behaviour	55	6
Development (including speech and hearing)	26	3
Maternal problem (for example, depression, anxiety)	12	1
Social problem	7	1
Immunization	255	28
Miscellaneous (including neonatal jaundice, meningitis, hypothyroidism, urinary infection, epilepsy, whooping cough, injuries)	30	3

of the corridor while waiting to see the health visitor or doctor — hence complaints about waiting were few.

Personality factors, such as attitudes to authority and medical services, may play a part in whether parents choose to attend clinics, and in a survey of reasons for non-attendance in Oxfordshire a third of non-attending parents either disliked the staff or found the clinic unhelpful, while others had transport difficulties or diffuse social problems (J.A. Macfarlane, personal communication).

Some of the more innovative approaches to child health service provision are reported by Dowling (1983); these include mobile clinics, evening clinics, clinics situated in shopping centres, and those based on other centres that children attend (such as nursery schools). Some of the most successful clinics are those based on children's centres where social and educational needs of children can be met, but these centres are few and far between. The crucial factor is that provision is made for parents' as well as children's needs. Any health centre or children's centre has the potential to become a focal point for community activities and self-help groups, hence providing support for both parents and children.

Even the more traditional child health clinics can, with imagination and flexibility, go some way towards meeting some needs of young families. Without much in the way of extra resources, groups can be run (often by health visitors or parents) such as single-parent groups, mother and toddler clubs, keep fit classes, health education groups, and so on. Toy libraries, even on an occasional basis, are a valuable extra resource, and links with other agencies, such as educational home visiting schemes, language schemes, and so on, can all enhance the child health clinic as a community resource.

General practitioner usage

In the Thomas Coram study, a large number of different general practitioners, many in single-handed practices, were responsible for the primary care of the children in the survey areas. In Camden 548 children seen in the course of the study were registered with 72 general practitioners, while in Westminster 322 children were registered with 80 general practitioners. No single general practitioner had more than 17% of the sample as patients, while many had only one or two of the children on their lists. Four per cent of the Camden children and 2% of those in Westminster were not registered with a general practitioner.

At that time there were only two practices with attached health visitors, and only one practice ran a child health clinic.

These findings illustrate the fragmentary nature of the general practitioner service typical of many inner city areas at the time of the study (1975–1980), which has not substantially changed in the two study areas since then. It also illustrates the immense difficulties of ensuring effective communication between the different members of primary care services regarding the children with whom they come into contact.

This is in marked contrast to many other areas of the country, where primary health care teams headed by general practitioners are becoming increasingly common. They are providing child health surveillance for the children on their lists, and in some rural areas with stable populations they are likely to cover relatively defined geographical areas, ensuring cover of a total child population.

More general practitioners in both urban and rural areas are working in group practices and, where the group is large enough, will have attached health visitors. There is an increasing tendency to provide a wide range of services and clinics, and scope for combining child health clinics with antenatal, postnatal or family planning clinics, a service which is popular with mothers. Many general practices are sensitive to the needs of the consumers and are aware of the need to provide good services in order to attract patients.

Table 10.4 Average number of GP consultations per child per year.

	Camden	Westminster	England and Wales		GLC
			NMS 1970/71	GHS 1971/72	
Age	0–4½	0–4½	0–4	0–4	0–4
Mean no. of visits	2.7	2.3	3.7	4.6	5.2

NMS: National Morbidity Statistics; GHS: General Household Survey; GLC: Greater London Council.

General practitioner consultation rates

The average number of consultations for zero- to four-year-olds in England and Wales in 1970–1971 was 3.7 and in the GLC area at around the same time was 5.2. At this time, just before the start of the study and the setting up of the child health clinic service in Camden and Westminster, the mean number of GP visits in the past year for all the children (aged 0 to four and a half) was 2.5 (Table 10.4), a somewhat lower rate. This may be explained by the fact that many of the GPs in the study area were single-handed with restricted surgery hours and relying on relief services for out-of-hours calls. Parents often found it easier to take their child to the nearest accident and emergency department than to call out a relief doctor. This is true of many inner urban areas, particularly where there is easy access to a hospital, but may not be the case for more rural areas.

During the study period, over 80% of children attended their general practitioner at least once a year from birth to four and a half years, around two-thirds of children made one to five visits per year, while 15% attended on six or more occasions. There were no significant age or area differences in general practitioner attendance, although children under two years old were somewhat more likely to attend their general practitioner than children over two. The mean number of attendances was 2.8 per year.

Reasons for consultation

Parents were asked the reasons why they had consulted the general practitioner with their child and in a subsample this was cross-checked against general practitioner records and found to be substantially accurate. Only a few consultations (1%) were said to be for developmental or behavioural reasons, although we know that these form a high proportion of any paediatric workload.

This is in marked contrast to reasons for attending the child health clinic, where 17% of consultations were regarding children's development, and 13% for concerns regarding behaviour. In addition behaviour and development were discussed at every routine visit.

There were no associations between level of general practitioner usage and sex of child, birth order, birthweight or method of feeding. There were social class differences, however; children of manual workers were twice as likely to have made six or more visits in a year as those in non-manual groups, and this may be partly accounted for by the increased incidence of respiratory and other illnesses in the children of manual workers.

Use of hospital services

The use made of any hospital service is dependent to a large extent on the geographical proximity of the hospital, as well as factors such as quality and availability of the general practitioner service. Where hospitals are close by, and general practitioners are single-handed with evening and weekend deputizing services, families are likely to choose to use accident and emergency departments for their primary care.

The children in the two areas studied made high use of both out-patient and accident and emergency departments at the local hospitals. In both study areas there were several hospitals within walking distance, and in Westminster the Children's Hospital accident and emergency department is open 24 hours a day and has traditionally been used by some members of the local community for primary care.

By the age of one year, 40% of children had attended hospital out-patient or accident and emergency departments at least once and 30% had attended more than once. By the age of three years, 60% of Camden children and 52% of Westminster children had attended out-patients at least once.

Quite a large proportion of children were admitted to hospital and, as with out-patient and accident and emergency attendance, hospital admissions were more frequent in the first year of life. Eighteen per cent of Camden children and 10% of those in Westminster had received in-patient care by the age of 12 months, and by the age of four and a half one-third of all children had received in-patient care, while 6% had had three or more admissions. Three-quarters of all admissions were for medical reasons, and one-quarter for surgical operations of various types.

The rates of out-patient attendance and hospital admissions were higher than in the British Birth Study (1970 cohort) (Chamberlain & Simpson, 1979) and considerably higher than earlier cohort studies.

This reflects both the close proximity of several hospitals to the areas studied, and the lack of group practices providing 24-hour cover for their patients. There is some evidence too that hospital admission rates for children are continuing to rise despite adequate primary care, possibly reflecting increasing expectations from both parents and professionals, and an unwillingness to risk caring for an ill child at home.

Day-care provision

In western societies for a very long time the attitude of society and successive governments towards women with children returning to employment has been critical and unsympathetic. While this has changed dramatically in the past two decades, particularly in Sweden and the USA, the UK still lags far behind, and this is reflected in the lack of state provision of child care and support for women returning to work. Provision for under-fives is patchy and developed by historical accident rather than by any rational look at needs.

Overall, one in six women returns to employment within six months of having their first baby and one in four returns by 12 months. Much larger numbers of women want to return to work, but are deterred by the difficulty of finding appropriate and affordable child care.

Nationally, of children under two, only 1% will be able to take up places in day nurseries and only a further 2% will find places with registered child-minders. For the three- to four-year-olds the situation is somewhat better, with 10% of children having access to nursery schools, and 12% having access to play-groups or crèches.

It is interesting to see how poorly Britain compares with other European countries in this respect. In Belgium 95% of three- to five-year-olds have access to child-care services and in France it is over 75%; the Swedish government in 1985 introduced a bill which entitled all children between 18 months and school age to municipal child care.

In spite of considerable research demonstrating the need and desire for improved state provision of services (Hughes *et al.*, 1980; Martin & Roberts, 1984; Moss, 1986) and much campaigning from pressure groups such as the National Childcare Campaign, little has changed in the last decade. The prevailing government attitude is that women should stay at home with their young children and that the state has no responsibility for child-care provision. Proposals to pass a law relating to parental leave, following an EEC directive in 1985, were rejected with little constructive debate.

As a result of society's indifference, parents are left to make child-care arrangements in an almost entirely private market, with the state offering extremely limited support. For the majority of children child-care arrangements are made within the family, with relatives, particularly grandmothers, providing care. One survey found that, of under-one-year-olds, two-fifths of children were cared for by relatives, with friends and neighbours also fulfilling an important role.

Women in high-status jobs who wish to return to work have more choices and some are likely to employ nannies or au pairs, but these options are expensive and only open to parents who are high-wage earners. Those returning to low-paid jobs are most likely to use relatives to provide child care.

Although a small proportion of fathers do participate in selecting and arranging child care, the reality is that mothers often have the sole responsibility for doing this. A recent London study found that 81% of placements were made by the mother alone, while for 14% of children both parents shared in the making of child-care arrangements (Moss, 1986).

Research and statistics strongly support the notion that women do indeed want some sort of flexible day-care arrangements for their children; over 50% of mothers would like day care for their under-three-year-olds, while over 90% want nurseries or other provision for their three- to five-year-olds. Clearly a balance must be struck between providing child care for women who want or need to work, and supporting women who want to stay at home and look after their young children.

Many of the arguments put forward for providing nurseries focus on the needs of the child, and the contribution that good day care can make to children's social and intellectual development; a further argument is that the majority of women want and need nursery provision. Here as elsewhere it is fallacious to argue the interests of the child and of the parent as separate issues — the two are closely interrelated, and the topic of day care should be addressed as an integrated issue.

For some women child-rearing is an immensely satisfying and fulfilling experience, but for many it can be an unsatisfactory experience which makes great demands on inner resources and is frequently stressful. This is not to say that they do not love and enjoy their children, but the constant demands and frustrations of looking after children and housework unremittingly can be overwhelming.

A woman at home all day with young children may become depressed, and this is particularly so if she does not have a supportive partner around to share some of the load. Research has shown that even part-time work away from home can help in preventing depression (Brown & Harris, 1978). Day-care facilities for children even on the basis of a few hours a day can be a lifeline, enabling a parent to cope with the demands of child-rearing in a way which is more positive for both parent and child.

The old argument that mothers should stay home and care exclusively for their children in the first few years can still be heard and reflects the view of women that a male-dominated society still largely holds. These views were reinforced by Bowlby's early theory of maternal deprivation, but the pertinence of this has been firmly rejected by more recent researchers in the field of child development (Rutter, 1982; O'Connell, 1983; Tizard, 1986).

However, health care professionals were profoundly influenced by some of Bowlby's ideas, and it is quite common for mothers still to receive conflicting advice about the effects of child-care provision outside the home from any professionals they consult, not to mention their own relatives and friends. Similar ambivalence is reflected in the views of both the popular and the professional press. As Scarr & Dunn (1987) say in their useful book which discusses the issue, 'much current advice is out of step with the times and with recent research on maternal employment and child care'.

In the rest of this chapter we consider some of the options open to parents wishing to use day-care facilities for their children, the health service input into the various types of day care and the possible implications for the children's health and well-being. Our own role as paediatricians to the two children's centres that were part of the Thomas Coram study is also considered.

Child-minders

A recent national survey suggested that around 23% of under-fives whose mothers work full-time are looked after by child-minders, but only a small proportion of these are registered (OPCS Survey, *Women and Employment*, 1980; Martin & Roberts, 1984). The total availability of full-time care for zero- to four-year-old children is only 4% nationally for day nurseries and registered minders combined.

Child-minders provide the cheapest day-care option for local authorities and for parents, and the DHSS currently recommends child-minding to working mothers as the best solution for child care.

Much of the earlier research on child-minding in the 1960s and 1970s painted a gloomy picture of the quality of care, with stories of under-stimulated, depressed children being minded in unsuitable and often overcrowded environments (Mayall & Petrie, 1983). In the past decade local authorities have made great efforts to support child-minders, and there has consequently been a vast improvement in the facilities open to minders, in terms of training, loan equipment, and access to social centres. As well as this an active organization, the National Childminders' Association, has grown up to promote and campaign for better conditions and more recognition for minders.

A child-minder is anyone who in his or her own home looks after a child under compulsory school age for a period of more than two hours in any six days (Nursery and Childminders Act, 1948). The local authority keeps, by law, a register of child-minders and has an obligation to ensure certain minimum standards. The child-minder's home will be visited to assess size and suitability of accommodation, a question-naire relating to family circumstances and the minder's health has to be completed and references from both a doctor and social services are required. A list of local child-minders is available from social services offices. Unfortunately, however, many child-minders do not become registered, so for them there can be no control of standards.

The Childminders Act is open to interpretation by each local authority and hence there are some variations, but usually the maximum number of children allowed per minder is three under-fives including the minder's own children, only one of whom may be under one year old. A member of the local social services under-fives team is then empowered to visit on a regular basis, and will normally encourage the minder to join the National Childminders' Association (NCMA).

This Association has a growing membership of now well over 10 000 and carries out regular surveys of its members. In the 1985 survey it was found that facilities for minders varied considerably; 55% of responders reported attending local child-minders' groups, 45% had access to an equipment loan scheme (for such items as stair-guards, etc.), and 26% had access to drop-in centres. Only 23% of minders reported that they had ever attended a child-minders' course, a disappointingly small proportion. Child-minders on the whole work long hours for low pay — 52% of minders surveyed worked a 40-hour week or more, and charges ranged from 50p to £1 per child per hour including meals. Thirty-one per cent of minders cared for only one child, with smaller percentages caring for two or three children. Almost all these minders were providing this service for working parents and 3.5% were caring for a handicapped child.

As facilities for training and supporting child-minders in their jobs improve, so should the quality of care that they provide. Particularly for children below the age of three this can be a satisfactory and stimulating form of child care, enabling the child to form a secure and warm attachment to another adult as well as to the other children cared for, and to the minder's own family. This is particularly advantageous for the single child of a single parent.

Clearly parents ought to exercise discretion in their choice of minder, and should spend some time talking to a prospective minder and seeing the quality of care in her own home. Reassurance will be needed about the level of warm affection and stimulation that the child will receive, and a discussion of aspects such as outings provided, the amount of time spent watching television, and access to facilities such as libraries or toy libraries is helpful. It is also important, as in any day-care facility, that the child is settled in gradually, with several visits accompanied by a parent before being left for a number of hours. The age of the child needs to be borne in mind when settling in; a two-year-old will normally take longer to feel comfortable about being left with a new adult than a child of three or over.

Problems clearly can arise if a child is insecure or unhappy, or inadequately stimulated by play and conversation. It is important that parent and minder continue to make time to communicate with each other, and do not try to hide any worries about the child's behaviour or development. Often a child-minder will be quite prepared to take a child to the doctor or clinic when necessary for a parent who has difficulty taking time off work (obviously permission from the parent is needed) and avenues of communication must remain open. Health visitors would expect to visit any children they were responsible for at the minder's home, although this should in no way be a substitute for the local authority social services representative visiting regularly. One of the negative findings from the NCMA survey was that in 1985 nearly one-fifth of minders had not been visited by social services in the past 12 months or more.

Although as stated earlier the research from the early 1970s regarding the quality of child care and child-minders made gloomy reading, recent research is much more positive. Ongoing studies are in progress in both the USA and the UK which should answer some questions about children's social and cognitive development in different types of day care. Clearly the effects on development of day care need to be disentangled from effects which could be due to the child's home environment, as well as to the child's individual temperament and genetic disposition. Early results from the USA suggest that the crucial factor in determining outcome related to child-minding is the level of interest and training in child care of the care-giver. Several years' experience of looking after babies and young children was not found to contribute to improved child care, but knowledge of child development did. Child-minders who were well trained were found to be more likely to praise, respond to, question and instruct young children than child-minders with minimal training, and, interestingly, the number of years of formal education of the minder did not influence outcome. It would appear, then, that it is the quality of the individual that is the most important variable when considering the influence of child-minders.

This has implications for social services policy; further emphasis must be put on ensuring training for *all* child-minders rather than the minority as at present. Health professionals can help by encouraging minders to participate in classes run at local clinics and adult education establishments and by reinforcing the valuable contribution that child-minders can make to an individual child's development.

Day nurseries

Local authority day nurseries are run by social services departments, and applications for a place are made either to the social services or to a health visitor. A health visitor's report is normally required, and this is usually quite influential when applications are being considered. Day nurseries potentially provide long hours of care, being open from 8.00 a.m. to 6.00 p.m., and remaining open during school holidays. The age range of children in day nurseries varies from district to district, with some districts offering places to babies as young as six months and others having a policy of admitting only children over one year old. On the whole, social services departments encourage parents to make other arrangements until the child is at least 12 to 18 months old.

Staff in day nurseries all have Nursery Nurse Examination Board (NNEB) certificates or equivalent training, and there are recommended staff ratios of one member of staff to five children over the age of two, and one to every three children under the age of two. Because of the high staff ratio needed for under-twos most local authority nurseries have only a few places for this age-group. Places in day nurseries are available only to priority groups and their availability differs widely in different parts of the country.

Priority groups include children with special needs such as those with developmental disorders or stressful homes or who are considered at risk of non-accidental injury or neglect; and sometimes children of single parents who are working. While some nurseries are extremely good, the quality of care does vary. In many day nurseries more attention is paid to the physical needs of the child than the emotional needs, and parents are not always encouraged to participate.

Increasingly, though, the wider needs of the child are being recognized and catered for, and more day nurseries are becoming family-centred.

Other nurseries may be available in a neighbourhood, such as workplace nurseries, community nurseries and private nurseries. All nurseries are required to be registered with social services departments, and hence are subject to inspections to ensure adequate facilities and safety standards.

Fees vary enormously and so does the quality of the nursery, the latter not necessarily bearing much relationship to the former.

Some of the best nurseries are very often community nurseries, usually set up in response to local initiative and local need and often receiving funds from government or local authority as well as charitable organizations. The management commmittee usually consists of parents and staff, and parents in these nurseries are much more involved in the planning and organization of their child's nursery. Because they normally service a geographical catchment area rather than only pro-viding for 'priority ' children, community nurseries can in principle be used by any family within that catchment area.

THE EFFECTS OF DAY CARE

Children go to nurseries for a variety of reasons, and good nurseries provide many opportunities for children which might not otherwise be available to them. These include the possibility of peer-group friendships and support, relationships with other adults, and a wide range of play opportunities including safe supervised outdoor play space. This is particularly advantageous in urban areas; the Thomas Coram study found that 48% of families with preschool children had no garden.

Nurseries too can encourage the development of social, self-help, and cognitive skills, and foster independence and maturity, and perhaps more attention should be paid to these positive effects. Data from the USA Headstart programmes demonstrated gains in children's social and intellectual skills and, although these were most striking in the short term, long-term gains were also measurable.

There is no support from recent research studies for the view that attendance at day nurseries is likely to have adverse effects on children's social and emotional development, despite arguments to this effect in the 1950s and 1960s. However, the *quality* of day care is crucial and, where researchers have looked at outcome in nurseries with poor staff:child ratios and large groups of children, adverse findings have been reported.

It must be remembered that evidence of this sort may be affected by the nature of the mother's employment, as the type and duration of work undertaken are also likely to influence the child's emotional and social development. A mother who is in a job which is physically demanding may come home exhausted and lack the energy to meet her child's demands for attention, whereas a mother in a more rewarding job which improves her self-esteem and is less tiring may have more to give her child at the end of the working-day.

There is no doubt that in this country children attending social services day nurseries do have high rates of health, developmental and behaviour problems compared with children who are attending play-groups or nursery schools. Frost & Downham (1979) reported a high incidence of speech and language delay, failure to thrive, and other previously unsuspected health problems among children attending one day nursery (there was no control group) and suggested that a high level of medical input was necessary in day nurseries. A later study in Inner London (Spies, 1980) found rates of hearing problems, speech and language delay and behaviour problems to be considerably higher among three-year-olds attending day nurseries than among other three-year-olds.

Recently further research on children's behaviour in different types of preschool setting has found significantly higher rates of behaviour problems among children aged two to five in day nurseries compared with children attending either play-groups or nursery schools (McGuire & Richman, 1986). The prevalence of behaviour problems was 34% among their day-nursery sample, and again rates of both speech and language delay and health problems were very much higher among these children than among those attending the other forms of day care. In this study those children with a health problem or speech and language delay also had significantly higher rates of behaviour problems, confirming again the interrelationship between health, development and behaviour (see also Chapters 8 and 9).

In all three settings boys showed more problem behaviour than girls. As these authors state, the findings in day-nursery children are unsurprising, in that

> they are likely to form a group of children most at risk of behavioural or emotional disturbance by virtue of the admission criteria for day nurseries...reasons for admission to day nurseries now more often focus upon the presence of non-accidental injury, inadequate parenting, poor home conditions or handicap, so that staff are dealing with large numbers of children who are difficult to manage.

Interestingly, there was only limited overlap between behaviour as reported by the parents and behaviour problems in the nursery, although the findings were inconclusive since many parents did not complete the questionnaires. Behaviour in young children is very often situation-specific and, as McGuire & Richman point out, some behaviours such as aggression may be displayed more in a group setting. This study highlights the need for staff working in preschool settings to be adequately trained to deal with the emotional needs of children and with difficult behaviour, and also points to the importance of closely integrated health services in day-care settings.

As with other research in this field, the evidence is not that placement in a day nursery *causes* developmental or behaviour problems, but that the children selected for admission to day nurseries are a high-risk group for these disorders. In many ways day nurseries are an inappropriate setting for caring for such children, because their wider needs are seldom met, and the parents are all too often excluded from the care offered to the child. Family centres where the team of staff includes social workers and psychologists would be more appropriate for many day-nursery children and their families, but few such centres exist and then predominantly in deprived inner-city areas with long waiting-lists for admission.

In Scandinavia and North America, where nurseries cater predominantly for children of working mothers rather than 'priority' children, studies have not found that day-care children have more social or emotional problems than home-reared children, although certain differences have been noted, day-nursery children being more sociable than others and co-operating better with their peer groups.

The organization of individual day nurseries is likely to have considerable influence, for example group size, staff familiarity with individual children, staff turnover, layout and size of rooms, play materials, and group constancy. In some nurseries staff turnover is high; sickness rates among day-nursery staff are also very high. This reflects the poor status given to those who work in child care, with low pay and poor career structure as well as insufficient staff support and back-up and stressful working conditions. Attention to these issues would greatly enhance the quality of care afforded to the children.

Play-groups

Most play-groups are affiliated with the Pre-school Playgroups Association; this organization runs training courses for group leaders and encourages mothers to participate in planning and running the groups.

Play-groups are used nationally by around 14% of children over the age of three years, but do not provide day care for children of working mothers. Most sessions are for two to three hours, and many play-groups only operate three or four days a week, usually in the mornings. The underlying philosophy is not so much educational as encouraging mothers to participate in their children's play, increasing their confidence in their own caring abilities and providing a mutually enjoyable experience.

There is enormous variety among play-groups over such issues as fees charged, degree of parental participation, and organization. Some are set up and run in parents' own homes, others in church halls or community centres, and variation is also found in the range of activities and equipment available. Attendance at play-groups is normally a beneficial experience for a child, providing (as in any day-care setting) that staff are sensitive to the child's individual needs and stage of development, that group size is not too large, and that the care is both affectionate and responsive.

Nursery schools

These are run by the local education authority and cater for children between the ages of three and five years. Some are organized as nursery classes within primary schools, while others are separate and not linked to any particular school. They are part of the state schooling provision and are free of charge, with the same hours and holiday periods as primary schools. The majority of children are offered part-time places, particularly in the younger age groups, but a proportion of children (usually over the age of four) attend for a full day. The availability of full-time places will depend on locality and demand, which varies greatly from district to district. Nationally, around 40% of children will have attended some form of nursery school or class before the age of five. The teachers in nursery schools are highly trained, and children are offered a wide range of activities and experiences, the underlying philosophy being implicitly educational. Attendance at a local nursery school or play-group enables children to form friendships with children living in the same locality and is often a route for parents too to form friendships and build up supportive local networks. There is some evidence that children who have attended nursery schools or play-groups have less difficulty settling into school than children who have remained at home during the preschool years. This is likely to relate to the social skills that are fostered and valued in preschool settings.

An argument is often put forward that attendance at a nursery school (or similar setting) will encourage language development in a child who may have some speech and language delay. The main stimulus to language development, however, comes from a one-to-one relationship with a familiar adult who is sensitive to the child's experience and who can interpret and discuss the child's conversation in relation to both past and future events in that child's life. Tizard & Hughes (1984) in their elegant study of London four-year-olds in two different settings found that a child's language experience was very much richer when the child was at home with a parent than when at nursery school.

The findings from this study do not deny the importance of nursery schools but highlight the fact that adult : child interactions in such settings are considerably more limited than in the home environment. It follows that, in selecting the type of preschool provision, the child's individual needs and temperament are of paramount importance. Unfortunately the limited availability of preschool provision means that decisions about placement are most often made for practical rather than ideological reasons.

Health services in day-care settings

During the time of our research study we were fortunate in being able to work in two children's centres which were the focal points of the catchment areas. These were the Thomas Coram Children's Centre in Camden, and the Dorothy Gardner Centre in Westminster. Both these preschool centres aim to meet children's needs by the provision of nursery-school facilities alongside day-care facilities, and aim to break down the traditional barriers between 'care' and 'education'. Both centres offer flexibility in the range of service and hours provided to meet the individual needs of children and their families. Regular health surveillance of all children took place in the centres, and the health input by paediatricians and health visitors was an integral part of the service.

In our view a strong health service input to preschool day-care settings is beneficial to children, parents and staff. Unfortunately, in most health districts the input is fairly minimal, and is not based on the assessed health needs of the children concerned. From our studies of the health of preschool children in the two centres, and our experience of working in other less privileged day-care settings, we are convinced that the preschool services which work best are those where educational, social services and health inputs are combined, with the breaking down of traditional barriers between services.

We are all concerned with providing a service to families with young children which is flexible, appropriate to their needs, and both helpful and acceptable to the consumers. The high take-up of service during the Thomas Coram Study illustrates that health services can be acceptable to families and the interview data supported a positive view of the child health service offered. It is important to note that the child health service was not working in isolation, but was closely integrated with other preschool services offered by the children's centres, and in our view it is this combined approach to service provision which is most beneficial to young children and their families.

In deciding what health input is needed to day-care settings, there are four main points to consider:

1   There is a close interrelationship of health, development and behaviour in preschool children (see Chapter 11). A disorder in any one aspect of the child's functioning can affect other aspects, and it is essential to review the whole child. Services which attempt to 'fragment' the child (e.g. referring behaviour problems directly to psychologists without considering health and other background factors) are potentially disastrous, as underlying causal factors may remain undetected.

2   Although health and developmental problems can be detected in any setting, behaviour in children is often situationally determined. Thus a child may exhibit disturbed behaviour in a nursery setting while not causing any particular concern at home. It is generally more helpful, then, to review children with their parents and the staff in the day-care setting that the child attends rather than in a child health clinic or general practitioner's surgery.

3   Children attending day nurseries constitute an at-risk group with high rates of health, developmental and behavioural problems. It is essential that adequate health visitor and community paediatric time and expertise is available to these children and their families.

4   Children's needs cannot be seen in isolation from those of their parents. Day-care provision should be flexible enough to respond to parents' needs, which may be to work full-time, or perhaps to be nurtured in a day-care setting themselves. The health input must also be flexible and respond to parental need, with liaison to other community resources and agencies as appropriate.

Finally, some consideration should be given to the needs of staff in day-care settings for preschool children. They are undervalued in our society and underpaid, yet committed to the welfare of the children they look after. They deserve support, information and encouragement in the valuable role they play. Time must be set aside to listen to what staff have to say about the health and behaviour of children in their care, for they are acute observers. They should also be given information about the children's health which is relevant to their functioning, bearing in mind issues of confidentiality.

We have avoided prescribing a 'model' health service input to any particular day-care setting, but stress the importance of evaluating the needs of the children, parents and staff and planning a service sensitive to these. Greater priority should be given to the health visitor's role in the various day-care settings, and an adequate community paediatric presence should be allowed for. Close links are needed with all the other relevant agencies, particularly speech therapy and child psychiatry and psychology services, and close communication between all those concerned with promoting the health and development of children must be maintained at all times.

References

Acheson, D. (1981) *Primary Health Care in Inner London*. London Health Planning Consortium, London.

Alpert, J.J., Kosa, J. & Haggerty, R.J. (1967) Medical help and maternal nursing care in the life of low income families. *Pediatrics*, **39**, 749–55.

Barber, J.H. (1982) Pre-school developmental screening – the results of a four year period. *Health Bulletin*, **40** (4), 170–8.

Brown, G.W. & Harris, T. (1978) *Social Origins of Depression: a Study of Psychiatric Disorders in Women*. Tavistock Publications, London.

Burke, P. & Bain, J. (1986) Paediatric developmental screening: a survey of general practitioners. *Journal of the Royal College of General Practitioners*, **36**, 302–6.

Chamberlain, R.N. & Simpson, R.N. (1979) *The Prevalence of Illness in Childhood*. Pitman Medical, London.

Cox, A.D. (1988) Maternal depression and impact on children's development. *Archives of Disease in Childhood*, **63**, 90–5.

Crouchman, M., Gazzard, J. & Forester, S. (1986) A joint child health clinic in an inner London general practice. *Practitioner*, **230**, 667–72.

Curtis Jenkins, G., Collins, C. & Andren, S. (1978) Developmental surveillance in general practice. *British Medical Journal*, **1**, 1537–40.

Dowling, S. (1983) *Health for a Change*. Child Poverty Action Group, London.

Frost, G.J. & Downham, M.A.P.S. (1979) Child health in a day nursery. *Journal of Maternal and Child Health*, **4**, 418–27.

Graham, H. (1979) Women's attitude to the child health service. *Health Visitor*, **52**, 175–8.

Graham, H. (1984) *Women, Health and the Family*. Wheatsheaf Books, Brighton.

Graham, H. & Stacey, M. (1984) Socio-economic factors related to child health. In *Progress in Child Health*, vol. 1 (ed. Macfarlane, J.A.). Churchill Livingstone, London 167–77.

Hart, H., Bax, M. & Jenkins, S. (1981) The use of the child health clinic. *Archives of Disease in Childhood*, **56** (6), 440–5.

Hughes, M., Mayall, B., Moss, P., Perry, J., Petrie, P. & Pinkerton, J. (1980) *Nurseries Now*. Penguin Books, London.

McGuire, J. & Richman, N. (1986) The prevalence of behavioural problems in three types of preschool groups. *Journal of Child Psychology and Psychiatry*, **27** (4), 455–72.

Martin, J. & Roberts, L. (1984) *Women and Employment: a Lifetime Perspective*. HMSO, London.

Mayall, B. (1986) *Keeping Children Healthy*. Allen & Unwin, London.

Mayall, B. & Grossmith, C. (1985) Keeping children healthy. *Health Visitor*, **58** (11), 317–20.

Mayall, B. & Petrie, P. (1983) *Childminding and Day Nurseries: What Kind of Care?* Heinemann Educational, London.

Moss, P. (1986) *Child Care in the Early Months*. Occasional Paper No. 3, Thomas Coram Research Unit, University of London.

National Children's Bureau (1987) *Report of the Policy and Practice Review Group. Investing in the Future: Child Health Ten Years after the Court Report*. National Children's Bureau, London.

O'Connell, J.C. (1983) Children of working mothers: what the research tells us. *Young Children: Research in Review*, **38**, 63–70.

Rutter, M. (1982) *Maternal Deprivation Reassessed*, 2nd edn. Penguin Books, London.

Scarr, S. & Dunn, J. (1987) *Mother Care/Other Care*. Penguin Books, London.

Spencer, N.J. (1984) Parents' recognition of the ill child. In *Progress in Child Health*, vol. 1 (ed. Macfarlane, J.A.). Churchill Livingstone, London.

Spies, J. (1980) *Child Health Surveillance Survey*. Chelsea and Westminster Area Health Authority, Kensington (unpublished).

Tizard, B. (1986) *The Care of Young Children: Implications of Recent Research*. Occasional Paper No. 1, Thomas Coram Research Unit, University of London.

Tizard, B. & Hughes, M. (1984) *Young Children Learning*. Fontana, London.

The Intimate Relation of Health, Development and Behaviour — and the Doctor

I N THIS FINAL CHAPTER we first review the relationship which we have emphasized throughout this book between health, development and behaviour in the young child, and in the light of this we then discuss the organization of periodic examinations of the child and the doctor's role in treatment and management of the common disorders of childhood. The latter involves not only the proper treatment of specific conditions, which we have described in relevant sections of the book, but also the management and counselling of families where a condition exists which is not amenable to treatment. We have not included here a full account of the important role of our health visitor colleagues, but we reaffirm that the health visitor is the linchpin of the child health service.

The relationship of health, development and behaviour in the young child

The doctor in primary care is uniquely placed to study the way in which the child's physical health and unfolding development affect the way he behaves and relates to those around him. The social and physical environment in which the child is brought up can affect his development and health. The way the environment affects development is complex. Children not exposed to language will not talk, although the effect of less extreme deprivation on language development is not clear. Chronic handicapping conditions, particularly neurological ones, are often associated with slow development, which is partly an integral feature of the condition and partly the result of restricted environmental experience. An adverse physical environment can also cause ill health. Thus it has long been known that respiratory illness is commoner in social class V families, and the way this effect is mediated has now been studied: poor housing, poor nutrition and smoking have all been incriminated. The social environment also affects health, and problems such as unemployment, poverty and mental illness (in the parents) may be associated with frank child abuse or neglect — factors which obviously can profoundly affect the child's health.

That the health of a child can affect behaviour has also been firmly established for many years, particularly with chronic illness in the older child. The Isle of Wight study (Rutter *et al.*, 1970) showed that children with conditions such as cerebral palsy and other disabilities involving the central nervous system had four or five times the rate of behaviour disturbances of ordinary children. The situation in relation to intercurrent illness in the preschool child has been less clear-cut. That stress can affect health is also well known. Haggerty (1980) and his colleagues (see Chapter 5) showed that stressful life events could lead to illness and emphasized the importance of social support systems for sick children.

In our own studies we were able to look at the relationship between development, health and behaviour in geographically defined populations. The details of the rates of abnormalities found have been discussed throughout the text. Table 11.1 repeats the rates of common respiratory illness in the different age-groups. Table 11.2 records the prevalence of the commonest developmental disorder, which was speech and language delay, and Table 11.3 gives the assessment of behaviour problems as the doctors rated the children and their families when they saw them. In Chapter 9 we described what these problems were. In the younger child sleep disturbances are common but by the age of

Table 11.1 History of respiratory illness in different age groups.

	Age group (%)			
	0–1 year	1–2 year	2–3 year	3–4.5 year
URTIs > once a month	14	14	16	9
LRTI at least once in last year	13	10	11	9
Otitis media at least once in last year	15	16	15	24
Total *n* =	274	280	329	274

Table 11.2 Percentage of children with abnormal speech and language.

	Age (%)					
Speech and language	2 year	(*n*)	3 year	(*n*)	4.5 year	(*n*)
Possibly abnormal	17	(50)	12	(38)	7	(19)
Definitely abnormal	5	(14)	8	(25)	5	(13)
n =	296		323		269	

Table 11.3 Prevalence of problems by age.

	6 week		6 month		1 year		18 month		2 year		3 year		4.5 year	
	n	%	*n*	%	*n*	%	*n*	%	*n*	%	*n*	%	*n*	%
Parents worried about behaviour	22	6	11	3	23	8	15	6	34	11	48	15	35	13
Behaviour problem on doctor's assessment	14	4	8	2	16	6	15	6	32	11	55	17	33	12
n =	352		331		278		251		302		327		276	

three difficulties in management such as temper tantrums were the most important issues parents told us about.

How do these findings interrelate? Consistent relationships can be demonstrated: for example, at the age of two the incidence of ear infections was significantly related to speech and language delay and at three years there were twice as many children with speech and language delay who had a history of ear infections as there were without such infections. Just as physical health can affect development, it can also affect behaviour. Then there are significant relationships between night-waking and ear infections and similarly between management and temper tantrums later. Behaviour and speech and language delay are also significantly interrelated (as has been shown in several studies) and Table 11.4 gives our findings with regard to two-, three- and four-and-a-half-year-olds. The relationship is highly significant at two and four and a half, and just fails to reach this level at three.

The purpose of this present discussion therefore is to emphasize how important it is to view the child as a whole and not simply be concerned with his present illness or his parents' worry about development or complaints about his temper tantrums. A doctor assessing a young child must bear in mind continually that he cannot simply be concerned with one aspect of the child but must also be aware of this intimate relationship between health, development and behaviour in the young child. The primary care doctor must consider how the child's situation relates to that of the family. In Chapters 8 and 9 we note the fact that depression or stress affects young mothers very frequently. Stress tends to be commoner for example in mothers whose babies have had bronchitis and in the mothers of children who have frequent temper tantrums. Again the family doctor is in a good position to integrate all aspects of the child's care within the family.

Table 11.4 Relationship between speech and language and behaviour problems.

	Normal	Possibly abnormal	Definitely abnormal
Speech and language at 2 years			
No problem	219	41	4
Mild problem	12	5	4
Moderate/severe problem	1	2	6
		$P < 0.001$	
Speech and language at 3 years			
No problem	221	30	18
Mild problem	31	4	5
Moderate/severe problem	8	4	2
		$P < 0.05$	
Speech and language at 4½ years			
No problem	214	15	7
Mild problem	13	3	4
Moderate/severe problem	8	1	2
		$P < 0.001$	

Routine health checks in the young child

The tradition of a health service periodically reviewing children's health and development extends in the UK back to before the First World War. The aims of such activities are to promote children's health, to help families with the common difficulties of child-rearing and to identify children with health, developmental or behaviour problems which require further treatment and management. Given skilled and informed staff, parents use a child health clinic as an easily accessible source of advice and expertise, for they know that familiar and friendly staff will be regularly present to meet these needs.

Routine health checks (we prefer the word 'checks' to surveillance) have been much discussed in recent years. They are health service-initiated and not client-initiated, that is to say we ask the family to bring their child for a check. These checks have often been referred to as 'screening' of the child, but the use of the word in this context is wrong. Screening is a test which simply sorts the child into one category or another, whereas what actually happens in a routine check is that the child is examined and an assessment made of his health, development and behaviour. This may lead to referral to a secondary source, usually a hospital doctor, but more often the primary care physician and other health staff will, on the basis of their assessment, plan the extent to which they need to help to provide assistance or treatment for the child. This also involves knowledge of local resources for young children and liaison with social and educational services.

In books and articles about preschool children, authors often consider only one aspect of need and suggest different timings as appropriate for seeing the child. Thus developmentalists are concerned with the variance in children's achievement, immunologists with the best time for immunization and psychiatrists about the timing of intervention over behaviour problems. Less attention has been given to the role of the child's so-called illnesses but it has been shown that demands on acute services can be reduced if these health problems are discussed at regular times when the child is being seen in the relaxed atmosphere of a health check.

Thought should also be given to the needs and anxieties of the parents and other family members, which will vary depending on social environment and in relation to a range of other factors. A single mother bringing up her first child in an inner city and living in a hotel room will need to be seen more often than the mother with a second or third child living in reasonable housing with an adequate income and possibly support available from grandparents and others with experience of young children. It is the parents who are first monitors of the child's health and development and one of the tasks of the primary health care team is to see that parents are provided with information so that they can themselves identify normal development and distinguish between the less severe infections and potentially serious illness. They also want information about the social and emotional development of a child which will allow them to understand some of the difficult behaviours which may appear at different ages.

Despite these parental resources, we believe that most parents welcome the opportunity for regular meetings with a trained doctor or nurse and the question remains as to how frequently it is worth doing this. During the years when we carried out systematic studies, the doctor regularly saw the children at six weeks, six months, one year, 18 months, two, three and four-and-a-half years. Obviously this was a research study and the frequency related more to our data require-ments rather than to a defined policy of how often regular checks should be done. Indeed, we had anticipated that we might have had some difficulty in getting good attendance for these clinic visits, but in practice we achieved over 98% attendance from the population at all our checks. This partly reflected the interest and commitment of our research health visitors and our own paediatric experience, which meant that we probably had more specialist knowledge than most clinic doctors, but it also reflects the parents' recognition of the value of regular health checks of their child.

Another issue which has been the subject of much debate is which member of the primary health care team, doctor or nurse, should see the family on these routine occasions. The DHSS has recommended that the doctor should do the six-week and the three-year check and the health visitor should be responsible for the others. We'd like to feel that a much more flexible approach was possible, reflecting the individual interests of the members of the team, and the needs of different children and their parents. Clearly where a problem or anxiety is voiced by a parent or by a health visitor or nursery nurse there must be ready access to trained medical personnel.

It is important that both the doctor and the nurse who are going to undertake primary care should have thorough knowledge of child development and have had experience of routine examination at all ages in the preschool period. It is not very reassuring to a health visitor when she realizes that the doctor knows less about normal child development than she does. Thus the doctor must take every opportunity to examine many children at all ages to acquire the necessary skills. Another attribute of the team is that they know their families, so that when a child does present with a problem the parents have confidence in members of the health care staff. If a doctor has not seen the child since the age of six weeks and is suddenly confronted with a major behavioural problem, he will find himself dealing with a family with whom he is not familiar and who don't know him and may be anxious and unwilling to share fully their concerns about their child. Clearly a general practitioner may have seen the family more frequently than a clinic doctor. In inner urban areas with high mobility the weekly child health clinic may see more of a young couple with a baby than the doctor would at routine surgeries (see Chapter 1 for a discussion of this). The establishment of a child health clinic where doctors and nurses have time to talk to families about the problems of their children and where other facilities are available, ranging from booklets about child-rearing to simple pharmaceuticals and play materials, will create a facility where parents will regularly bring their babies and young infants. We would stress too the continuing availability of the clinic, so that parents will continue to come throughout the toddler years.

We dislike being proscriptive about 'times' that a service should be offered — the service is a clinical one designed to meet needs. Quite often we suggest that the baby is weighed on a weekly basis for the first six weeks of life, thereafter on a fortnightly basis until three months, and then monthly until six months, when weighing can be more intermittent. The family with a new baby will become used to attending the clinic on a regular basis during the early months of life and a decision is then necessary about when to make a more formal assessment of the child. Dates and times need not be rigorously adhered to, so that the family and the staff may decide that it is not necessary to keep the next pre-set appointment, because an assessment has been carried out on the occasion of a special visit.

The baby, usually born nowadays in an obstetric unit, will have had a full examination on the neonatal ward and a full re-examination is not necessary early after discharge. On the other hand, immediate contact with the family from the local child health clinic is very important so that a relationship can be established and any early child-rearing or management difficulties dealt with. Early health visitor contact can improve the rate of breast-feeding (for discussion of this see Chapter 6) and parents should be encouraged to bring the child to the clinic regularly. The traditional date of six weeks seems to us to be a reasonable one for the first formal check on the child. Some of the early rearing difficulties should have settled and a more stable pattern of management established for many infants. Persistent feeding difficulties are more likely therefore to be cause for concern and occasionally may result in failure to thrive, etc. Nine out of ten babies will be smiling and the social relationships between the mother (and father) and the child should be well established. Physical examination at this age includes the important check for congenital dislocation of the hips, which most people believe should be repeated at every check until the child is walking well.

The next occasion for a check is often the first time an immunization is given (the DHSS recommended ages are set out in Chapter 6). At the three month injection stage, hip location is re-examined. The next injection is usually given at four and a half months as outlined in Chapter 6. If (as often happens) injections become delayed, try to be a little flexible. With families who are poor clinic attenders, the opportunity should be taken to immunize their children whenever they present.

In terms of child-rearing, four to four and a half months sees the introduction of mixed feeds and is often an occasion when the family will want to discuss the child's progress, as well as being the time that the second immunization is due. The child is usually sitting with support, and beginning to grab for objects and hold on to them, and showing an interest in the environment. The colicky baby will be at the height of his problems at around the three-month stage. Health visitors will often see the baby at these ages.

Any time after six months is a good age for the next examination. Hearing can now be tested clinically, and this should be done as early as possible. Hips and testicles should be re-examined on this occasion

and the findings noted in discussing present development and behaviour. Developmentally the baby will be just about sitting unsupported and one can usually feel quite happy about gross motor
development and also observe fine motor development at this age.
Vocalization is becoming more complex. It is an age at which families
usually have fewest problems with their children's behaviour although
sleep disorders may cause anxieties. The child will more than likely
have had the first upper respiratory tract infection and discussion of
management of minor illness is something which can appropriately be
undertaken at this age.

Between ten months and a year the next check can be associated
with the giving of the third immunization. From the development
point of view recognition of the beginning of the first words and an
increasing consonantal vocabulary are reassuring. A second hearing
check can be performed and is particularly desirable if there is concern
about the child's language and there have been ear infections. In
addition more serious sleep and feeding problems may begin to emerge.

At thirteen to fifteen months many clinics will give the measles,
mumps and rubella injection. This is not a very profitable age to look
at the child's development as he is in a rather 'betwixt and between'
stage. Eighteen months is a suitable age to get a good, clear account of
developing language and symbolic play. In addition, non-walkers
should be identified and fully assessed. At this age the highest rate of
sleep disturbances occurs and management problems are beginning to
show themselves. Height and weight progress should be reviewed at
all ages.

At two years, speech and language should be firmly established
and this is the age at which the child who is likely to be late can be
picked out for interval surveillance before the next formal check at
three years. This is also the time when the non-talking, exploring 15-
to 18-month-old has changed to the much more participating two-
year-old and the parents usually welcome the opportunity to discuss
child-rearing practices at this age. Incidentally, around this age a
second sibling most commonly arrives and this also raises issues for
discussion. As at all other ages if anxieties exist about the child's
development a check before the next planned one at three years should
be arranged.

By three, the child has some cognitive functions which can be
assessed. He should be copying, reasonable hand function should be
observed, sentence structure should be well developed and he should
be a participating and socially amenable member of the family group.
It is at this age that the most difficult preschool management problems

arise (see Chapter 9) and intervention may be indicated. Parents will often wish to discuss anxieties about their children's health, particularly the common coughs and colds. At three, visual acuity can be clinically tested for the first time, although some children will resist monocular occlusion at this age and will have to have their visual acuity assessed again six months later.

Given the normal, reasonably behaved child of this age, we do not believe that it is necessary for a health check to be made again until the child is seen at four and a half to five as he enters school. By this time other cognitive functions have emerged and a careful neuro-developmental examination will serve to identify those children who are at risk for later school difficulties (Bax & Whitmore, 1987). Some will say that in a child population which has been adequately assessed earlier, a three-year examination will serve to identify all the children who need further examination around five. This may be so in a settled community but, given the amount of movement within most urban societies particularly by young parents of children, we believe that the advantages of carrying out examination of all children at school entrance are numerous.

Treatment, counselling and management

Some of the diseases and disorders discussed in this book are amenable to medical treatment, for example, a known bacterial infection can be effectively treated with an antibiotic. We can offer rational plans of management for sleep disorders and we can certainly make useful suggestions about approaches to the language-delayed child. Often, however, the problem which the family present to the doctor about a young child will not be amenable to medical treatment or management in a formal way, and the doctor can only offer counselling to the family.

'Counselling' has a huge (and often rather jargony) literature associated with it. However, Hobson (1978) has usefully defined the ways in which we can help people. They are:
1 *Direct action*. Taking action yourself to provide or meet somebody's needs (this would include giving them medicines).
2 *Giving advice or making suggestions* about a course of action a person can or possibly should take (telling them how to manage a sleep or a feeding problem).
3 *Teaching*. This is helping someone acquire knowledge and skills which you think they need and which they do not have. This could be providing a young family with books about child development and

child-rearing and encouraging them to find out about the processes.
4 *Counselling.* This is helping people to explore a problem so that
they can decide themselves what to do about it.

Counselling has been defined as a process through which one
person helps another by purposeful conversation in an understanding
atmosphere; its basic purpose is to assist the individual to make his or
her own decisions from the choices available. Parents vary widely in
the way they wish to bring up their children. Some, for example, are
happy to live with boisterous children who are not conventionally
well-mannered at the table and whose regular involvement in all
parental activities is encouraged. Other parents expect to see a much
more regularized pattern of behaviour in their young child — waiting
for a meal quietly and 'being seen and not heard' — and will not want
young children to obtrude at adult meal-times. Obviously these are
stereotypes of attitudes but different families have very different styles
of living and it is certainly none of our purpose to suggest which are
right and wrong. But when the family are having difficulties with their
children, or the children are having difficulties with their family, it is
the job of the health professional to counsel parents and children
about these issues.

Counselling was classically described by Karl Rogers as having
three elements: empathy, warmth and genuineness. Empathy involves
understanding what the other person is feeling and that means sometimes accepting emotions which are alien to oneself. Warmth requires
one to be a friendly and sympathetic listener to the person, but genuineness also requires one to provide honest information and reasonable
criticism if that seems appropriate.

There are two basic techniques by which information may be
elicited in a counselling situation — the directive and the non-directive.
In general, doctors are trained to use the directive approach — 'has he
been sick, how is he feeding, how is he sleeping?' and so on. The
second technique, the non-directive approach, involves asking very
general questions and allowing the information to be divulged by the
patient. Open-ended questions like 'how are things going, are you
having any difficulties at the moment?' may be used in non-directive
counselling, which is very time-consuming so that the doctor may be
forced to use directive techniques in order to deal with a particular
problem. But directive techniques tend to discourage conversation and
merely to elicit information, whereas the non-directive technique is at
the heart of ordinary converse between friends. On the other hand if
the doctor seems rushed and hurried the parent may not respond to
non-directive questions. We often try and open our interviews in the

child health clinic with some non-directive questions, but realize the value of the directive technique too in identifying particular issues, providing we use a reasonably systematic approach. Thus, if we see a mother in the afternoon and ask her if she has any worries, she may say no, but, when specifically asked about sleep in the night, she suddenly may remember what she has sublimated for the moment, the appalling nights that the family are having because of the child's sleeping behaviour.

Again, counselling should be shared by all members of the primary health care team and is not simply the responsibility of the doctor. Medical students, we believe, do not receive as much training in these techniques as they should. Any doctor who spends time listening and talking to families with young children will find that his skills as a counsellor will develop and he may wish to proceed further and study these techniques in more detail.

Conclusion

In this book we have tried to deal with the issues of primary health care for the child of under five and his family from the doctor's perspective. We are aware that the level of service we propose is probably greater than is being offered in many parts of the UK at the moment. We make no apology for this for as a society we should be ashamed of the poor level of health service we offer to young children and their families. We believe it is a mark of a civilized community that it takes good care of its children.

References

Bax, M. & Whitmore, H. (1987) The medical examination of children on entry to school. The results and use of neurodevelopmental assessment. *Developmental Medicine and Child Neurology*, **29**, 40−55.

Haggerty, R.J. (1980) Life stress: illness and social supports. *Developmental Medicine and Child Neurology*, **22**, 391−400.

Hobson, B. (1978) Counselling. *Nursing Times*, **74**, 12 January 1978.

Rutter, M., Graham, P. & Yule, W. (1970) *A Neuropsychiatric Study in Childhood*. Spastics International Publishing Co, Heinemann: London.

Appendices

A1 Growth Charts

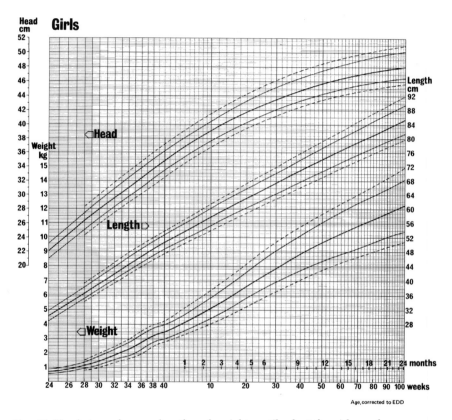

Fig. A1 Head circumference, length and weight centile chart for girls aged 0−2 years (courtesy of Castlemead Publications).

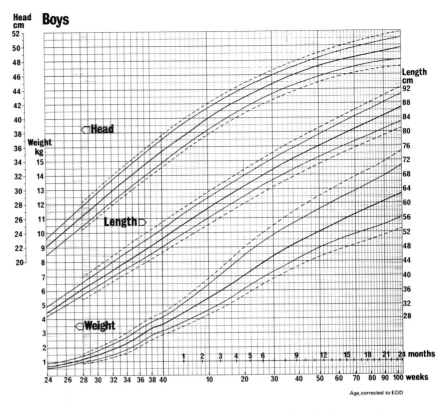

Fig. A2 Head circumference, length and weight centile chart for boys aged 0–2 years (courtesy of Castlemead Publications).

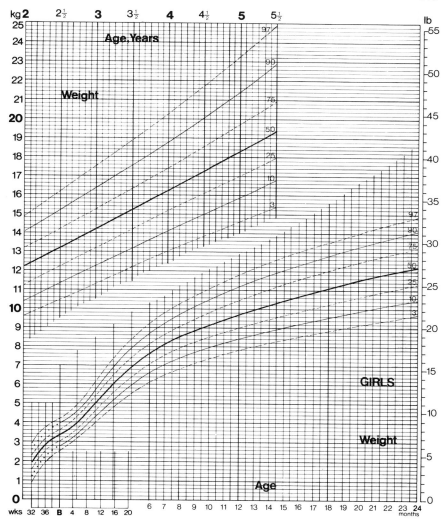

Fig. A3 Weight standard chart for girls aged 0–5 years (courtesy of Castlemead Publications).

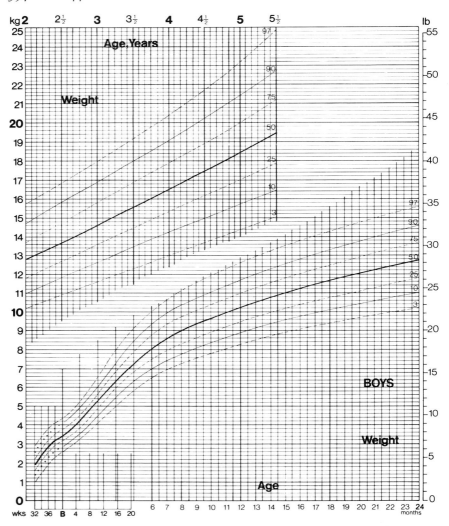

Fig. A4 Weight standard chart for boys aged 0–5 years (courtesy of Castlemead Publications).

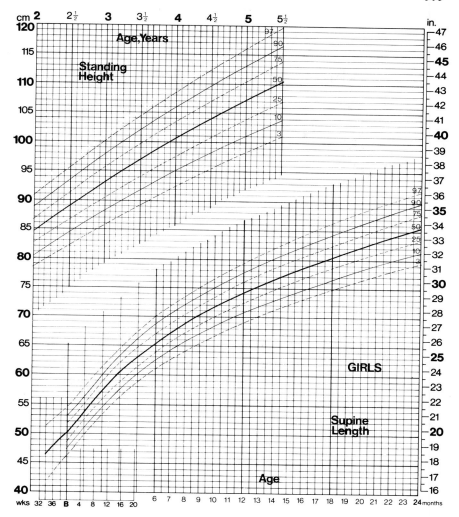

Fig. A5 Length and height standard chart for girls aged 0–5 years (courtesy of Castlemead Publications).

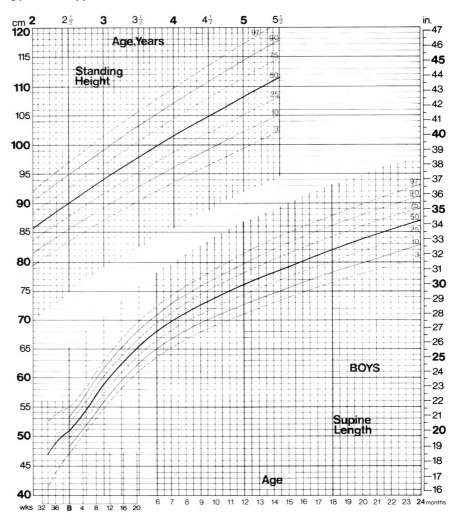

Fig. A6 Length and height standard chart for boys aged 0–5 years (courtesy of Castlemead Publications).

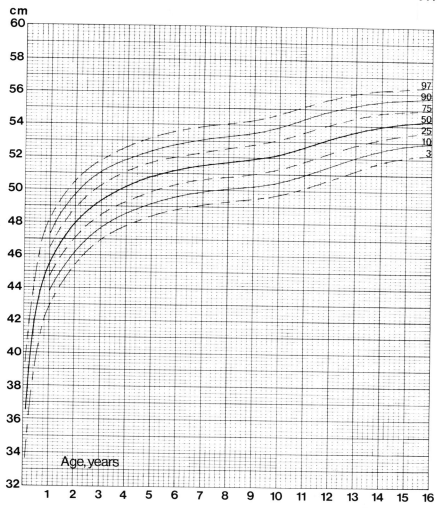

	Percentiles					
	10		50		90	
Age (year)	(in)	(cm)	(in)	(cm)	(in)	(cm)
0.25	15.0	38.1	15.6	39.7	16.1	40.9
0.50	16.2	41.2	16.9	42.9	17.4	44.2
0.75	17.0	43.2	17.6	44.6	18.1	46.2
1	17.5	44.4	18.0	45.7	18.6	47.2
2	18.1	46.2	18.9	48.0	19.4	49.3
3	18.5	47.1	19.4	49.2	19.9	50.5
4	18.9	48.0	19.6	49.9	20.2	51.4
5	19.1	48.6	19.8	50.4	20.4	51.9

Fig. A7 Head circumference for girls aged 0–18 years (courtesy of Castlemead Publications).

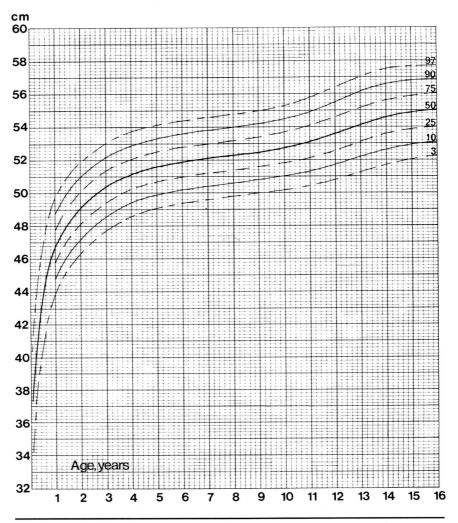

	Percentiles					
	10		50		90	
Age (year)	(in)	(cm)	(in)	(cm)	(in)	(cm)
0.25	15.5	39.3	16.0	40.6	16.6	42.1
0.50	16.5	42.0	17.2	43.8	17.7	45.0
0.75	17.1	43.6	18.0	45.7	18.6	47.2
1	17.5	44.5	18.4	46.8	19.1	48.5
2	18.5	47.1	19.3	49.1	20.0	50.9
3	19.0	48.2	19.8	50.2	20.5	52.0
4	19.3	48.9	20.0	50.8	20.7	52.5
5	19.4	49.4	20.2	51.3	20.9	53.0

Fig. A8 Head circumference for boys aged 0–18 years (courtesy of Castlemead Publications).

A2 The Feelings and Behaviour of Parents of Handicapped Children*

This article was first published nearly twenty years ago. Nevertheless it still seems to us the best short account of the feelings of parents who have a disabled child. Over the years some attitudes (and the words we use) have changed. The article reflects some of these swings and opinions. It is not now common for a child to be placed in residential care for example. These changes in practice do not affect the basic approaches that the late Dr Ronald MacKeith set down.

The behaviour of parents of handicapped children derives from many factors. These include cultural and social-class attitudes to children in general, to handicapped people and to teachers, social workers and to doctors and medical care in general. But to a major degree, their behaviour derives from their feelings about having a handicapped child.

Whatever the handicap, the reactions of parents to all the varieties of handicapped children have much that is similar.

The reactions will be influenced by whether the handicap is evident at birth or becomes evident later, after the parents have 'fallen in love' with the child. They will be influenced by whether there is a prospect of severe mental handicap or not. They will be influenced by whether the handicap is obvious to other people, and by the attitudes of other people — including lay people, teachers, social workers and doctors — to handicap and to handicapped people.

Parents' feelings

What may be the reaction of parents who find their child is handicapped? What will the feelings (and hence the behaviour) be of a couple who find themselves in what may be called a 'classical' or typical situation? Consider the reactions of a young couple who have as their first child one with Down's syndrome or spina bifida — handicaps which are evident at birth. They have not yet 'fallen in love' in a way that means the child is part of them whatever happens to him. Their feelings will be mixed ones.

1 *Two biological reactions*: protection of the helpless; revulsion at the abnormal.
2 *Two feelings of inadequacy*: inadequacy at reproduction; inadequacy at rearing.

* Reprinted from MacKeith, R.C. (1973) *Developmental Medicine and Child Neurology*, **15**, 524–7.

3 *Three feelings of bereavement*: at the loss of the normal child they expected, with almost infinite potentialities: (a) anger; (b) grief; and (c) adjustment, which takes time.
4 *Feeling of shock*.
5 *Feeling of guilt*, which is probably less common than many writers state.
6 *Feeling of embarrassment*, which is a social reaction to what the parents think other people are feeling.

Parents' behaviour

1 (a) The biological reaction of protectiveness towards the helpless infant will tend to produce 'maternal' behaviour in both the mother and the father: (i) frequently there is *warm normal care*; or (ii) there may be *highly protective care*. Labelling highly protective care as overprotection is not an observation but a judgement and should involve the mother's need to behave in this way and the child's need to be highly protected.

(b) The biological reaction of revulsion at the abnormal is a normal reaction, even if in our culture it is frowned upon. It will produce rejection of the child. Rejection may show itself as: (i) *cold rejection*; (ii) *rationalised rejection*, the parents suggesting that the child should be 'in a home with specially trained people to care for him'; (iii) *dutiful caring* without warmth; or (iv) *lavish care* from over-compensation of the feeling of rejection.

2 (a) Feelings of inadequacy at reproduction can strike deep at a person's self-respect and may produce *depression*.

(b) Feelings of inadequacy at rearing can produce *lack of confidence and hence inconsistency of rearing*.

3 (a) The anger of bereavement may cause *aggressive behaviour* towards those who are trying to help the parents.

(b) The grief may cause *depression*.

(c) The *adjustment* may come fairly quickly and though often stable is not always so in face of problems that arise later.

4 The sense of shock may cause *disbelief* and *a succession of consultations at other clinics in the search for better news*.

5 Guilt is frequently written about but it is not felt by all parents. It is a complex feeling with understones, for example of punishment. It can produce *depression*.

6 Embarrassment can lead to *withdrawal from social contacts* and consequent social isolation.

The feelings and behaviour of professional advisers

Nurses, social workers, teachers, therapists and doctors faced with a handicapped person are often disturbed, as are most adults. As with parents, their behaviour will be influenced by their feelings. Social workers and doctors can feel revulsion at the abnormal and, having these feelings, show them in *recommending the parents to put the child away into a home* when this is not what the parents would choose. The family's advisers may be over-solicitous about the child and *forget the needs of the rest of the family*.

Doctors may reveal their own feelings of inadequacy at caring for the child by *brusque dismissal of the child and parents*. Doctors may also reveal their sense of inadequacy by objecting to the parents 'shopping around' for a further opinion. A doctor who feels he is reasonably competent and who has given adequate attention and time to the parents may regret that he has failed to meet their needs, but he will understand why they feel they must ask for a further opinion. He may wonder where he failed them, but he will convey his understanding of their desire and will help them to see another physician. He will also convey very clearly that he is willing to accept them back again at any time.

Should the child go away from home?

Sometimes parents ask for this when they first know — at the birth of the child — that he is lastingly handicapped. It seems best to convey that there is no urgency to make a permanent decision. They may leave the child in hospital and later take him home, or they may take him home earlier with the knowledge that the physician will re-admit the child to hospital at any time.

Later on, the decision will depend on three principles which are presented to the parents.
1 In our culture, most people live with their families and do better if they do so.
2 People go away from home if thereby they are able to get treatment and education which are better — and sufficiently better to outweigh the disadvantages of being away from home.
3 People go away from home if other people in the family are suffering from their continued presence.
These general principles can be conveyed over the years, long before any decision is urgently needed.

Crisis periods during the growth of the handicapped child

Crisis periods are important to know about, for the professional adviser can himself be prepared to act to diminish the difficulties of parents at these times. Furthermore, at the times of crisis, parents are often more open to receiving helpful guidance.
1 *When parents first learn about or suspect handicap* in their child. Until their anxieties are (to some extent) dealt with by full assessment and explanation, their child is 'not a person but a question mark'. This is a doctor's job.
2 When, *at about age five*, a decision has to be reached as to whether the child will be able to go to ordinary school, which would be a 'certificate' that he is more or less normal. The decision is reached by psychologists, educationalists and doctors in collaboration.
3 When the handicapped person comes to *the time of leaving school*: both the

parents and the handicapped person realize that cure is never going to happen and they wonder whether he or she will be independent and able to work, while the handicapped person wonders whether he or she will be able to meet girls or boys, make love and marry. Some of the explanation will fall on the employment services, some on social workers and some on doctors.

4   *When the parents become older* and are unable to care for their handicapped child. Parents will look ahead anxiously and they deserve to be reminded that there are statutory services which will give help.

Support for the parents

Support for the parents is one of the major needs that therapists, teachers, social workers and doctors have to provide. Perhaps the support given in the earliest days and months is of crucial importance for long-term acceptance by the parents. Their questions must be answered but they will also be greatly helped if they are shown how they themselves can be helping their child every day to move towards achieving full potential.

For the community, there are economic benefits to be gained from giving full support and help to the parents but, more important, this is a compassionate and necessary part of the care of the handicapped person and his family.

A3 Summary of Development

Summary of development

Gross motor

NEWBORN

Prone: arms and legs flexed, pelvis high, knees under abdomen
Ventral suspension: head held just below body
Supine: arms and legs semiflexed, head to one side
Pull-to-sit: complete head lag
Held upright: legs extended, stepping and placing reflex

4 WEEKS

Prone: pelvis lower, lifts head off couch
Ventral suspension: lifts head momentarily
Supine: arms and legs semiflexed
Pull-to-sit: lifts head momentarily
Held sitting: rounded back, lifts head momentarily
Held upright: stepping and placing reflex, legs extended

6 WEEKS

Prone and ventral suspension: holds head in line with body for a few seconds
Supine and pull-to-sit: holds head up for a few seconds, intermittent ATNR
  posture

12 WEEKS

Prone: lifts head and upper chest off couch, pelvis flat, legs extended
Ventral suspension: maintains head 45–90° to body
Pull-to-sit: little or no head lag
Held sitting: lumbar curve still present, some head wobble
Held upright: sags at knees, stepping and placing reflex disappeared

Fine motor

4 WEEKS

Grasp reflex
Drops object immediately
Hands mainly fisted
Sweeping movements towards objects

12 WEEKS

Little or no grasp reflex
Opens and closes hands
Watches objects for few seconds
Holds bottle for a few moments, but seldom capable of regarding it at same time
Hand regard begins — watches movement of own hands

20 WEEKS

Accurate reaching
Palmar grasp on ulnar side of hand
Hand regard ceases

Language

4 — 6 WEEKS

Coos, gurgles
Phonemes — oo, ugh

12 WEEKS

Long streams of babble
Conversations with mother

16 — 24 WEEKS

Babbling — ebe, ele, da, ba, ka, mum

Social behaviour and understanding

4 WEEKS

Can imitate tongue protrusion
Gazes at bright lights, faces, coloured objects
Recognizes mother

12 WEEKS

Laughs at playful activities
Recognizes familiar situation — bathing, feeding
Dislikes being left

20 WEEKS

Looks for dropped toy
Holds bottle
Smiles at mirror image

Vision

4 WEEKS

Pupils react to light

Focuses at 9 inches away
Looks at faces, bright light, coloured objects
Prefers mother's face to stranger's
Appreciates depth
Follows moving objects and faces up to 45° from midline

12 WEEKS

Visually very alert
Looks at small objects
Smooth convergence and binocular vision developed
Discriminates between colours
Follows moving objects through 180° vertically and horizontally

Hearing

4 WEEKS

Turns eyes and head to sound
Prefers voice sounds to pure tones
Startles, blinks, cries to loud sounds
Quietens to mother's voice or rattle
Recognizes mother's voice

12 WEEKS

Eyes and head move together to sound

5–6 MONTHS

Downward localization of sound

Six months

Gross motor

Supine — raises head in anticipation of being picked up
Prone — lifts head, chest and upper abdomen off couch with extended arms
Held standing bears weight on legs and bounces up and down
Sits with minimal support, head firmly erect
Rolls front to back
Hand regard ceased

Fine manipulation and vision

Picks up cube with palmar grasp, places in mouth
Transfers objects from one hand to the other
Looks at pellet — attempts to scoop up with palmar grasp
Holds bottle
Visually very alert
Follows dropped toy to the ground

Follows object at three feet through 180° arc
Looks at one-quarter inch mounted ball at 3 m

Vocalization and hearing

Vocalizes tunefully using consonants, e.g. da, mum, nan
Localizes sound to left and right
In response to sounds at 45° turns head, horizontally and then towards sound

Social behaviour and play

Friendly towards strangers
Excited by approach of familiar people
Laughs at peep-bo game
Smiles at mirror image

One year

Gross motor

Rises from lying to sitting
Crawls on hands and knees
Pulls himself to standing
Walks with one hand held

Fine manipulation and vision

Points at objects with index finger
Picks up pellet with pincer grasp between thumb and tip of index finger
Compares (matches) two objects
Releases toy on request
Watches and follows mounted one-eighth inch ball at 3 m

Language and hearing

Long tuneful babble in sentence-like pattern
Imitates sound
First naming words
Understands several words, e.g. dog, dad, teddy
Understands simple commands if accompanied by gestures, e.g. waves bye-bye
Localizes sounds above and below ear level

Social behaviour and play

Imitates sounds and actions, e.g. claps hands
Drinks from cup
Eats food with fingers
Looks for hidden toy
Wary of strangers, closely attached to familiar adult

18 **months**

Gross motor

Walks (from 13 months) with feet slightly apart
Holds arms nearly to sides (low guard)
Runs

Fine manipulation and vision

Picks up one-eighth inch pellet with neat pincer grip
Casting and mounting ceased
Builds tower of three or four cubes
Feeds self with spoon
Drinks from cup unaided
Identifies small detail in pictures

Language and hearing

Identifies familiar objects by use, e.g. toothbrush, comb
Identifies familiar objects when named
Obeys simple instructions
Points to part of body
Uses 6–20 recognizable words
Possibly four-animal Stycar picture hearing test

Social understanding and play

'Domestic mimicry' — copies mother's actions
Meaningful play with toys
Plays with toys alone but near familiar people
Emotionally dependent on familiar adult
Likes sitting on knee and looking at books for a few minutes

Two years

Gross motor

Runs
Kicks ball

Goes up and down stairs (on standard six- to eight-inch treads) holding rail or hand (two feet per step)

Fine manipulation and vision

Builds tower of six or seven cubes
Holds pencil in fist and draws circular scribble
Handedness developing
May recognize and name familiar in pictures at 3 m
May perform Stycar matching-toy vision test

Language and hearing

Obeys simple commands
Identifies common objects and parts of body
Uses 50 or more words
Starting to use two- or three-word phrases
Identifies named toys in hearing test

Social behaviour and play

Plays make-believe games with toys etc., makes cup of tea
Plays near other children but not with them
Constantly demands parents' attention
Tantrums when unable to make himself understood and when demands are refused
Puts on and takes off shoes and socks
Clean and dry by day

Three years

Gross motor

Goes upstairs one foot per step, downstairs two feet per step
Stands on one foot momentarily
Rides tricycle

Fine manipulation and vision

Builds tower of nine cubes
Copies train made of cubes
Imitates bridge
Holds pencil in preferred hand with tripod grip
Copies circle and imitates cross
Threads large beads on shoe-lace

Cuts with scissors
Performs Stycar five-letter vision test at 3 m

Language and hearing

Large vocabulary
Holds conversation
Uses sentences with most prepositions and personal pronouns
Uses why, where, who
Knows names and sex
Still has some consonantal omissions and substitutions
(Stycar high-frequency pictures and Reed-hearing test)
Performs speech discrimination test
(Kendal or McCormick toy test)

Social behaviour and play

Eats with fork and spoon
Dresses himself, except buttons
Plays imaginative games with other children
Dry at night
Able to be left in familiar surroundings — understands mother's temporary absence

Four and a half years

Gross motor

Goes downstairs one foot per step
Walks along narrow line
Hops on each foot (may need hand held)

Fine manipulation and vision

Guesses — copies steps
Mature tripod grip of pencil
Copies cross and square
Draws a recognizable man with six parts
Stycar seven-letter test, each eye in turn at 6 m

Language and hearing

Long sentences grammatically correct
Phonetically correct excepts s, f, th, r
Repeats a short story

(Hearing: 12 high-frequency picture test and Reed hearing test.)
Kendal toy test/co-operates with audiogram

Social behaviour and play

Complicated make-believe play alone and with other children
Dresses himself fully
Appreciates meaning of time of day

Index